Standards in Pediatric Orthopedics

TABLES, CHARTS, AND GRAPHS ILLUSTRATING GROWTH

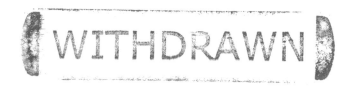

403p.

Standards in Pediatric Orthopedics

TABLES, CHARTS, AND GRAPHS ILLUSTRATING GROWTH

Robert N. Hensinger, M.D.

Co-Editor
JOURNAL OF PEDIATRIC ORTHOPEDICS

Professor
Department of Surgery
Section of Orthopedic Surgery
University of Michigan Medical Center
Ann Arbor, Michigan

Raven Press ■ New York

225 81

71.00

This book is dedicated to all the "controls"
that make up the data contained herein and to
my three faithful and usually uncomplaining
"controls", Missy, Laura and Michael

Raven Press, 1140 Avenue of the Americas, New York, New York 10036

Made in the United States of America

Library of Congress Cataloging-in-Publication Data

Hensinger, Robert N.
  Standards in pediatric orthopedics.

  Includes bibliographies and index.
  1. Pediatric orthopedia—Tables. 2. Pediatric
orthopedia—Charts, diagrams, etc. 3. Children—
Growth—Tables. 4. Children—Growth—Charts, diagrams,
etc. I. Title.
RD732.3.C48H46   1986   617'.3   86-450
ISBN 0-88167-183-5

The material contained in this volume was submitted as previously unpublished material, except in the instances in which credit has been given to the source from which some of the illustrative material was derived.

Great care has been taken to maintain the accuracy of the information contained in the volume. However, Raven Press cannot be held responsible for errors or for any consequences arising from the use of the information contained herein.

Preface

This began as a simple project: to compile a few graphs and charts that are particularly helpful in the day-to-day practice of pediatric orthopedics. Growth curves, bowleg/knock-knee charts, the Green and Anderson growth-arrest chart for the distal femur and proximal tibia, Colin Mosley's modification, and the like, which are essential but not always accessible during a busy clinic. I had expected to find 60, at the most 80, items; however, that amount grew rapidly like Jack's beanstalk. A great deal of information has been published, and more than 400 illustrations have been included here.

The focus of this volume has been narrowed to the speciality of pediatric orthopedics and to material that has been published in journals and older texts that are no longer readily accessible. The criterion for inclusion was relevance to the clinical assessment of our patients or as a possible aid in future research; thus the emphasis on the joints of the extremities and spine and measurements of joint function, bone growth, bone strength, and changes in hand and foot. Where available, I have included longitudinal data that illustrate abnormal growth, such as achondroplasia. Similarly, the effect of growth following the treatment of orthopedic problems is dealt with in a chapter we have termed "remodeling." (An example is the change in femoral head and acetabulum following successful reduction of a congenitally dislocated hip.) Also, the data had to encompass an adequate sample of children and represent a longitudinal assessment to demonstrate the influence of growth on the measurement. The material had to have been published in a journal; occasionally we used material from a book if it was adequately documented.

I have made a sincere effort to include the most recent charts or tables, particularly those which combine the older literature to form a more comprehensive chart. Several authors have performed an extraordinary service in combining bits and pieces of information that have accumulated over the years into very excellent and illustrative charts and graphs. In these situations, I have noted the related references but have avoided reprinting the older material.

I was impressed in preparing this material by the many children who have had roentgenographic surveys, measurements, and testing (prodding and poking); what we typically refer to as the "controls." The controls have provided us with a great deal of information, which should now allow us to limit that type of testing and exposure in the future, to hone in on areas of need, and to avoid repeating what has been adequately done in the past.

This is the effort of one group, and is, as a consequence, limited. A number of valuable items may have been overlooked. To that end, I want to encourage the readers to contribute and to help me improve the material, since we plan to update this volume on a regular basis. Similarly, a goal of this publication is to stimulate further investigation to broaden or clarify the material. I am hopeful that this volume will in fact become the "standard in pediatric orthopedics." If there is great interest and continuing updating, this document can become an invaluable tool in the management of the orthopedic problems in children.

This volume will be of interest to physicians, health professionals, and all persons interested in the growth and development of children.

ROBERT N. HENSINGER

Acknowledgments

I would like to thank the people who have been instrumental in this initial effort. Susan B. Lillie, whose dedication and giving of her time at a busy time, deserves special praise. Carmen Elston, who came aboard for this project, proved to be a tenacious pursuer of references and photographs and is now completely familiar with the University of Michigan Libraries. I also thank Thomas F. Kling for his advice and my Co-editor, Lynn T. Staheli, and Kathy Alexander in the Seattle office of the *Journal of Pediatric Orthopedics*, for their encouragement, kindness, and forebearance.

Contents

GAIT

BIOMECHANICS

REMODELING

UPPER EXTREMITY

HEIGHT AND WEIGHT

HAND

LOWER EXTREMITY

FOOT

GROWTH AND MATURATION

NEUROMUSCULAR DEVELOPMENT

SPINE AND SKULL

Head Circumference: Normal

TABLE 1. *Mean head circumferences of 43 infants from birth to 16 weeks of age according to gestation*

Age	Head circumferences (cm)		
	Gestation 30–33wks (healthy)	Gestation 34–37wks (healthy)	Gestation various (sick)
≤24hrs	27·0 ± 0·7	32·0 ± 0·7	30·9 ± 0·9
1wk	28·2 ± 0·7	32·7 ± 0·9	31·3 ± 1·0
2wks	29·5 ± 0·8	33·8 ± 0·8	31·7 ± 0·8
3wks	30·8 ± 0·8	35·0 ± 0·7	32·0 ± 0·8
4wks	32·0 ± 0·9	35·8 ± 0·8	32·4 ± 0·7
6wks	34·4 ± 0·7	37·1 ± 0·8	32·7 ± 0·8
8wks	35·8 ± 0·8	38·5 ± 1·0	33·3 ± 0·9
12wks	38·4 ± 1·1	40·3 ± 1·1	34·0 ± 0·9
16wks	40·2 ± 1·0	41·8 ± 0·9	34·5 ± 0·9

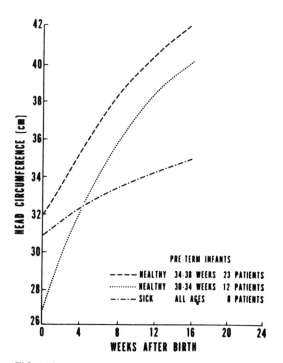

FIG. 1A. *Velocity Curves for Preterm Infants*
This graph is based on gestational age and medical status and is a graphic representation of the data in Table 1.

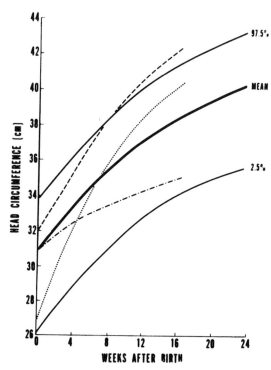

FIG. 1B. *Head Circumferences of Preterm Infants*
Head circumferences of preterm infants (Table 1) superimposed on data of O'Neill (—); note that the healthy preterm infants appear to cross percentiles. (O'Neill EM. Normal head growth and the prediction of head size in infantile hydrocephalus. *Arch Dis Child* 1961;36:241.)

Source: Sher PK, Brown SB. A longitudinal study of head growth in preterm infants.
I. Normal rates of head growth. *Dev Med Child Neurol* 1975;17:705–10.

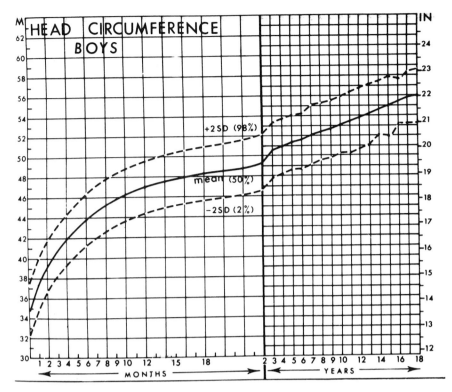

FIG. 1C. *Normal head circumferences of males from birth to 18 years*

The mean and standard deviations for age and sex were calculated from pooled variances of those reports of head circumferences published in the world literature since 1948, which provided the appropriate data (i.e., the sex and number of children measured at the specific age and values in terms of the mean and standard deviations). The head circumferences reported in these studies signified the measurement obtained when the tape was applied over the greatest frontal (i.e., supraorbital and occipital) protuberances.

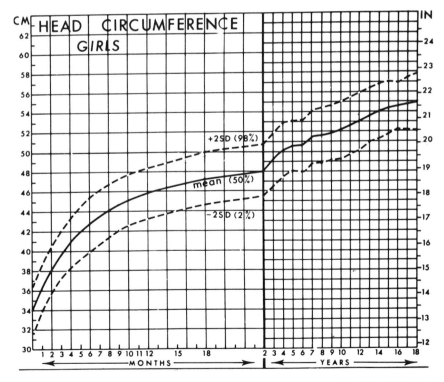

FIG. 1D. *Normal head circumferences of females from birth to 18 years.* See Fig. 1C for background on data calculations.

Source: Nellhaus G. Head circumference from birth to 18 years. *Pediatrics* 1968;41:106–14.

Head Circumference: Achondroplasia

Head circumferences for males (**top**) and females (**bottom**) with achondroplasia (stippled area) compared to normal male and female head circumferences. Only those individuals satisfying the strict diagnostic criteria (clinical and radiological) were included in this study.

Source: Horton WA, Rotter JL, Rimoin DL, Hall JG, Scott CI. Standard growth curves for achondroplasia. *J Pediatr* 1978;93:483.

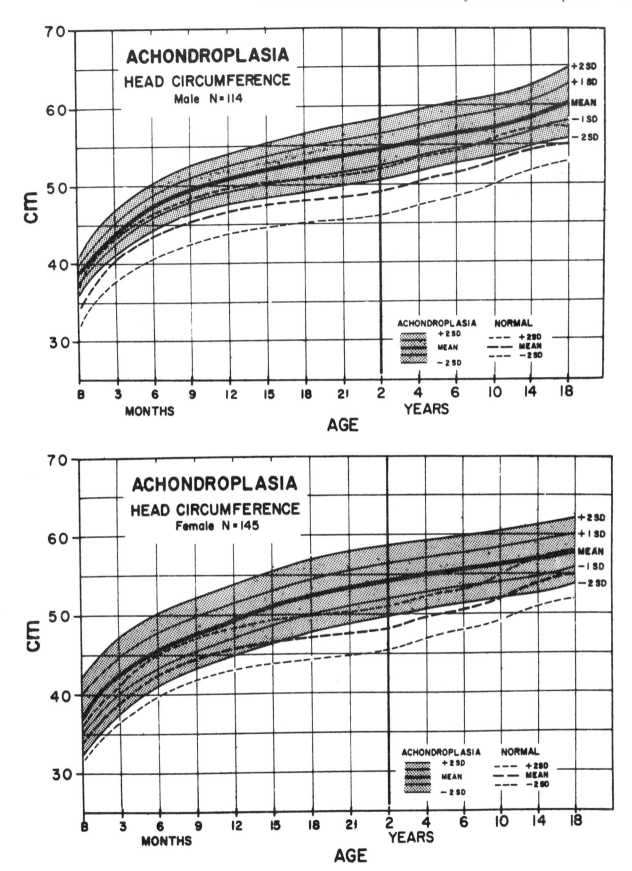

FIG. 2. Head circumferences for males and females with achondroplasia from birth to 18 years.

Time Spectrum of Neural Tube Development in Human Embryos

The estimated gestational age is based on data derived from Iffy et al. and Nishimura et al.; meningeal development data are from Sensenig:

Iffy LT, Shephard TH, Jakobovits A, Lemire RJ, Kerner P. The rate of growth in young embryos of Streeter's horizons XIII–XXIII. *Acta Anat (Basel)* 1967;66:178–86.

Nishimura H, Takano K, Tanimura T, Yasuda M. Normal and abnormal development of human embryos: First report of the analysis of 1,213 intact embryos. *Teratology* 1968;1:281–90.

Sensenig EC. The early development of the meninges of the spinal cord in the human embryo. *Carnegie Inst Contrib Embryol* 1951;34:145–57.

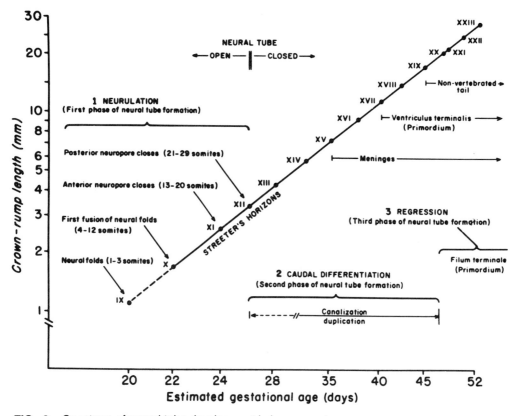

FIG. 3. Spectrum of neural tube development in human embryos.

Source: Lemire RJ. Variation in development of the caudal neural tube in human embryos (horizons XIV–XXI). *Teratology* 1969;2:361–70.

Normal Width of Cranial Sutures

Skull films from 107 normal neonates were used to determine the normal range of cranial sutures between 0 and 45 days of age. Assessment was based on the lateral view and evaluates both coronal and lamboid sutures, as well as the degree of V shape of the coronal sutures. The upper normal limits for the measurements of the V shape are along the horizontal axis (C1 + C2) − (C3 + C4) and sum of the suture width along the vertical axis (C1 + C2 + C3 + C4 + L1 + L2). The *dotted area* represents values between +2 and +3 SD.

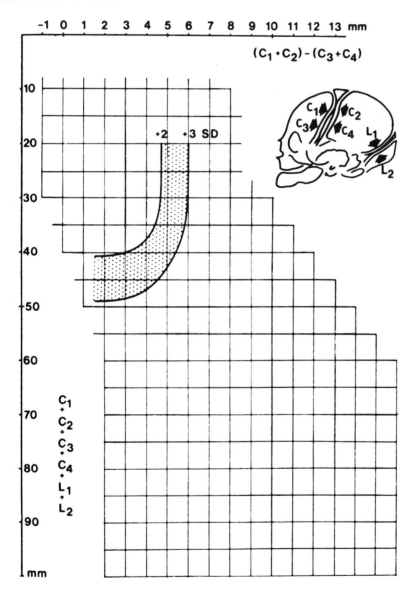

FIG. 4.   Normal width of cranial sutures.

Source: Erasmie V, Ringertz H. Normal width of cranial sutures in neonates and infants. *Acta Radiol Diagnosis* 1976;17:572–95.

Vertebral Ossification

TABLE 2A. *Time of ossification of the vertebral arches*

Embryo No.	202	274	263,b2	266	263,b1 right	263,b1 left	272	J	I	282	K	284	288b	M	N	300	O	S	306c	Q	306a	306b	P	R
Crown-rump length (mm)	30	31	32	33	34	34	34	36	41	42	53	54	57	69	70	73	73	75	75	81	100	105	105	110
Probable age of embryo (days)	55	56	56	57	58	58	58	60	64	65	72	73	75	83	83	85	85	87	87	90	100	105	105	110
Arches of the vertebrae[a] 1					*	*	*	*	*	*	*	*	*	*	*	*	*	*	*	*	*	*	*	*
2		*			*	*	*	*	*	:	*	*	*	*	*	*	*	*	*	*	*	*	*	*
3						*	*	*	*	*	*	*	*	*	*	*	*	*	*	*	*	*	*	*
4							*	*	*	*	*	*	*	*	*	*	*	*	*	*	*	*	*	*
5							*	*	*	*	*	*	*	*	*	*	*	*	*	*	*	*	*	*
6							*	*	*	*	*	*	*	*	*	*	*	*	*	*	*	*	*	*
7				*			*	*	*	*	*	*	*	*	*	*	*	*	*	*	*	*	*	*
8		*		*		*	*	*	*	*	*	*	*	*	*	*	*	*	*	*	*	*	*	*
9				*		*	*	*	*	*	*	*	*	*	*	*	*	*	*	*	*	*	*	*
10						*	*	*	*	*	*	*	*	*	*	*	*	*	*	*	*	*	*	*
11						*	*	*	*	*	*	*	*	*	*	*	*	*	*	*	*	*	*	*
12							*	*	*	*	*	*	*	*	*	*	*	*	*	*	*	*	*	*
13							*	*	*	*	*	*	*	*	*	*	*	*	*	*	*	*	*	*
14							*	*	*		*	*	*	*	*	*	*	*	*	*	*	*	*	*
15							*	*	*		*	*	*	*	*	*	*	*	*	*	*	*	*	*
16							*	*	*		*	*	*	*	*	*	*	*	*	*	*	*	*	*
17							*	*	*		*	*	*	*	*	*	*	*	*	*	*	*	*	*
18							*	*	*		*	*	*	*	*	*	*	*	*	:	*	*	*	*
19							*	*	*		*	*	*	*	*	*	*	*	*	*	*	*	*	*
20									*		*	*	*	*	*	*	*	*	*	*	*	*	*	*
21									*		*	*	*	*	*	*	*	*	*	*	*	*	*	*
22									*		*	*	*	*	*	*	*	*	*	*	*	*	*	*
23											*	*		*	*	*	*	*	*	*	*	*	*	*
24											*			*		*	*	*	*	*	*	*	*	*
25											*					*	*	*	*		*	*	*	*	*
26											*					*						*		*
27											*													*
28																								?

[a]Asterisk indicates that the bone listed in the first column is ossified.

TABLE 2B. *Time of ossification of the vertebral bodies*

Embryo No.	202	274	263,b,2	266	263,b,1	272	282	284	288,b	M	N	300	O	S	306,c	Q	306,a	306,b	P	R
Crown–rump length (mm)	30	31	32	33	34	34	42	54	57	69	70	73	73	75	75	81	100	105	105	110
Probable age of embryo (days)	55	56	56	57	58	58	65	73	75	83	83	85	85	87	87	90	100	105	105	110
Bodies of the vertebrae[a] 1																				
2											*	0			*				*	*
3											*	0	*		*		*		*	*
4										*	*	0	*	*	*	*	*	*	*	*
5										*	*	0	*	*	*	*	*	*	*	*
6									*	*	*	0	*	*	*	*	*	*	*	*
7									*	*	*	0	*	*	*	*	*	*	*	*
8								*	*	*	*	0	*	*	*	*	*	*	*	*
9								*	*	*	*	0	*	*	*	*	*	*	*	*
10						*	*	*	*	*	*	0	*	*	*	*	*	*	*	*
11						*	*	*	*	*	*	0	*	*	*	*	*	*	*	*
12						*	*	*	*	*	*	0	*	*	*	*	*	*	*	*
13						*	*	*	*	*	*	0	*	*	*	*	*	*	*	*
14						*	*	*	*	*	*	0	*	*	*	*	*	*	*	*
15						*	*	*	*	*	*	0	*	*	*	*	*	*	*	*
16						*	*	*	*	*	*	0	*	*	*	*	*	*	*	*
17						*	*	*	*	*	*	0	*	*	*	*	*	*	*	*
18						*	*	*	*	*	*	*	*	*	*	*	*	*	*	*
19						*	*	*	*	*	*	*	*	*	*	*	*	*	*	*
20						*	*	*	*	*	*	*	*	*	*	*	*	*	*	*
21						*	*	*	*	*	*	*	*	*	*	*	*	*	*	*
22						*	*	*	*	*	*	*	*	*	*	*	*	*	*	*
23						*	*	*	*	*	*	*	*	*	*	*	*	*	*	*
24						*	*	*	*	*	*	*	*	*	*	*	*	*	*	*
25						*	*	*	*	*	*	*	*	*	*	*	*	*	*	*
26							*	*	*	*	*	*	*	*	*	*	*	*	?	*
27							*	*	*	*	*	*	*	*	*	*	*		*	*
28								*		*	*	*	*				*			*
29											*						*			

[a]Asterisk indicates that the bone listed in the first column is ossified.

Source: Mall FP. On ossification centers in human embryos less than 100 days old. *Am J Anat* 1906;5:433–58.

TABLE 3A. *Time of ossification of the primary ossification centers of the neural arches of the vertebrates*

1 CENTERS	2 SMALLEST SPECIMEN(S) WITH CENTER PRESENT (mm CR)[1]	3 SPECIMEN(S) OF A CR LENGTH AFTER WHICH CENTER ALWAYS OBSERVED	4 SPECIMENS BETWEEN THOSE LISTED IN COLUMNS 2 AND 3 WITH THE BONE OSSIFIED	5 DATA IN LITERATURE IN MM CR
Cervical 1	45(1,2,4)	49	48(1)	34(M),50–60(T)
Cervical 2	40(3)	45(1,2,4)	44(1,2)	33(M),51–60(T)
Cervical 3–7	38(4)	45(1,2,4)	40(3),44	34(M),51–60(T)
Thoracic 1	38(4)	45(1,2,4)	40(3,4),44(2)	33(M),51–60(T)
Thoracic 2	38(4)	45(1,2,4)	40(3),44(2)	34(M),51–60(T)
Thoracic 3	40(3)	52	44(2),45(1,2,4),48(1,2),49	34(M),51–60(T)
Thoracic 4–5	40(3)	60(1,2)	44(2),45(1,2,4),48(1,2),49, 52,53,54,56(1,2),57	34(M),51–60(T)
Thoracic 6	40(3)	60(1,2)	44(2),45(1,4),48(1,2),49, 52,53,54,56(1,2),57	34(M),51–60(T)
Thoracic 7	45(1,4)	60(1,2)	48(1,2),49,52,53,54, 56(1,2),57	34(M),51–60(T)
Thoracic 8	45(1,4)	60(1,2)	48(1),52,53,54,56(1,2),57	34(M),51–60(T)
Thoracic 9	45(1,2,4)	60(1,2)	48(1),52,53,56(1,2),57	34(M),51–60(T)
Thoracic 10	45(1,2,4)	60(1,2)	48(1),52,53,56(1,2)	34(M),51–60(T)
Thoracic 11	45(1,4)	60(1,2)	48(1),52,53,56(1,2)	34(M),51–60(T)
Thoracic 12	45(1,4)	60(1,2)	48(1),52,53,56(1,2)	34(M),52–60(T)
Lumbar 1	45(1,4)	60(1,2)	48(1),52,53,54,56(1,2)	41–53(M),51–60(T)
Lumbar 2	45(1)	60(1,2)	48(1),56(1,2)	41–53(M),51–85(T)
Lumbar 3	45(1)	68(2)	56(1,2),60(1,2),61(1),62, 65(1,2,3),67	41–53(M),55–91(T)
Lumbar 4	45(1)	68(2)	60(1,2),61(1),62,65(1,3), 67	53–69(M),58–91(T)
Lumbar 5	60(1,2)	69(1,2)	61(1),62,65(1,3),67,68(2)	53–69(M),60–93(T)
Sacral 1	65(3)	76	68(2),69(1,2),71	53–81(M),75–110(T), 65–120(O),65–128(Ad)
Sacral 2	102(1,2)	127(2)	108,110,112,113(2), 115(1,2),116(1,2), 120(1,2,3),124(2), [69(1,2)][1]	53–110(M),80–139(T), 115–155(O), 65–150(Ad)
Sacral 3	102(2)	161	110,116(2),120(2,3), 127(2),134,135,139(1,2), 140,141,143,147(1,2),148	53–110(M),135–170(T), 127–155(O), 100–170(Ad)
Sacral 4	135	161	139,147(2),148(1)	139–205(T),127–220(O), 130–170(Ad)
Sacral 5	163(2)	173		170–350(T), 190–newborn (O)

Human embryos (136) ranging in crown-rump length from 14 to 235 mm were cleared with potassium hydroxide and their bones stained with alizarin red.

Numbers in parentheses refer to specimens in which that specific center apparently appears precociously.

Letters in parentheses refer to previously published reports: (Ad): Adair FL. The ossification centers of the fetal pelvis. *Am J Obstet Dis Women Child* 1918;78:175–99; (M): Mall FP. On ossification centers in human embryos less than 100 days old. *An J Anat* 1906;5:433–58; (O): Obata R. Die Knochenderene des fetalen menschlichen Beckens. *Z Geburtsh Gynakol* 1912;22:533–74; (T): Tessandier J. L'ossification des Cotes et de la Colonne Vertebrale Chez le Foetus Humain [Thesis]. Paris: Faculté de Medicine, 1944.

TABLE 3B. *Time of appearance of the primary ossification centers of the vertebral center*

1 CENTERS	2 SMALLEST SPECIMEN(S) WITH CENTER PRESENT (mm CR)[1]	3 SPECIMEN(S) OF A CR LENGTH AFTER WHICH CENTER ALWAYS OBSERVED	4 SPECIMENS BETWEEN THOSE LISTED IN COLUMNS 2 AND 3 WITH THE BONE OSSIFIED	5 DATA IN LITERATURE IN MM CR
Cervical 1	135	161		165–195(T)
Cervical 2	69(1)	120(2,3)	76, 83(1), 85, 86, 91, 94, 97(2), 102(1,2), 104, 108, 110, 112, 113(1,3), 115(1,2), 116(1)	70–105(M), 75–130(T)
Cervical 3	69(1)	102(1,2)	76, 83(1,2), 84(1), 85, 86, 88, 91, 94, 95, 97(1,2)	70–105(M), 75–105(T)
Cervical 4	57	85	69(2,3), 76, 78, 83(1,2), 84(1)	69–75(M), 75–105(T)
Cervical 5	57	71	61(1), 65(1), 67, 69(1,3)	69(M), 65–91(T)
Cervical 6	52	71	57, 60(1), 61(1), 65(1), 67, 68(1,2), 69(1,2,3)	57(M), 65–80(T)
Cervical 7	52	68(1)	56(1), 57, 60(2), 61(1), 65(1,2,3), 67	57(M), 60–80(T)
Thoracic 1	52	69(1,2,3)	54, 56(1), 57, 60(1,2), 61(1,2), 65(1,2,3), 67, 68(2)	54(M), 57–72(T)
Thoracic 2	52	57	54, 56(1)	54(M), 57–65(T)
Thoracic 3	48(1)	57	52, 54, 56(1)	34(M), 54–60(T)
Thoracic 4	48(1)	57	52, 54, 56(1)	34(M), 51–60(T)
Thoracic 5–7	40(3)	52	45(4), 48(1)	34(M), 51–60(T)
Thoracic 8	40(3)	52	45(4), 48(1), 49	34(M), 51–60(T)
Thoracic 9	40(3)	52	45(1,4), 48(1), 49, 50	34(M), 51–60(T)
Thoracic 10–12	40(3)	52	44(2), 45(1,4), 48(1), 49, 50	34(M), 43–60(T)
Lumbar 1	40(3)	52	44(2), 45(1,4), 48(1), 49, 50	34(M), 43–55(T)
Lumbar 2	45(1,4)	52	48(1), 49, 50	34(M), 51–56(T)
Lumbar 3	45(1,4)	52	49, 50	34(M), 51–56(T)
Lumbar 4	45(1,4)	54	52	34(M), 51–65(T)
Lumbar 5	45(1)	57	52, 54, 56(1)	34(M), 57–85(T), 50(O), 51–60(Ad)
Sacral 1	52	65(1,2,3)	56, 57, 60(1,2), 61, 62	54(M), 59–93(T), 65(O), 60–65(Ad)
Sacral 2	60(1,2)	68(2)	61, 62, 65(1,2), 67	54(M), 59–93(T), 65–120(O), 65–128(Ad)
Sacral 3	60(1,2)	97(3)	61(1), 62, 65(3), 67, 68(2), 69(1,2,3), 71, 72, 76, 78, 83, 84(1,2), 85, 86, 88, 91, 94, 95	57–110(M), 82–170(T), 102–155(O), 77–170(Ad)
Sacral 4	84	143	88, 95, 97(3), 102(1,2), 108, 110, 113(1,2), 115(1), 116(1,2), 120(1,2,3), 127, 133, 134, 135, 139(1,2), 140, [62, 69(1)][2]	70–after 110(M), 107–350(T), 155–230(O)
Sacral 5	135	after 175	148, 163(2), 235, [62]	

Human embryos (136) ranging in crown-rump length from 14 to 235 mm were cleared with potassium hydroxide and their bones stained with alizarin red. Numbers in parentheses refer to specimens in which that specific center apparently appears precociously.

Letters in parentheses refer to previously published reports: (Ad): Adair FL. The ossification centers of the fetal pelvis. *Am J Obstet Dis Women Child* 1918;78:175–99; (M): Mall FP. On ossification centers in human embryos less than 100 days old. *An J Anat* 1906;5:433–58; (O): Obata R. Die Knochenderene des fetalen menschlichen Beckens. *Z Geburtsh Gynakol* 1912;22:533–74; (T): Tessandier J. L'Ossification des Cotes et de la Colonne Vertebrale Chez le Foetus Humain [Thesis]. Paris: Faculté de Medicine, 1944.

Source: Noback CR, Robertson GG. Sequences of appearance of ossification centers in the human skeleton during the first five prenatal months. *An J Anat* 1951:89:1–27.

Development of Cervical Spine

The illustrations in Section 6 are based on the study of roentgenograms of the cervical spine from approximately 100 normal children ranging from newborn to 14 years of age. The children had no history of trauma.

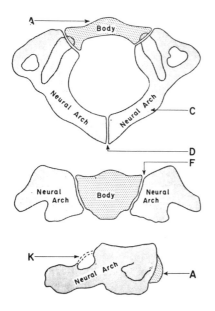

FIG. 5A. *First cervical vertebra (atlas)*
(A) Body. Not ossified at birth; the center (occasionally two centers) appears during the first year after birth; the body may fail to develop, and forward extension of neural arches may take its place. *(C) Neural arches.* Appear bilaterally at approximately the seventh fetal week; most of the anterior portion of superior articulating surface is usually formed by the body. *(D) Synchondrosis of spinous processes.* Unites by the third year. Union may rarely be preceded by the appearance of a secondary center within the synchondrosis. *(F) Neurocentral synchondrosis.* Fuses at approximately the seventh year. *(K) Ligament surrounding the superior vertebral notch.* May ossify, especially later in life.

FIG. 5B. *Second cervical vertebra (axis or epistropheus)*
(A) Body. One center (occasionally two) appears by the fifth fetal month. *(C) Neural arches.* Appear bilaterally by the seventh fetal month. *(D) Neural arches* fuse posteriorly by the second or third year. *(E) Bifid tip of spinous process.* Occasionally a secondary center is present in each tip. *(F) Neurocentral synchondrosis.* Fuses at 3 to 6 years. *(G) Inferior epiphyseal ring.* Appears at puberty and fuses at approximately 25 years. *(H) "Summit" ossification center for odontoid.* Appears at 3 to 6 years and fuses with the odontoid by 12 years. *(I) Odontoid (dens).* Two separate centers appear by the fifth fetal month and fuse with each other by the seventh month. *(J) Synchondrosis between odontoid and neural arch.* Fuses at 3 to 6 years. *(L) Synchondrosis between odontoid and body.* Fuses at 3 to 6 years. *(M) Posterior surface of body and odontoid.*

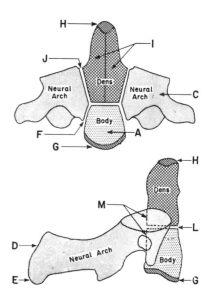

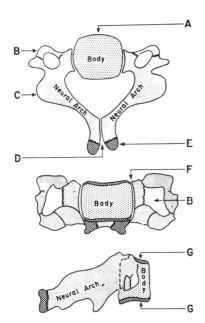

FIG. 5C. *Typical cervical vertebrae C3 to C7*
(A) Body. Appears by fifth fetal month. *(B) Anterior (costal) portion of transverse process.* May develop from a separate center that appears by the sixth fetal month and joins the arch by the sixth year. *(C) Neural arches.* Appear by seventh to ninth fetal week. *(D) Synchondrosis between spinous processes.* Usually unites by second or third year. *(E) Secondary centers for bifid spine.* Appear at puberty and unite with spinous process at 25 years. *(F) Neurocentral synchondrosis.* Fuses at 3 to 6 years. *(G) Superior and inferior epiphyseal rings.* Appear at puberty and unite with body at approximately 25 years. The seventh cervical vertebra differs slightly because of a long, powerful nonbifid spinous process.

Source: Bailey DK. The normal cervical spine in infants and children. *Radiology* 1952;59:712–9.

Radiographic Determination of Lordosis, Kyphosis, and L5-S1 Angle in Normal and Scoliotic Children

Kyphosis was measured from the superior aspect of T5 to the inferior aspect of T12 and lordosis from the superior surface of L1 to the inferior surface of L5 vertebral bodies both by the Cobb method. The L5-S1 angle is the angle between the inferior endplate of the fifth lumbar vertebra and superior aspect of the sacrum. Differences in spinal measurements in the normal and scoliotic groups were tested for use of the Mann–Whitney tests for group data. There were no significant relationships among the radiographic measurements of kyphosis, lordosis, or L5-S1 angle with the attributes of age, height, or weight.

TABLE 4. *Summary of distributions of lordosis, kyphosis, and L5-S1 angle*

	Lordosis[a]		Kyphosis[b]		L_5-S_1 angle[c]	
	Normal	Scoliotic	Normal	Scoliotic	Normal	Scoliotic
Median	40	48.5	27	28	12	10.5
25–75%	31–49.5	40–55	21–33	16.5–36	9–16	6–14.5
10–90%	22.5–54	33.5–61.5	11.5–39.5	9–53	5–21	4–18

Data are degrees. Patients: 104, normal; 114, scoliotic.
[a] Mann-Whitney: $z = -4.81$; $p < 0.0001$.
[b] Mann-Whitney: $z = 0.13$; $p = 0.90$.
[c] Mann-Whitney: $z = 2.46$; $p = 0.014$.

Source: Propst-Proctor SL, Bleck EE. Radiographic determination of lordosis and kyphosis in normal and scoliotic children. *J Pediatr Orthop* 1983;3:344–6.

Spina Bifida Occulta

All subjects were Japanese who had been residents of Hiroshima City at the time of the examination (1953). They constitute part of the population sample under study for biologic effects of exposure to the atomic bomb.

Roentgenographic diagnosis of spina bifida occulta was made only in the presence of a distinct unossified space or gap between the lamina and the neural arch. Statistical analysis of the data indicates that sex and age differences exist in the incidence of spina bifida in both pediatric and adolescent age groups.

TABLE 5. *Incidence of spina bifida occulta of fifth lumbar vertebra*

Age Group, Yr.	No.	Male w/Defect	%	No.	Female w/Defect	%	No.	Total w/Defect	%
7-8......................	86	19	22.09	69	6	8.70	155	25	16.13
12......................	44	7	15.91	51	3	5.88	95	10	10.53
16-18......................	48	6	12.50	60	2	3.33	108	8	7.41
Adults.....................	79	3	3.80	103	1	0.97	182	4	2.20

TABLE 6. *Incidence of spina bifida occulta of first sacral vertebra*

Age Group, Yr.	No.	Male w/Defect	%	No.	Female w/Defect	%	No.	Total w/Defect	%
7-8......................	86	40	46.51	69	40	57.97	155	80	51.61
12......................	44	21	47.73	51	21	41.18	95	42	44.21
16-18......................	48	25	52.08	60	18	30.00	108	43	39.81
Adults.....................	79	21	26.58	103	27	26.21	182	48	26.37

TABLE 7. *Incidence of spina bifida occulta of fifth lumbar or first sacral vertebra*

Age Group, Yr.	No.	Male w/Defect	%	No.	Female w/Defect	%	No.	Total w/Defect	%
7-8......................	86	50	58.14	69	41	59.42	155	91	58.71
12......................	44	24	54.55	51	22	43.14	95	46	48.42
16-18......................	48	26	54.17	60	20	33.33	108	46	42.59
Adults.....................	79	23	29.11	103	28	27.18	182	51	28.02

Source: Sutow WW, Pryor AW. Incidence of spina bifida occulta in relation to age. *J Dis Child* 1956;91:211–7.

Thoracic Spine Length

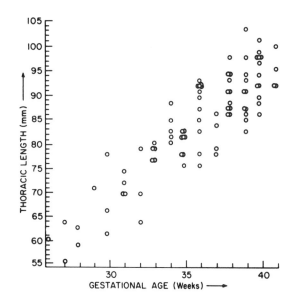

FIG. 6. Relationship of the thoracic spine length and birth weight in 88 newborn infants of 26 to 41 weeks gestational age. Thoracic spine length was plotted against gestational age according to maternal history, from the top of T1 to the bottom of T12.

Source: Kuhns L, Holt JF. Measurement of thoracic spine length on chest radiographs of newborn infants. *Pediatr Radiol* 1975;116:395–7.

Vertebral Growth

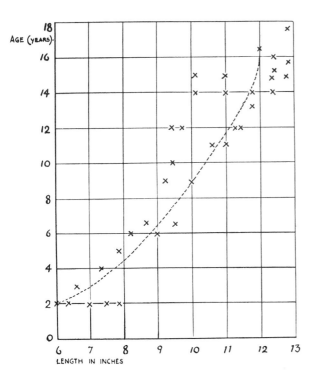

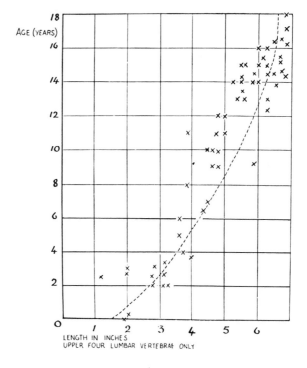

FIG. 7. *Normal growth curve for the thoracic spine*
Measurements were made on radiographs obtained with standard technique. The authors did not include the relative height of the patient or the degree of kyphosis or lordosis.

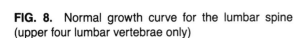

FIG. 8. Normal growth curve for the lumbar spine (upper four lumbar vertebrae only)

Source: Roaf, R. Vertebral growth and its mechanical control. *J Bone Joint Surg (BR)* 1960;42:40–59.

Atlantodental Interval

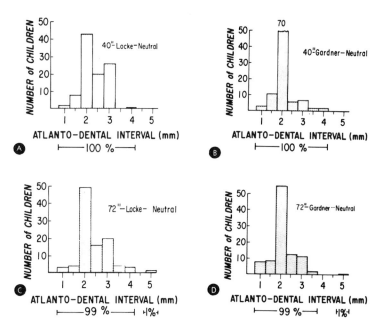

FIG. 9. Atlantodental interval determined from lateral roentgenograms of the cervical spine in 200 normal children 3 to 15 years of age. The lower limit of 3 years was selected because the summit of the epiphysis of the odontoid process is not present earlier, and adequate roentgenograms are more difficult to obtain in the younger children. One hundred studies were done in the upright position using a 72-inch tube-to-film distance and were interpreted by one examiner **(A, B)**. Another 100 studies were done at a 40-inch tube-to-film distance with the patient supine and the film exposed with the horizontal beam and again read by one examiner **(C, D)**. These positions were selected because supine studies are usually utilized in trauma investigations, whereas children with inflammatory disease are examined upright.

Source: Locke GR, Gardner JL, Van Epps EF. Atlas-dens interval (ADI) in children: A survey based on 200 normal cervical spines. *AJR* 1960;97:135–40.

Sagittal Diameter of the Normal Cervical Canal

Twenty-five normal infant spines were obtained at postmortem examination. In none of the cases was the cause of death attributable to deformity or disease of the central nervous system or of the vertebral column. Anteroposterior and lateral rentgenograms were obtained of the whole spine *(W)* at 90 cm using nonscreened films. Then, 11 spines were dissected *(D)*; the radiographs were repeated and compared (Fig. 11) to the whole spine *(W)*.

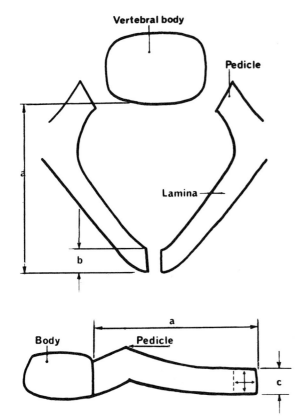

FIG. 10. Method of measuring the sagittal diameter: *a* is the distance from posterior border of vertebral body to the tip of the spinous process, *b* the thickness (on dissected specimen) of the spinous process, and *c* the height (on lateral radiograph) of the spinous process. At this age, *b* = *c*, and the sagittal diameter in the radiographs is equal to *a* − *c*.

Source: Naik DR. Cervical spinal canal in normal infants. *Clin Radiol* 1970;21:323–6.

		C2	C3	C4	C5	C6	C7
1.	W	12.5	12.0	12.0	13.5	14.0	14.0
	D	12.5	12.5	12.5	12.5	13.0	13.5
2.	W	13.0	13.0	12.0	14.0	13.0	13.0
	D	12.0	11.5	11.5	12.0	11.5	11.5
3.	W	10.0	9.5	10.0	11.0	11.0	11.0
	D	10.0	9.0	9.0	9.0	10.0	9.0
4.	W	14.0	13.0	12.0	13.5	13.5	14.0
	D	13.0	12.0	11.0	11.5	11.5	12.5
5.	W	13.0	12.5	12.0	12.5	13.0	13.0
	D	11.0	11.0	10.0	12.5	13.5	11.5
6.	W	12.5	13.0	13.0	13.0	13.5	14.5
	D	12.0	11.5	11.0	11.0	11.5	12.5
7.	W	13.0	12.0	13.5	12.0	13.0	12.0
	D	13.5	12.5	12.5	12.5	12.0	12.0
8.	W	13.0	12.5	13.5	12.0	13.0	11.5
	D	12.5	10.5	11.5	10.5	11.5	10.5
9.	W	13.0	11.0	10.5	11.5	11.0	11.5
	D	13.0	11.0	11.0	10.5	10.0	9.5
10.	W	10.0	8.0	9.0	9.5	10.0	8.0
	D	10.0	10.0	10.0	11.0	10.5	10.0
11.	W	13.0	10.0	10.5	12.0	13.5	12.5
	D	12.0	12.0	11.5	12.0	12.0	11.5

FIG. 11. Comparison of radiographs of the whole spine and the dissected vertebrae

Note that the difference between the actual diameter (D) and that derived from the method described in Fig. 10, indicated as whole spine (W), is never more than 2 mm.

Source: Naik DR. Cervical spinal canal in normal infants. *Clin Radiol* 1970;21:323–6.

Sagittal Diameter of Bony Cervical Spinal Canal

The data are based on studies of lateral roentgenograms of the cervical spine in 120 normal children between 3 and 14 years of age. The sagittal diameter of the spinal canal was measured from the middle of the posterior surface of the vertebral body to the nearest point on the ventral line of the cortex seen at the junction of the spinous process and lamina.

TABLE 8. *Sagittal diameter of the bony cervical spinal canal in 120 normal children: relation to age*

Age group	3 – 6 years			7 – 10 years			11 – 14 years		
Sex	Boys	Girls	Total	Boys	Girls	Total	Boys	Girls	Total
n	20	20	40	20	20	40	20	20	40
	Mean mm	Mean mm	Mean/SD mm	Mean mm	Mean mm	Mean/SD mm	Mean mm	Mean mm	Mean/SD mm
C1	20.2	19.6	19.9 ± 1.3	20.5	20.6	20.6 ± 1.3	21.2	21.4	21.3 ± 1.4
C2	18.2	17.6	17.9 ± 1.3	18.8	18.9	18.8 ± 1.0	19.3	19.5	19.4 ± 1.1
C3	16.3	15.8	16.0 ± 1.3	17.3	17.2	17.2 ± 1.0	17.8	17.7	17.8 ± 1.0
C4	16.0	15.6	15.8 ± 1.3	17.0	16.9	16.9 ± 0.9	17.3	17.2	17.3 ± 0.9
C5	15.9	15.5	15.7 ± 1.3	16.7	16.6	16.7 ± 0.9	17.1	16.9	17.0 ± 0.9
C6	15.8	15.3	15.6 ± 1.2	16.5	16.3	16.4 ± 0.9	16.8	16.6	16.7 ± 0.9
C7	15.6	15.0	15.3 ± 1.1	16.1	15.9	16.0 ± 0.9	16.3	16.2	16.2 ± 0.9

TABLE 9. *Sagittal diameter of the bony cervical spinal canal in 120 normal children: relation to height*

Height (cm)	Age (years)	n (Boys and Girls)	C1 Mean mm	C2 Mean mm	C3 Mean mm	C4 Mean mm	C5 Mean mm	C6 Mean mm	C7 Mean mm
91–100	2.84– 4.41	12	19.0	17.2	15.3	15.0	14.9	14.8	14.6
101–110	3.13– 5.78	13	19.9	17.7	15.9	15.6	15.5	15.4	15.3
111–120	4.04– 7.48	16	20.6	18.5	16.8	16.5	16.4	16.1	15.7
121–130	5.44–10.50	20	20.5	18.8	17.2	16.9	16.6	16.4	16.0
131–140	7.79–11.51	18	20.7	18.9	17.3	17.0	16.7	16.4	16.1
141–150	8.83–13.50	19	21.2	19.2	17.6	17.2	16.9	16.6	16.0
151–160	11.22–14.39	14	21.3	19.5	17.8	17.2	17.1	16.8	16.5
161–170	13.09–14.48	8	21.4	19.6	17.9	17.5	17.2	16.9	16.4

Source: Markuske H. Sagittal diameter measurement of the bony cervical spinal canal in children. *Pediatr Radiol* 1977;6:129–31.

Tolerance Limits for Sagittal Diameters

Measurements were made on 333 films taken on the Bolton–Broadbent cephalometer from 48 white children aged 3 to 18 years (chronological age) at annual intervals. No child had been followed the entire 15 years.

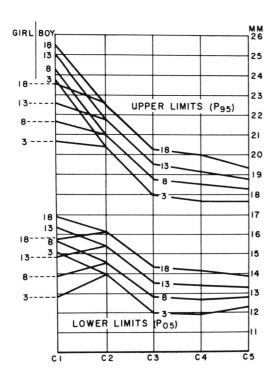

FIG. 12. Ninety percent tolerance limits for sagittal diameters in C1 to C5 in boys and girls 3 to 18 years of age.

FIG. 13. Ninety percent tolerance limits for sagittal diameter differences between adjacent vertebrae, C1 to C5, in boys and girls from 3 to 18 years of age

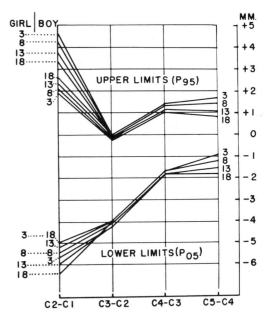

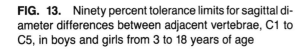

Source: Hinck VC, Hopkins CC. Savara BS. Sagittal diameter of cervical spine canal in children. *Radiology* 1962;79:97–108.

TABLE 10. *Tolerance ranges for normal boys and girls: C1 to C5*

Diameter	Sex	Age	Mean	S.D.	90% Tolerance Range	
					Lower Limit (P_{05})	Upper Limit (P_{95})
C-1	Boys (N = 27)	3	19.5	1.7	15.2	23.8
		8	20.0	1.7	15.7	24.3
		13	20.7	1.7	16.4	25.0
		18	21.3	1.7	17.0	25.6
	Girls (N = 21)	3	16.8	1.5	12.9	20.7
		8	17.8	1.5	13.9	21.7
		13	18.8	1.5	14.9	22.7
		18	19.7	1.5	15.8	23.6
C-2	Boys and Girls (N = 48)	3	17.2	1.5	14.0	20.4
		8	17.8	1.5	14.6	21.0
		13	18.6	1.5	15.4	21.8
		18	19.4	1.5	16.2	22.6
C-3	Boys and Girls (N = 48)	3	15.0	1.4	12.0	18.0
		8	15.8	1.4	12.8	18.8
		13	16.6	1.4	13.6	19.6
		18	17.3	1.4	14.3	20.3
C-4	Boys and Girls (N = 48)	3	14.8	1.3	11.9	17.7
		8	15.6	1.3	12.7	18.5
		13	16.3	1.3	13.4	19.2
		18	17.1	1.3	14.2	20.0
C-5	Boys and Girls (N = 48)	3	15.0	1.2	12.3	17.7
		8	15.6	1.2	12.8	18.3
		13	16.1	1.2	13.3	18.8
		18	16.7	1.2	13.9	19.4

These figures were used to create the graph in Fig. 12.

TABLE 11. *Tolerance ranges for measurement differences between adjacent vertebrae in normal boys and girls*

Difference	Sex	Age	Mean	S.D.	90% Tolerance Range	
					Lower Limit (P_{05})	Upper Limit (P_{95})
C-2–C-1	Boys (N. = 27)	3	−1.9	1.5	−5.7	+1.9
		8	−1.7	1.5	−5.5	+2.1
		13	−1.4	1.5	−5.2	+2.3
		18	−1.2	1.5	−5.0	+2.6
	Girls (N. = 21)	3	−0.2	1.9	−5.0	+4.7
		8	−0.5	1.9	−5.4	+4.3
		13	−1.0	1.9	−5.9	+3.8
		18	−1.5	1.9	−6.4	+3.4
C-3–C-2	Boys and Girls (N. = 48)	3	−2.2	0.9	−4.2	−0.2
		8	−2.1	0.9	−4.1	−0.1
		13	−2.1	0.9	−4.0	−0.1
		18	−2.0	0.9	−4.0	−0.0
C-4–C-3	Boys and Girls (N. = 48)	3	−0.2	0.8	−1.7	+1.4
		8	−0.2	0.8	−1.7	+1.3
		13	−0.3	0.8	−1.8	+1.2
		18	−0.3	0.8	−1.8	+1.1
C-5–C-4	Boys and Girls (N. = 48)	3	+0.4	0.6	−0.9	+1.7
		8	+0.1	0.6	−1.2	+1.4
		13	−0.2	0.6	−1.5	+1.1
		18	−0.6	0.6	−1.8	+0.8

These figures were used to create the graph in Fig. 13.

Sagittal Diameter of the Spinal Canal in Normal Subjects by Age

The sagittal diameter of the spinal canal was measured at the level of each lumbar vertebra. The sagittal diameter was the shortest midline perpendicular distance from the vertebral body to the inner surface of the neural arch.

TABLE 12. *Age-group means and standard deviations, by sex (mm)*

Vertebra	Male N	Mean	S.D.	Female N	Mean	S.D.	Male N	Mean	S.D.	Female N	Mean	S.D.
	Age 3, 4, 5 years						Age 6, 7, 8 years					
L1	15	20.3	1.8	9	19.8	1.2	14	20.3	1.9	10	19.3	2.6
2	15	19.6	1.2	9	18.9	1.4	15	19.9	1.7	9	19.5	1.6
3	15	18.4	1.4	9	18.1	1.4	15	19.1	1.8	10	18.4	1.6
4	15	18.8	1.1	9	18.0	1.5	15	19.0	1.7	10	19.1	1.8
5	14	19.0	1.6	9	17.5	1.4	15	19.0	2.4	10	19.1	2.3
	Age 9, 10 years						Age 11, 12 years					
L1	8	20.1	1.0	4	19.8	1.9	5	22.6	2.0	11	19.6	1.1
2	8	19.6	1.0	5	19.6	1.7	5	21.2	2.7	11	18.9	1.7
3	8	18.8	1.6	5	18.9	1.3	5	19.9	2.9	11	18.4	1.4
4	8	18.6	1.7	5	18.6	1.2	5	18.8	3.0	11	19.1	1.7
5	8	19.1	1.9	5	18.9	1.1	5	19.7	2.7	11	19.8	2.4
	Age 13, 14 years						Age 15, 16 years					
L1	14	20.5	1.5	10	20.8	1.4	10	21.6	2.2	18	21.6	2.2
2	14	19.7	1.4	10	20.1	0.9	11	20.8	2.1	18	20.9	1.8
3	14	18.9	1.7	10	20.0	1.3	11	20.5	1.6	18	20.7	1.6
4	14	20.4	4.1	10	20.2	2.5	11	20.0	1.7	18	21.0	2.1
5	14	20.8	4.2	10	20.1	3.2	10	20.1	2.9	18	20.8	3.4
	Age 17, 18 years						Adult					
L1	11	23.9	1.9	17	21.7	1.7	22	22.2	3.1	25	21.3	2.3
2	11	22.4	2.3	17	21.3	1.9	23	22.3	2.7	26	21.2	2.1
3	12	22.6	2.3	18	22.0	3.1	23	21.7	2.6	26	21.3	2.1
4	12	22.9	2.8	18	21.9	2.6	23	21.8	2.4	26	21.3	1.9
5	12	22.6	3.4	18	21.4	2.2	21	22.6	2.7	25	20.4	2.4

Source: Hinck VC, Hopkins CE, Clark WM. Sagittal diameter of the lumbar spinal canal in children and adults. *Radiology* 1965;85:929–37.

Sagittal Diameter of Lumbar Spine

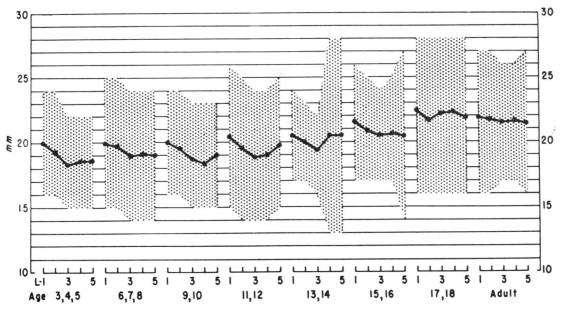

FIG. 14. Age-group means and 90% tolerance limits for the sagittal diameter of the spinal canal of each lumbar vertebra, male and female combined

TABLE 13. *Data for sagittal diameter of the lumbar spine*

Vertebra	N	Mean	S.D.	90% Tolerance Min.	90% Tolerance Max.	N	Mean	S.D.	90% Tolerance Min.	90% Tolerance Max.
		Age 3, 4, 5 years					Age 6, 7, 8 years			
L1	24	20.1	1.6	16	24	24	19.9	2.2	15	25
2	24	19.4	1.2	16	24	24	19.7	1.7	15	25
3	24	18.4	1.3	15	22	25	18.8	1.7	14	24
4	24	18.6	1.2	15	22	25	19.1	1.7	14	24
5	23	18.6	1.5	15	22	25	19.0	2.3	14	24
		Age 9, 10 years					Age 11, 12 years			
L1	12	20.0	1.3	16	24	16	20.6	2.0	15	26
2	13	19.6	1.2	16	24	16	19.6	2.3	14	25
3	13	18.8	1.4	15	23	16	18.9	2.0	14	24
4	13	18.6	1.5	15	23	16	19.0	2.1	14	24
5	13	19.0	1.6	15	23	16	19.8	2.4	15	25
		Age 13, 14 years					Age 15, 16 years			
L1	24	20.6	1.4	17	24	28	21.6	2.2	17	26
2	24	19.9	1.2	17	23	29	20.9	1.9	17	25
3	24	19.4	1.6	16	22	29	20.6	1.6	17	24
4	24	20.4	3.5	13	28	29	20.7	2.0	17	25
5	24	20.5	3.7	13	28	28	20.6	3.2	14	27
		Age 17, 18 years					Adult			
L1	28	22.5	2.1	16	28	47	21.8	2.7	16	27
2	28	21.7	2.1	16	28	49	21.7	2.5	16	27
3	30	22.2	2.7	16	28	49	21.5	2.3	17	26
4	30	22.3	2.7	16	28	49	21.6	2.2	17	26
5	30	21.9	2.8	16	28	49	21.4	2.7	16	27

These are the data from which the graph in Fig. 14 was prepared, including age-group means, standard deviations, and 90% tolerance limits for each lumbar vertebra (sagittal), male and female combined.

Source: Hinck VC, Hopkins CE, Clark WM. Sagittal diameter of the lumbar spinal canal in children and adults. *Radiology* 1965;85:929–37.

Extreme Upper Size of Interpediculate Spaces

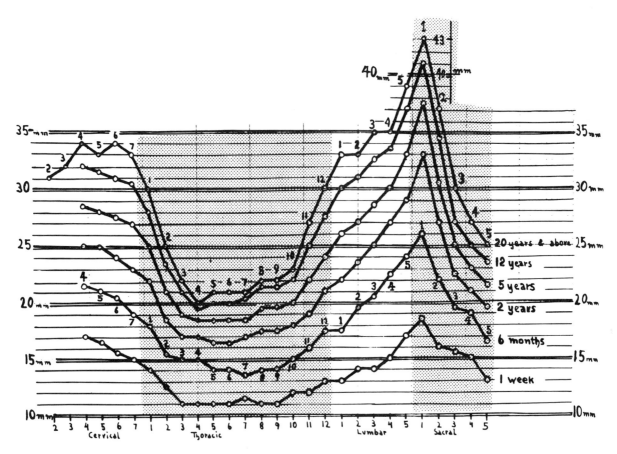

FIG. 15. This composite graph contains a family of curves delineating the largest normal measurement for any vertebra from C4 to S5 inclusive. Curves selected were for the following ages: 1 week or less; 6 months; and 2, 5, 12, and 28 years or older. The last curve (*top curve* on the graph) is that of Ellsberg and Dyke except for the sacral measurements, which were obtained by Schwarz. Selection of ages was solely based on convenient spacing of the curves for best legibility and does not reflect any inherent law of nature.

Sources: Ellsberg CA, Dyke CG. Diagnosis and localization of tumors of the spinal cord by means of measurements made on X-ray film of vertebrae and correlation of clinical and X-ray findings. *Bull Neurol Inst NY* 1934;3:359–94.

Schwarz GS. The width of the spinal canal in the growing vertebra with special reference to the sacrum, maximum interpediculate distances in adults and children. *AJR* 1956;76:476–81.

Spinal Canal Width

A method is presented for comparing the width of the spaces between the vertebral pedicles on radiographs of infants, children, and adults by means of simple line drawings on transparent material portraying the average normal values of persons of similar age and height. The set of transparencies marked with simple linear figures provides such a standard for comparison. The appropriate transparency is selected according to the thoracic height of the individual and is superimposed on the radiograph for direct comparison. The thoracic height is defined as the distance measured on the radiograph from the cervical thoracic junction to the thoracolumbar junction.

TABLE 14. *Average measurements for standard thoracic height at various ages*

Average Age→		23 days	10 months	2 years	4.5 years	10 years	Adults (18 to 78 years)		
Average Thoracic Height→		10 cm.	13 cm.	16 cm.	19 cm.	25 cm.	29 cm.	31.5 cm.	34 cm.
C	2	...	16 mm.	19 mm.	20 mm.	28.3 mm.	27 mm.	28.8 mm.	29.5 mm.
	3	12.0 mm.	18.0	19.3	21.8	28.5	26.0	27.4	28.8
	4	14.5	19.0	20.0	22.6	29.0	28.0	28.6	30.0
	5	14.6	19.0	21.0	23.5	30.3	29.0	30.0	30.6
	6	15.0	19.0	20.8	23.8	27.8	27.0	29.4	30.6
	7	14.8	18.0	20.5	23.4	27.1	26.2	28.0	28.6
TH	1	13.5	16.0	18.5	19.7	22.5	23.4	23.9	25.4
	2	11.8	14.7	16.2	17.1	19.5	19.9	20.8	21.7
	3	10.9	13.1	15.0	15.6	18.0	18.3	19.9	19.9
	4	10.7	12.7	14.5	15.3	17.2	17.1	18.0	19.0
	5	10.3	12.7	14.4	14.8	16.9	16.9	17.7	18.5
	6	10.4	12.7	14.5	15.0	16.8	16.8	17.5	18.4
	7	10.5	13.0	14.5	15.3	16.6	16.8	17.5	18.4
	8	10.6	13.0	14.8	15.3	16.7	17.1	17.6	19.2
	9	10.9	13.1	14.9	15.6	17.4	17.5	17.8	19.2
	10	10.8	13.3	14.9	15.6	18.0	18.1	18.3	19.8
	11	11.0	13.8	15.7	16.7	19.6	19.6	19.6	20.6
	12	11.9	15.1	17.3	18.7	22.3	22.6	22.8	23.7
L	1	12.5	15.7	18.0	19.7	23.1	23.1	24.9	25.9
	2	13.2	16.1	18.5	20.1	23.7	24.8	25.3	26.7
	3	13.5	16.7	19.5	20.8	25.0	25.7	26.5	27.4
	4	13.9	17.8	20.5	22.6	26.0	26.5	27.7	28.3
	5	14.6	20.5	24.5	25.1	28.6	29.5	30.3	31.0
S	1	15.2	23.6	28.7	32.5	33.6	33.1	33.7	36.9
	2	12.6	18.0	23.5	24.2	27.1	26.3	27.0	32.3
	3	10.6	16.0	20.0	21.0	23.0	22.0	23.4	26.1
	4	10.0	14.0	17.0	18.8	21.0	20.6	21.0	25.0
	5	10.0	12.0	16.0	17.3	18.0	18.3	18.0	21.0
Sample		17 infants newborn to 45 days	23 infants 2 to 12 months	22 children 13 to 35 months	35 children 3 to 7 years	33 children 8 to 14 years	31 adults thoracic height up to 30.4 cm.	33 adults thoracic height 30.5 to 32.9 cm.	36 adults thoracic height 33 cm. or more

Data are given in millimeters of average thoracic height.

Source: Haworth JB, Keillor GW. Use of transparencies in evaluating the width of the spinal canal in infants, children, and adults. *Radiology* 1962;79:109–14.

Tracings from radiographs of infants and children illustrate the relative widths of different portions of the spinal canal from the neonatal period to adolescence using thoracic height as noted in Table 14.

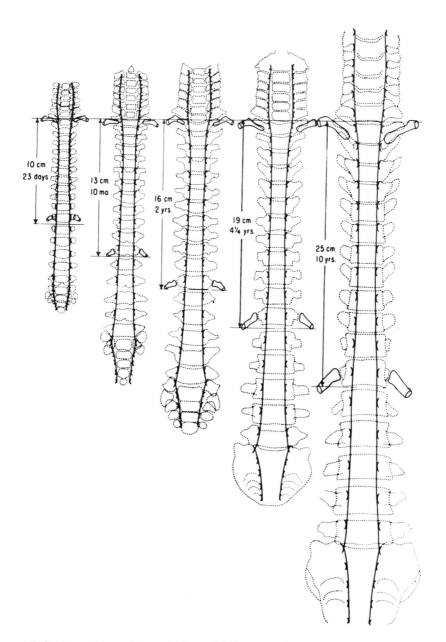

FIG. 16.   Shape of the spinal canal during growth

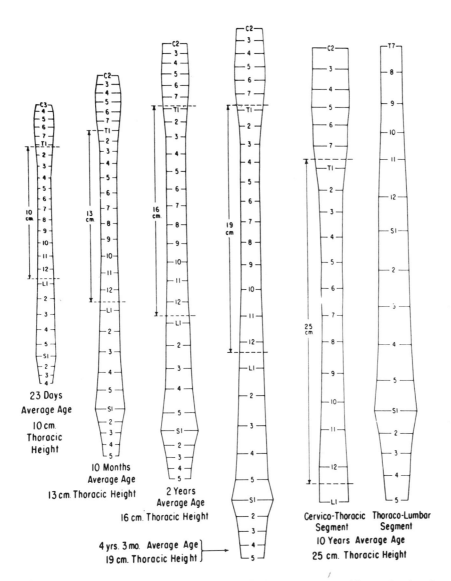

FIG. 17. Photographic reduction of the original 14 × 17 transparency used for evaluating the width of the spinal canal in infants and children. Measurements are derived from films exposed at a 40-inch tube–film distance and are corrected for divergent distortion.

Source: Haworth JB, Keillor GW. Use of transparencies in evaluating the width of the spinal canal in infants, children, and adults. *Radiology* 1962;79:109–14.

Intrapedicular Distances

Intrapedicular distances were measured on 474 roentgenograms, including 353 children (boys and girls under the age of 19 years) and 121 adults. The first two cervical vertebrae were excluded as unmeasurable, and the sacral measurements were omitted for want of an adequate sample. Because the roentgenograms had been taken for purposes other than this study, it was not possible in all cases to visualize the entire spine for measurement. Thus, there is a sample size variation from one vertebra to the next.

TABLE 15. *Mean interpediculate distance of each vertebra by age: males and females combined*

	3, 4, 5	6, 7, 8	9, 10	11, 12	13, 14	15, 16	17, 18	Adult
Age (yr.)	4.1	7.1	9.4	11.6	13.6	15.6	17.5	>18
Vertebra								
C3	23.9	26.0	26.4	26.2	27.2	27.1	27.7	28.0
4	24.9	26.8	26.9	27.0	28.3	28.2	28.7	28.8
5	25.3	27.2	27.1	27.4	28.6	28.6	29.1	29.4
6	25.3	27.6	27.0	27.3	28.5	28.2	29.1	29.3
7	24.4	26.4	26.2	25.9	27.2	26.9	27.6	28.0
T1	21.4	22.4	23.4	23.5	23.4	23.5	23.1	24.0
2	18.2	18.9	20.0	19.8	20.1	19.9	19.8	20.5
3	16.9	17.6	18.4	18.1	18.7	18.1	18.4	18.8
4	16.0	17.0	17.6	17.2	18.1	17.3	17.8	18.1
5	15.8	16.8	16.9	16.8	17.7	17.1	17.5	17.6
6	15.8	16.7	16.5	16.8	17.8	16.7	17.3	17.3
7	16.0	16.9	16.5	16.8	18.2	16.9	17.5	17.4
8	16.3	17.6	16.7	17.1	18.4	17.3	18.0	17.7
9	16.4	17.8	17.0	17.4	18.7	17.7	18.3	18.2
10	16.4	18.1	17.2	17.7	18.8	17.8	18.8	18.7
11	17.6	19.2	18.5	18.9	20.3	19.5	20.0	20.2
12	19.9	21.2	21.2	21.4	23.1	22.3	22.8	23.2
L1	20.5	21.8	23.0	23.0	23.7	23.9	24.5	25.0
2	20.4	21.9	23.2	23.1	23.4	23.9	24.4	25.5
3	20.8	22.4	23.8	23.6	24.0	24.6	24.8	26.0
4	21.7	23.3	24.8	24.9	25.7	25.6	26.1	26.9
5	24.5	26.5	28.3	28.7	29.1	29.1	29.6	29.7

Data are given in millimeters.

TABLE 16. *Mean interpediculate distance of each vertebra by age: males*

	3, 4, 5	6, 7, 8	9, 10	11, 12	13, 14	15, 16	17, 18	Adult
Age (yr.)	4.0	7.0	9.4	11.6	13.5	15.6	17.4	>18
Vertebra								
C3	24.3	26.3	26.9	26.0	26.9	27.9	28.6	28.6
4	25.5	27.4	27.3	27.8	28.0	28.8	29.5	29.5
5	26.1	27.8	27.5	27.0	28.4	29.3	29.9	30.3
6	25.8	28.2	27.3	27.2	28.4	29.2	30.1	30.2
7	24.8	27.1	26.2	26.0	27.3	28.0	28.8	29.3
T1	22.5	22.7	23.8	23.8	24.2	25.2	24.5	25.1
2	19.4	19.7	20.4	20.6	20.6	21.7	21.2	21.4
3	17.9	18.1	19.0	18.8	19.1	19.2	19.4	19.6
4	16.9	17.6	18.2	17.6	18.3	18.0	18.7	18.8
5	16.4	17.3	17.4	17.4	18.3	17.7	18.4	18.2
6	16.5	17.3	18.8	17.4	18.3	17.3	18.2	17.8
7	16.7	17.5	16.5	17.4	18.5	17.6	17.9	17.8
8	17.0	18.1	16.7	17.6	18.9	18.3	18.4	18.0
9	17.0	18.5	17.0	17.8	19.3	18.6	18.7	18.6
10	16.9	18.8	17.3	18.1	19.5	18.1	18.9	19.1
11	18.2	20.1	18.8	19.2	20.9	19.8	20.2	20.4
12	20.4	22.5	21.3	21.8	23.5	23.2	23.4	23.5
L1	20.7	22.5	23.3	23.9	23.8	24.5	25.1	25.9
2	20.7	22.4	23.5	24.2	23.3	24.6	24.8	26.5
3	21.2	23.0	24.1	24.6	23.6	25.1	25.2	26.8
4	21.9	23.6	24.8	23.6	24.7	26.0	26.6	27.6
5	24.7	26.9	28.4	28.9	28.0	30.1	29.9	30.7

Data are given in millimeters.

Source: Hinck VC, Clark WM, Hopkins CE. Normal interpediculate distances (minimum and maximum) in children and adults. *AJR* 1966;97:141–53.

TABLE 17. *Mean interpediculate distance of each vertebra by age: females*

	3, 4, 5	6, 7, 8	9, 10	11, 12	13, 14	15, 16	17, 18	Adult
Age (yr.)	4.2	7.2	9.6	11.6	13.7	15.5	17.6	>18
Vertebra								
C3	22.1	25.5	24.8	26.6	27.5	26.6	26.6	27.4
4	22.2	26.0	25.6	27.4	28.4	27.7	27.5	28.2
5	22.3	26.4	25.9	28.0	28.7	28.1	27.9	28.7
6	23.6	26.7	26.0	27.3	28.6	27.5	28.0	28.6
7	24.0	25.5	26.3	25.8	27.1	26.1	26.1	27.1
T1	19.8	22.1	23.1	23.0	22.6	22.3	22.4	23.1
2	16.6	18.2	19.7	18.8	19.6	18.9	19.1	19.8
3	15.2	17.0	17.9	17.5	18.3	17.6	17.9	18.2
4	14.6	16.3	17.1	16.6	17.8	16.9	17.4	17.4
5	14.6	16.3	16.6	16.0	17.2	16.8	17.1	17.1
6	14.5	16.1	16.3	15.9	17.4	16.5	16.9	16.9
7	14.7	16.3	16.5	16.1	17.8	16.6	17.4	17.0
8	15.0	16.9	16.6	16.4	18.0	16.8	17.8	17.4
9	15.1	17.1	16.9	16.8	18.1	17.3	18.2	17.9
10	15.4	17.3	17.1	17.1	18.2	17.7	18.7	18.4
11	16.5	18.0	18.2	18.4	19.8	19.2	19.9	20.0
12	19.1	20.2	21.1	20.9	22.8	21.7	22.5	22.9
L1	20.1	21.0	22.5	22.2	23.7	23.6	24.1	24.3
2	20.0	21.1	22.6	22.3	23.6	23.6	24.2	24.9
3	20.2	21.7	23.2	22.8	24.6	24.4	24.5	25.4
4	21.1	23.0	24.7	24.2	26.9	25.4	25.8	26.4
5	23.9	26.1	28.2	28.5	30.4	28.6	29.5	29.0

Data are given in millimeters.

Source: Hinck VC, Clark WM, Hopkins CE. Normal interpediculate distances (minimum and maximum) in children and adults. *AJR* 1966;97:141–53.

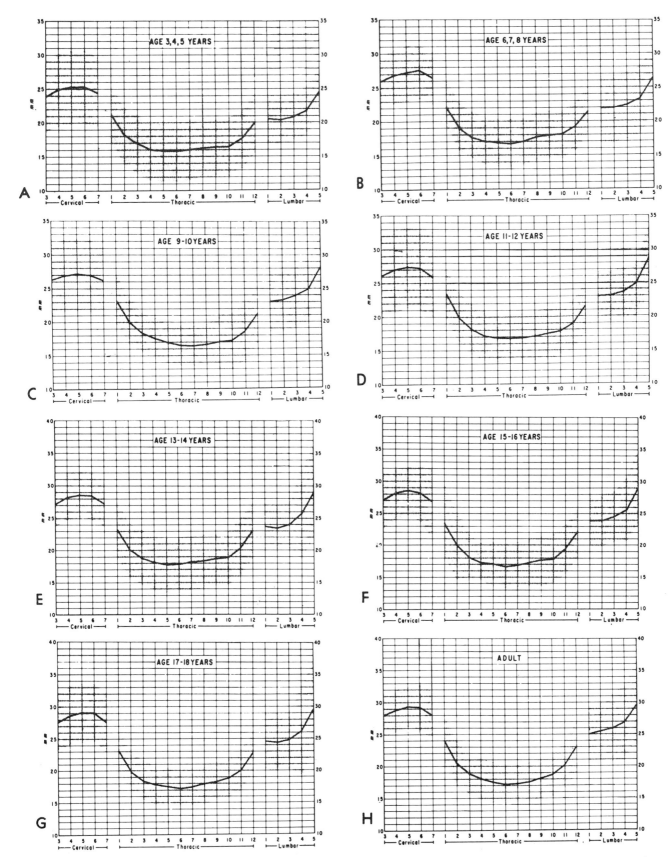

FIG. 18. *Tolerance range (90%) of the interpedicular distance in each vertebra: male and female combined.* **A:** Age 3–5 years. **B:** Age 6–8 years. **C:** Age 9–10 years. **D:** Age 11–12 years. **E:** Age 13–14 years. **F:** Age 15–16 years. **G:** Age 17–18 years. **H:** Adult.

TABLE 18. *Standard deviation of interpediculate distance of each vertebra by age: males and females combined*

	3, 4, 5	6, 7, 8	9, 10	11, 12	13, 14	15, 16	17, 18	Adult
				Standard Deviation in mm. (Sample Size, N)				
Age (yr.)	.09 (35)	.08 (52)	.05 (30)	.05 (46)	.05 (59)	.05 (63)	.05 (68)	— (121)
Vertebra								
C3	1.7 (8)	1.5 (18)	1.7 (8)	2.6 (18)	1.2 (22)	1.8 (17)	1.9 (21)	1.5 (36)
4	1.7 (8)	1.5 (18)	1.3 (8)	2.5 (18)	1.5 (23)	1.6 (18)	2.0 (22)	1.5 (43)
5	1.7 (8)	1.7 (18)	1.6 (8)	2.6 (19)	1.7 (23)	1.6 (18)	2.1 (22)	1.7 (44)
6	1.7 (9)	1.7 (18)	1.7 (8)	2.7 (20)	2.1 (23)	1.8 (20)	2.2 (24)	1.8 (50)
7	1.4 (9)	2.0 (19)	2.1 (8)	2.8 (21)	1.8 (25)	2.4 (21)	2.1 (24)	2.0 (60)
T1	2.5 (12)	1.9 (14)	1.4 (10)	2.2 (22)	1.5 (17)	2.3 (19)	1.6 (27)	1.8 (53)
2	2.2 (12)	1.6 (14)	1.2 (10)	2.0 (23)	1.8 (17)	2.4 (21)	1.4 (27)	1.7 (53)
3	1.6 (12)	1.5 (14)	0.9 (9)	1.6 (23)	1.6 (17)	1.5 (20)	1.3 (27)	1.5 (50)
4	1.5 (12)	1.4 (14)	1.0 (9)	1.7 (23)	1.8 (15)	1.3 (19)	1.3 (26)	1.6 (43)
5	1.4 (13)	1.2 (14)	0.8 (9)	1.6 (22)	1.8 (15)	1.4 (19)	1.3 (25)	1.7 (42)
6	1.6 (13)	1.2 (13)	1.0 (9)	1.5 (22)	1.8 (15)	1.3 (19)	1.6 (25)	1.5 (42)
7	1.6 (12)	1.2 (13)	1.3 (9)	1.4 (22)	1.9 (15)	1.6 (19)	1.5 (26)	1.5 (42)
8	1.6 (13)	1.4 (14)	1.0 (9)	1.5 (22)	1.9 (15)	1.6 (19)	1.5 (25)	1.5 (41)
9	1.5 (13)	1.3 (15)	1.3 (10)	1.6 (23)	1.8 (15)	1.8 (19)	1.6 (26)	1.5 (43)
10	1.3 (14)	1.4 (17)	1.6 (10)	1.7 (23)	2.0 (17)	1.6 (20)	1.5 (26)	1.6 (44)
11	1.5 (15)	1.9 (17)	1.8 (10)	1.8 (23)	2.3 (18)	1.7 (24)	1.7 (30)	1.8 (53)
12	1.5 (17)	2.1 (17)	1.6 (11)	1.8 (24)	2.3 (20)	1.7 (28)	1.7 (31)	2.0 (59)
L1	1.6 (26)	1.9 (33)	1.8 (20)	1.7 (26)	1.6 (35)	2.0 (40)	2.4 (37)	2.2 (59)
2	1.5 (26)	2.0 (32)	1.6 (20)	1.8 (25)	1.6 (35)	1.8 (40)	2.2 (36)	2.3 (57)
3	1.6 (26)	2.1 (33)	1.7 (20)	1.9 (25)	2.0 (35)	1.9 (40)	2.3 (36)	2.7 (53)
4	1.7 (26)	2.1 (33)	2.3 (20)	3.1 (24)	3.3 (34)	2.4 (39)	2.9 (36)	3.0 (52)
5	1.9 (26)	3.1 (33)	2.7 (20)	3.1 (23)	3.6 (34)	2.9 (38)	3.6 (35)	3.7 (50)

Sample size in parentheses; data are standard deviations in millimeters.

TABLE 19. *Tolerance range (90%) of interpediculate distance of each vertebra by age: males and females combined*

	3, 4, 5	6, 7, 8	9, 10	11, 12	13, 14	15, 16	17, 18	Adult
Vertebra								
C3	18–29	22–30	21–32	20–32	24–31	23–31	23–32	25–31
4	19–30	23–31	21–32	21–33	25–32	24–32	24–33	26–32
5	20–31	23–31	22–32	21–33	25–32	25–32	25–34	26–33
6	20–31	24–31	22–32	21–33	25–32	24–33	25–34	26–33
7	19–30	23–31	21–32	20–32	24–31	21–32	23–32	24–32
T1	17–26	19–26	20–27	20–27	19–28	18–29	20–26	20–28
2	14–22	15–22	17–24	16–24	16–24	14–25	17–23	17–24
3	13–21	14–21	15–21	14–22	15–23	15–22	15–21	16–22
4	12–20	14–21	15–21	14–21	14–22	14–20	15–21	15–21
5	12–20	13–20	14–20	13–21	14–22	14–21	15–21	14–21
6	12–20	13–20	14–20	13–20	14–22	13–20	14–20	14–20
7	12–20	13–21	14–20	13–20	14–22	13–21	15–21	14–20
8	12–21	14–21	14–20	13–21	14–23	14–21	15–21	15–21
9	12–21	14–21	13–21	14–21	15–23	14–22	15–21	15–21
10	12–21	15–22	13–21	14–21	15–23	14–22	16–22	16–22
11	13–22	16–23	14–23	15–22	16–25	16–23	17–23	17–24
12	16–24	18–25	17–25	18–25	19–27	18–26	20–26	19–27
L1	17–24	17–27	19–28	19–27	20–27	20–28	20–29	21–29
2	17–24	17–27	19–28	19–27	20–27	20–28	20–29	21–30
3	17–24	17–27	19–28	20–27	21–28	21–29	20–29	21–31
4	18–25	18–28	20–29	20–28	19–33	21–30	19–33	21–33
5	21–28	22–32	24–33	24–34	22–36	23–35	23–37	23–37

Data are given in millimeters.

These are the data from which the graphs in Fig. 18 were derived.

Source: Hinck VC, Clark WM, Hopkins CE. Normal interpediculate distances (minimum and maximum) in children and adults. *AJR* 1966;97:141–53.

Vertebral Bodies and Disc Spaces

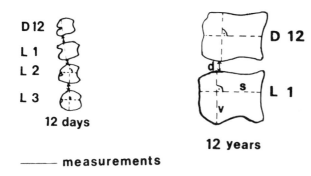

FIG. 19. *Method of measuring vertebral bodies and disc spaces.* Note that only the dotted lines were measurable. This method is used to form the indices, which include intervertebral body I_{vb}, the vertical diameter v divided by the sagittal diameter s; I_d is the intervertebral disc thickness d divided by the vertical vertebral diameter v.

$$\frac{v}{s} = I_{vb}$$

$$\frac{d}{v} = I_d$$

TABLE 20. *The ratio of the vertical divided by the sagittal diameter of various vertebral bodies*

Vertebral Body	Age Group	n	Mean v/s	s	Range $x \pm 2s$	p
D12	I	13	0.81	0.061	0.69–0.93	
	II	26	0.91	0.077	0.75–1.06	<0.005
	III	22	0.86	0.066	0.73–0.99	≅0.10
	IV f	18	0.86	0.062	0.74–0.98	
	IV m	35	0.78	0.052	0.67–0.88	<0.001
	V f	7	0.93	0.148	0.64–1.23	
	V m	20	0.84	0.116	0.60–1.07	<0.05
L1	I	16	0.87	0.060	0.76–0.99	
	II f	11	1.02	0.066	0.88–1.15	<0.001
	II m	16	0.96	0.043	0.87–1.05	<0.02
	II m+f	27	0.98	0.055	0.87–1.09	
	III	23	0.89	0.080	0.73–1.05	<0.001
	IV f	20	0.87	0.068	0.73–1.00	<0.001 (IV f/m)
	IV m	40	0.80	0.048	0.70–0.90	<0.001 (IV f/Vf)
	V f	19	1.03	0.095	0.88–1.22	<0.001 (IV m/Vm)
	V m	27	0.87	0.063	0.74–0.99	<0.001 (V f/m)
L2	I	10	0.92	0.060	0.80–1.04	
	II	21	1.01	0.090	0.83–1.19	<0.01
	III	20	0.91	0.060	0.79–1.03	<0.001
	IV	49	0.82	0.076	0.67–0.97	<0.001
	V f	15	1.03	0.096	0.84–1.22	<0.001
	V m	25	0.88	0.086	0.70–1.05	<0.001
L3	I	11	0.95	0.068	0.81–1.08	
	II	17	0.98	0.084	0.81–1.15	<0.25
	III	16	0.88	0.081	0.72–1.04	<0.005
	IV	35	0.79	0.072	0.67–0.91	<0.001
	V f	11	1.00	0.101	0.80–1.20	<0.001
	V m	17	0.87	0.094	0.68–1.03	<0.001

f, girls; m, boys; n = number; v/s = vertical/sagittal.

TABLE 21. *The ratio of the intervertebral disc thickness divided by the vertical vertebral diameters of various vertebral segments*

	Age Group	*n*	Mean *d/v*	*s*	Range *x* ± 2*s*	*p*
D 11/12	I	12	0.37	0.060	0.25–0.49	<0.005
	II	26	0.30	0.065	0.16–0.43	
	III	19	0.25	0.089	0.08–0.43	
	IV	49	0.24	0.053	0.13–0.34	≪0.001
	V	21	0.18	0.042	0.10–0.26	
D 12/L1	I	17	0.35	0.063	0.22–0.48	<0.01
	II	27	0.28	0.068	0.14–0.41	
	III	20	0.26	0.057	0.14–0.37	
	IV	53	0.25	0.050	0.15–0.35	≪0.001
	V	37	0.19	0.043	0.10–0.28	
L 1/2	I	15	0.35	0.046	0.26–0.44	<0.001
	II	26	0.26	0.073	0.12–0.41	
	III	19	0.27	0.055	0.15–0.38	>0.25
	IV	44	0.28	0.047	0.18–0.37	
	V	37	0.20	0.056	0.09–0.31	≪0.001
L 2/3	I	9	0.38	0.075	0.23–0.53	
	II	18	0.28	0.089	0.10–0.46	~0.01
	III	15	0.30	0.083	0.13–0.47	
	IV	32	0.30	0.049	0.20–0.40	
	V	22	0.21	0.051	0.11–0.31	≪0.001

d, disc thickness/vertical; s, sagittal; *n* = number; *d/v* = disc thickness/vertical; *s* = sagittal.

TABLE 22. *Age groups used in Tables 20 and 21*

Age	Age group
0–1 Month	I
2–18 Months	II
19–36 Months	III
4–12 Years	IV
13+ Years	V

Source: Brandner ME. Normal values of the vertebral body and intervertebral disk index during growth. *AJR* 1970;110:618–27.

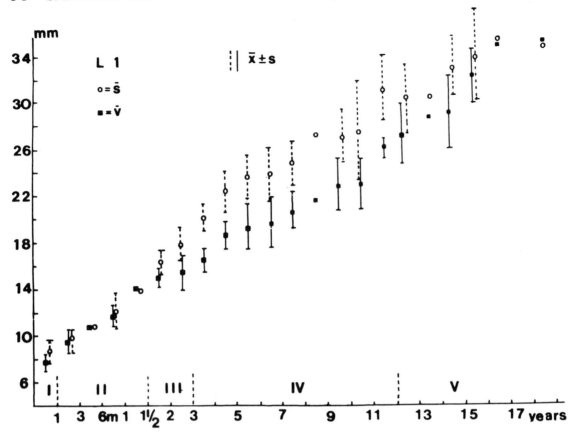

FIG. 20. Measured values of vertical (v) and sagittal (s) diameters of the first lumbar vertebral body in comparison to age

Source: Brandner ME. Normal values of the vertebral body and intervertebral disk index during growth. *AJR* 1970;110:618–27.

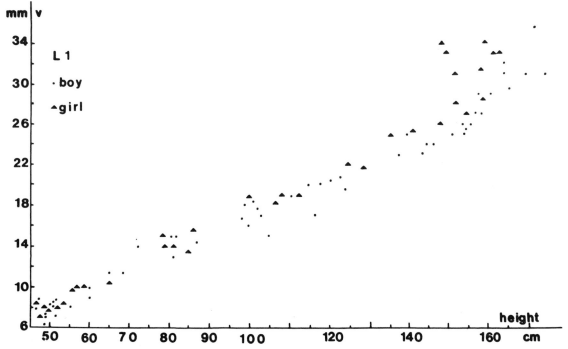

FIG. 21. Measured values of the sagittal diameter (s) of the first lumbar vertebral body as a function of the height of the children

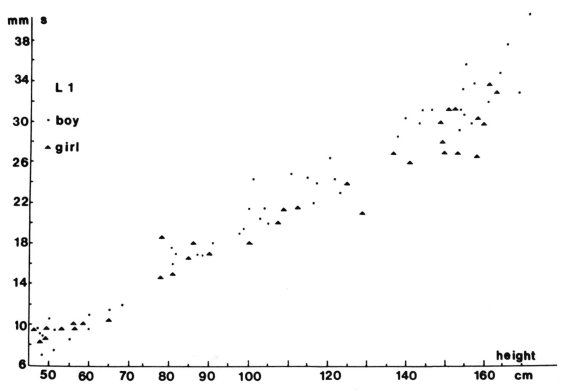

FIG. 22. Measured values of the vertical diameter (v) of the first lumbar vertebral body as a function of the height of the children

Measurement of Spinal Cord

A group of 110 normal air myelograms of children were reviewed. The spinal cord and subarachnoid space were measured in the sagittal diameter at the midvertebral level at right angles to the long axis of the cord and the transverse diameter at the interpedicular level. The ratio of the spinal cord width to the subarachnoid space width *(cord/SAS)* was calculated in both the sagittal and transverse planes. Values for this ratio were found to be independent of age and sex. The mean values at different vertebral levels are in close agreement with those previously reported for adults.

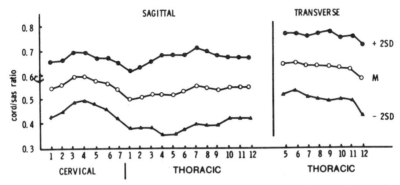

FIG. 23. Cord/SAS ratio in sagittal and transverse planes. The results are given as the mean values and 2 SD.

TABLE 23. *Spinal cord/SAS ratio*

	Ratio of sagittal diameters			Ratio of transverse diameters		
Level	n	x	S.D.	n	x	S.D.
C–1	44	0.56	0.06			
C–2	48	0.57	0.05			
C–3	51	0.61	0.05			
C–4	53	0.61	0.05			
C–5	54	0.59	0.05			
C–6	53	0.58	0.06			
C–7	51	0.55	0.06			
Th–1	24	0.51	0.06			
Th–2	19	0.52	0.07			
Th–3	16	0.53	0.07			
Th–4	17	0.53	0.08			
Th–5	16	0.53	0.09	5	0.66	0.07
Th–6	18	0.54	0.08	15	0.67	0.06
Th–7	23	0.57	0.08	21	0.65	0.06
Th–8	31	0.56	0.08	41	0.65	0.07
Th–9	44	0.55	0.07	56	0.65	0.07
Th–10	50	0.56	0.07	71	0.64	0.06
Th–11	54	0.56	0.06	71	0.64	0.07
Th–12	56	0.56	0.06	65	0.59	0.08

Number of measurements; *x*, mean value; S.D., standard deviation.

These are the data from which the graph in Fig. 23 was constructed.

Source: Boltshauer E, Hoare RD. Radiographic measurements of the normal cord in childhood. *Neuroradiology* 1976;10:235–7.

Length of Spinal Cord Segments

Length of spinal cord segments in 20 children with myelodysplasia and 15 normal children in the same age group. Small steel pins were passed directly through the posterior aspect of the spinal cord at the level between the egress of the dorsal root nerve fibers running to the spinal segments. X-rays of this preparation were obtained, and the distance between the center points of the pins was measured with fine calipers.

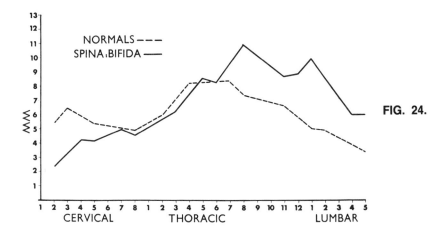

FIG. 24.

Source: Emery JL, Naik D. Spinal cord segment lengths in children with meningo-myelocele and the "Cleland–Arnold Chiari" deformity. *BJR* 1968;41:287–90.

Cervical Spine Mobility According to Age

Lateral upright roentgenograms with the head and neck in flexion, extension, and neutral position were obtained in 160 randomly selected children who had no history of symptoms of neck injury or recent upper respiratory infection. Ten children representing each year of age from 1 to 16 were studied.

TABLE 24.

Age (Years)	1	2	3	4	5	6	7	8	9	10	11	12	13	14	15	16	Total (1-16 Yrs.) (No.)	(Per cent)	Total (1-7 Yrs.) (No.)	(Per cent)
Anterior displacement C2–C3 (marked)	4	1	3	1	2	2	0	0	1	1	0	0	0	0	0	0	15	9	13	19
Anterior displacement C2–C3 (moderate)	1	2	1	3	2	2	4	1	1	2	3	1	1	0	0	0	24	15	15	21
Anterior displacement C2–C3 (total)	5	3	4	4	4	4	4	1	2	3	3	1	1	0	0	0	39	24	28	40
Measured anteroposterior movement 3 mm. and over	5	4	5	2	5	6	5	2	4	5	4	6	7	4	4	3	71	44	32	46
Number of children with measured anteroposterior movement over 3 mm. and observed anterior displacement at C2–C3	4	3	3	1	3	4	3	0	1	3	1	1	1	0	0	0	28	18	21	30
Anterior displacement C3–C4 †	3	2	1	1	2	4	1	0	2	2	2	1	1	0	0	0	22	14	14	20
Overriding of anterior arch of atlas relative to odontoid (extension views) ‡	2+	4++	3++	1	1+	3	0	1	0	0	0	0	0	0	0	0	14	9	14	20
Wide space between anterior arch of atlas and odontoid (flexion views)	2	2	3	2	2	2	1	0	0	0	0	0	0	0	0	0	14	9	14	20
																			Total (5-11 Yrs.) (No.)	(Per cent)
Presence of apical odontoid epiphysis	0	0	0	0	3	2	3	1	4	1	4	0	0	0	0	0	15	9	18	26
																			Total (1-5 Yrs.) (No.)	(Per cent)
Presence of basilar odontoid cartilage plate	10	9	9	6	4	0	0	0	0	0	0	0	0	0	0	0	48	30	38	76
Angulation at single level	1	4	1	1	3	3	2	0	1	2	1	2	2	1	2	0	25	16		
Absent lordosis in neutral position	3	0	0	0	0	0	0	1	2	1	3	2	2	5	1	2	22	14		
Absent flexion curvature C2–C7 in flexion view	1	2	1	6	4	1	0	0	2	3	1	1	1	1	2	0	26	16		

* Bold face numbers represent predominant age range for particular variable.
† Twenty of twenty-two children with anterior displacement at C3–C4 also had displacement at C2–C3.
‡ Presence of wide atlanto-odontoid space in same child (each + represents one child).

Source: Cattell HS, Filtzer DL. Pseudosubluxation and other normal variations in the cervical spine in children: a study of one hundred and sixty children. *J Bone Joint Surg (AM)* 1965;47:1295–1309.

Anterior Displacement of C2

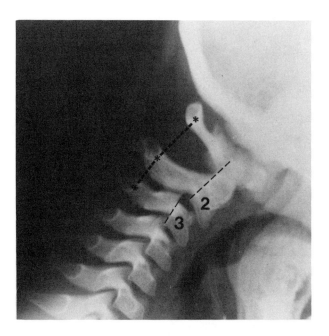

FIG. 25. In forward flexion, C2 slides forward so as to produce a variable degree of anterior offsetting of C2 on C3 *(anterior thin dotted lines)*. The posterior arch of C2 moves forward with the body of C2 and in so doing aligns itself in straight-line fashion with the posterior arches of C1 and C3 *(posterior thick dotted lines)*. This alignment is normal and as such constitutes the basis for the posterior cervical line proposed by Swischuk. These conclusions come from a review of all cervical spine radiographs in 500 children up to the age of 14 years from 1974 to 1975.

Source: Swischuk LE. Anterior displacement of C2 in children: physiologic or pathologic? A helpful differentiating line. *Radiology* 1977;122:759–63.

Development of the Sternum

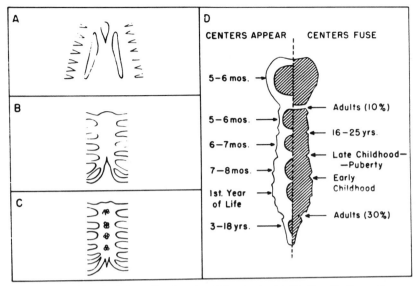

A—The Mesoblastic Primordia (2 Lateral Bands And A Median Rudiment)

B—Plate Of Hyaline Cartilage Originating From The Chondrification And Mid-Line Fusion Of The Primordia

C—Appearance Of Islands Of Hypertrophied Chondroblasts—The Future Ossification Centers

D—Ossification And Fusion Of The Various Sternebrae (Infant And Adult Sternum)

FIG. 26. Main stages of normal development of the sternum and its sutures. The true sternum originates from three agglomerations of mesoblastic cellular tissue embedded in the chest wall. **A:** Two lateral sternal bands, first visible at 6 weeks, and the anterior median rudiment, which appears slightly later. The sternal bands originate independently of the ribs; the medial element is embryologically related to the primordia of the shoulder girdle. **B:** As the embryo grows, the two sternal bands unite with the tips of the ribs, migrate forward with them, incorporate the median element, and finally fuse in the midventral line to form a single structure. All the mesenchymal primordia are rapidly converted to cartilage. **C:** Cartilage cells usually appear laterally in the sternal bands between ribs at the levels where the sternebrae will later develop. At 9 weeks, the sternum is uniformly cartilaginous and in shape resembles the future bone. It is still entirely unsegmented and solidly united with the ribs. A definite segmentation into the sternebrae is a late occurrence. **D:** Averge time at which the various segments of the sternum begin to ossify and the ages at which they fuse with each other. Multiple-ossification centers for each sternebra, especially in the gladiolus, are not uncommon.

Sources: Arey LB. *Developmental Anatomy*. Philadelphia: Saunders, 6th ed., 1954.

Bryson, V. Development of the sternum in screw-tail mice. *Anat Rec* 1945;91:119–41.

Cunningham DJ. *Textbook of Anatomy*. New York: Oxford University Press, 6th ed., 1931.

Currarino G, Silverman FN. Premature obliteration of the sternal sutures and pigeon-breast deformity. *Radiology* 1958;70:532–40.

Gladstone RJ, Wakeley CPG. Morphology of the sternum and its relations to the ribs. *J Anat* 1932;66:508–64.

Gray's Anatomy. Philadelphia: Lea & Febiger, 26th ed., 1954.

Hanson FB. Ontogeny and phylogeny of sternum. *Am J Anat* 1919:26:41–115.

Paterson AM. *The Human Sternum*. Liverpool: Williams & Norgate, 1904.

Warkany J, Nelson RC. Skeletal abnormalities in the offspring of rats reared on deficient diets. *Anat Rec* 1941;79:83–100.

HIP AND PELVIS

Center Edge Angle of Wiberg

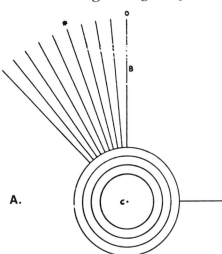

A.

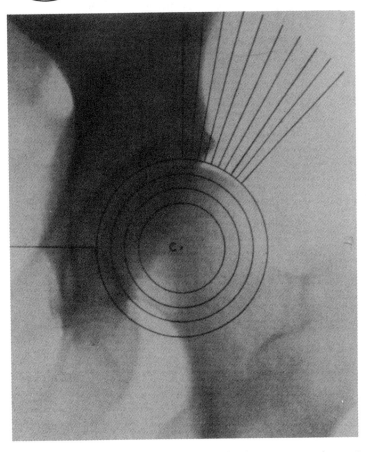

B.

FIG. 1.   Method for obtaining the center edge (CE) angle. **A:** A transparency is constructed by draw-ing four circles with a radius of 1.5 to 3 cm (0.5 cm between each) with India ink. From the center *(C)* a line *(A)* is drawn in the longitudinal axis of the film, and another line *(B)* is drawn perpendicular to A. Lines are then drawn from the center to form 5°, 15°, and so on up to 45° angles with B. **B:** The pattern so obtained is used in the following way. The circles are put over the femoral head in the roentgen plate under examination. One of the peripheries is fitted in parallel with the contour of the head, and through a small perforation in C the center of the head is marked with a pencil. The same is done with the femoral head on the other side. The lateral acetabular border *(E)* is marked on both sides. The pattern is placed over the film with C covering one of the head centers and line A running through the other. Thus for practical purposes line A goes through the center of the other head, and consequently line B lies parallel to the longitudinal axis of the body. E is the lateral edge of the ace-tabular roof, and the CE angle in this case is 14°.

TABLE 1. *Center edge angles in normal subjects*

Subjects	\multicolumn{11}{c}{No. of subjects with various center edge (C.E.) angles}

Subjects	20°	21°	22°	23°	24°	25°	26–30°	31–35°	36–40°	41–45°	46°+
Men	1	—	—	4	2	5	23	37	21	5	2
Women	—	—	2	—	3	1	31	29	23	10	1

Briefly summarizing the results of the investigation on normal series, CE angles below 20° may be considered definitely pathologic, indicating a defective development of the acetabular roof; values over 25° are definitely normal. Values between 20° and 25° are uncertain.

Source: Wiberg G. Studies on dysplastic acetabula and congenital subluxation of the hip joint. *Acta Chir Scand* 1939;(Suppl. 58)83:1–135.

Passive Range of Hip Motion in Normal Children

TABLE 2. *Range of hip motion in normal subjects*

Age	Flexion contracture (°) Mean	Range	"Frog leg" abduction (°) Mean	Range	Internal rotation (°) Mean	Range	External rotation (°) Mean	Range
Newborn[b]								
Male	28.0	20–75	76.7	50–90	60.8[a]	45–100[a]	87.5[a]	45–110[a]
Female	27.5	20–45	76.2	60–90	63.1[a]	35–90[a]	90.6[a]	60–110[a]
6 Weeks[c]	19	6–32			24	16–36	48	26–73
3 Months[c]	7	1–18			21	15–35	45	37–60
6 Months[c]	7	−1–+16			21	15–42	46	34–61
4 Years[d]					36		40	
9 Years[d]					26		36	

[a]Internal and external rotation were determined with the hip flexed 90°.
[b]Normal ranges of hip motion in the newborn. Hass SS, Epps CH, Adams JP. *Clin Orthop* 1973;91:114–18.
[c]Normal ranges of hip motion in infants–six weeks, three months, and six months of age. Coon V, Donato G, Houser C, Bleck EE. *Clin Orthop* 1975;110:256–60.
[d]Femoral torsion and its relation to toeing in and toeing out. Crane L. *J Bone Joint Surg (Am)* 1959;41:421–28. Note that these figures were estimated from a graph in Crane's paper.

Source: Chung, SMK. *Hip disorders in infants and children*, Philadelphia: Lea and Febiger, 1981.
Related References:
Engel GM, Staheli LT. Natural history of torsion and other factors influencing gait in childhood. *Clin Orthop* 1974;99:12.
Pitkow RB. External rotation contracture of the extended hip. *Clin Orthop* 1975;110:139.

Clinical Examination of Normal Infants

This study included 1,000 normal infants who were examined clinically and by X-ray at birth, 6 months, and 1 year of age.

TABLE 3. *Clinical findings and examination of skin folds in infants' hips to age three*

Parameter	White		Black	
	Male	Female	Male	Female
Total examined (no.)	267	268	217	242
Symmetrical folds (%)	50.0	55.0	49.0	51.0
Asymmetrical folds (%)	36.0	30.0	33.0	26.0
Extra folds (%)	14.0	15.0	18.0	23.0

TABLE 4. *Shortening and instability in newborn infants' hips*

Parameter	White		Black	
	Male	Female	Male	Female
Total examined (no.)	267	268	217	242
Apparent shortening (%)	1.0	0.0	0.5	0.4
Instability (%)	4.0	5.0	5.0	4.0

The relative length of the limb and the presence of instability as manifested by push/pull laxity or click or jerks were noted.

TABLE 5. *Degree of abduction at hips*

Parameter	White		Black	
	Male	Female	Male	Female
Total examined (no.)	269	269	220	242
Percent with angles				
Less than 45°	0.0	0.0	0.0	0.0
45° Bilateral	0.4	0.0	0.0	0.4
60° Bilateral	9.0	5.0	6.0	6.0
75° Bilateral	45.0	44.0	45.0	48.0
90° Bilateral	42.0	49.0	47.0	41.0
105° Bilateral	0.4	1.0	0.0	1.0
Abduction unequal	3.0	1.0	2.0	3.0

Source: Ryder CT, Mellun GW, Caffey J. The infant's hip—normal or dysplastic? *Clin Orthop* 1962;22:7–15.

Neck Shaft Angle

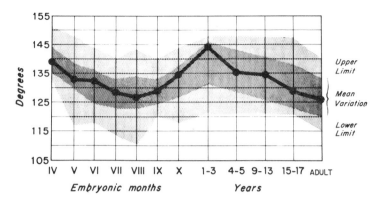

FIG. 2.   Variation of the neck shaft with age, starting with embryonic life and extending through to adulthood.

Source: Von Lanz T, Mayet A. Die gelenkorper des menschlichen hufgelenkes in der progredienten phase iherer umwegigen ausformung. *Z Anat* 1953;117:317–45.

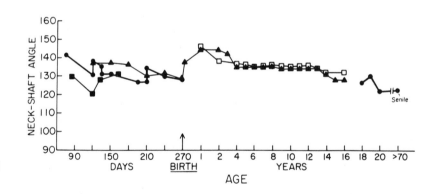

FIG. 3.   A composite graph of neck shaft angle from embryonic life to adulthood. (●) The angle of the neck with the shaft of the femur at different periods of life and under different circumstances. Humphrey, PR. *J Anat Physiol* 1889;23:273; (□) Die gelenkorper des menschlichen hufgelenkes in der progredienten phase iherer unwegigen ausformung. von Lanz T, Mayet AM. *Z Anat* 1953;117:317–45; (▲) Shands AR, Steele MK. Torsion of the femur. *J Bone Joint Surg (Am)* 1958;40:803; (■) Watanabe RS. Embryology of the human hip. *Clin Orthop* 1974;98:8–26.

Source: Chung SMK. *Hip disorders in infants and children*. Philadelphia: Lea & Febiger, 1981.

Measurement of Femoral Anteversion

The relationship between the various angles is given by the formula:

$$\tan A = \frac{\tan a \, \cos(i - \theta)}{\cos i}$$

in which

A = angle of anteversion
a = projected angle of anteversion
i = projected angle of inclination minus 90°
θ = angle of abduction used in making that view

This formula defines the relationships of the true angle of anteversion to the projected angles. The data contained in Fig. 4 were obtained by substituting all the various possible values for a and i, and solving for A in each case.

projected anteversion

inclination	0	5	10	15	20	25	30	35	40	45	50	55	60	65	70	75	80	85	90
80	0	3	7	12	16	20	24	29	33	38	43	47	53	59	65	71	77	84	
90	0	4	9	13	17	22	27	31	36	41	46	51	56	62	67	73	79	84	
95	0	5	9	14	18	23	28	32	37	42	47	52	58	63	68	74	79	85	
100	0	5	10	14	19	24	29	34	39	44	49	54	59	64	69	74	80	85	90
105	0	5	10	15	20	25	30	35	40	45	50	55	60	65	70	75	80	85	90
110	0	5	10	16	21	26	31	36	41	46	51	56	61	66	71	76	80	85	90
115	0	5	11	16	22	27	32	38	43	48	53	57	62	67	72	76	81	85	90
120	0	6	11	17	23	28	34	39	44	49	54	59	63	68	72	77	81	86	90
125	0	6	12	18	24	30	35	41	46	51	56	60	65	69	73	78	82	86	90
130	0	6	13	19	25	31	37	42	47	52	57	62	66	70	74	78	82	86	90
135	0	7	14	20	27	33	38	44	48	54	58	63	67	71	75	79	83	86	90
140	0	7	14	21	28	34	40	46	50	56	60	64	68	72	76	80	83	87	90
145	0	8	16	23	30	36	42	48	53	58	62	66	70	74	77	80	84	87	90
150	0	9	17	25	32	39	45	50	55	60	64	68	72	75	78	81	84	87	90
155	0	10	19	27	35	42	48	54	58	63	67	70	73	77	79	82	85	87	90
160	0	11	22	31	39	46	52	58	62	65	70	73	76	78	81	83	86	88	90
165	0	13	26	36	45	52	57	62	66	70	73	76	78	80	82	84	86	88	90
170	0	18	33	45	53	60	65	69	72	75	77	79	81	83	84	86	87	89	90
175	0	29	48	59	67	71	75	77	79	81	82	84	85	86	87	88	88	89	90
180	0	90	90	90	90	90	90	90	90	90	90	90	90	90	90	90	90	90	90

projected inclination (left axis) — ANTEVERSION (right axis)

FIG. 4. Ryder and Crane method.

Source: Ryder CT, Crane LL. Measuring femoral anteversion. *J Bone Joint Surg (Am)* 1953;35:324–8.

Figure 5 was prepared from the Webber formula No. 1 (below) in which the angle of abduction is 10°, which is the amount of abduction recommended for the lateral roentgenogram

$$\tan \theta = \tan \theta_2(\cos a - \cot B_2 \sin a)$$

where

θ = true angle of torsion
θ_2 = measured angle of torsion
a = angle of abduction
B = true angle of inclination
B_2 = measured angle of inclination

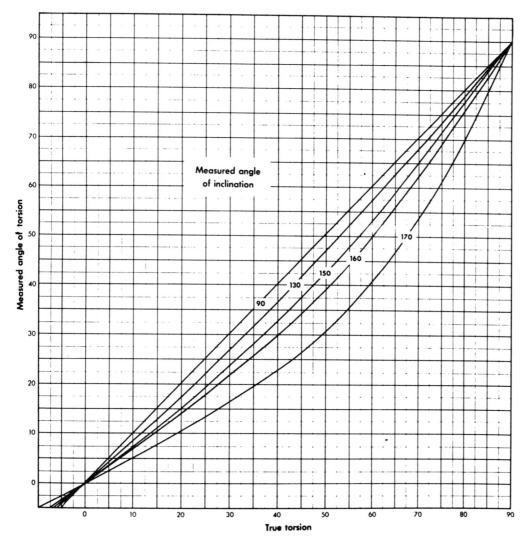

FIG. 5. Relationship of the true angle of torsion, measured angle of torsion, and measured angle of inclination from the roentgenograms, according to the K. Dunlap and A. R. Shands method.

Source: Dunlap K, Shands AR Jr, Hollister LC, Gaul JS Jr, Streit HA. A new method for determination of torsion of femur. *J Bone Joint Surg (Am)* 1953;35:289–311.

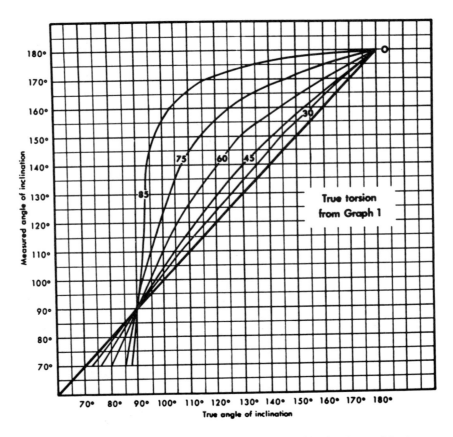

FIG. 6. Relationship of the true angle of inclination to the measured angle of inclination and the true angle of torsion; prepared from the Webber formula No. 2:

$$\cot B = \cot B_2 \times \cos \theta$$

Source: Dunlap K, Shands AR Jr, Hollister LC, Gaul JS Jr, Streit HA. A new method for determination of torsion of femur. *J Bone Joint Surg (Am)* 1953;35:289–311.

Femoral Anteversion

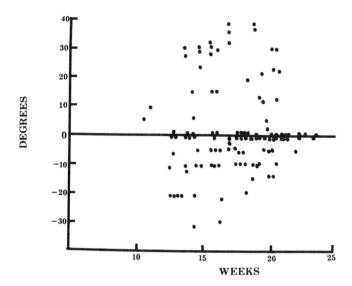

FIG. 7. Femoral anteversion versus weeks of embryologic development. These data are from a study based on the dissection and evaluation of 114 embryos and fetuses (288 hip joints).

Source: Watanabe RS. Embryology of the human hip. *Clin Orthop* 1974;98:8–26.

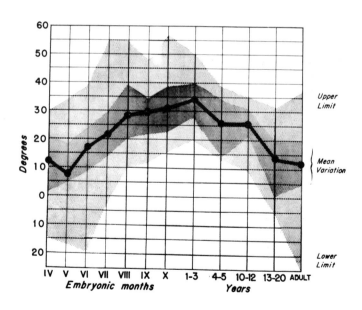

FIG. 8. Femoral anteversion from embryonic life to adulthood.

Source: Von Lanz T. Die gelenkorper des menschlichen hufgelenkes in der progredienten phase iherer unwegigen ausformung. *Z Anat* 1953;117:317–45.

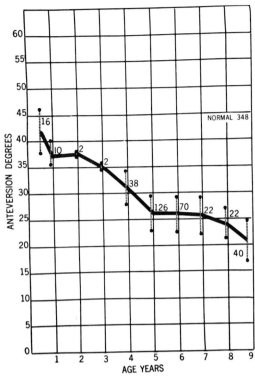

FIG. 9. Femoral anteversion versus age in normal children.

This chart was compiled from studies of 348 normal children. The dotted lines represent the standard deviation of the mean.

Source: Crane L. Femoral torsion and its relation to toeing in and toeing out. *J Bone Joint Surg (Am)* 1959;41:421–8.

TABLE 6. *Anteversion in 432 normal children*

Age (Yrs.)	No. of Studies	Average Anteversion* (Degrees)	Standard Deviation (Degrees)
1	96	31.13	8.936
2	74	29.96	8.486
3	66	26.71	7.260
4	78	26.17	7.770
5	66	26.70	7.401
6	68	26.60	7.189
7	52	23.19	6.976
8	40	24.40	6.523
9	42	21.26	5.504
10	54	20.89	6.598
11	40	20.60	7.534
12	38	19.87	6.427
13	48	19.98	6.104
14	34	14.53	8.554
15	42	15.36	8.021
16	26	15.35	7.647
Total	864		

*Average anteversion for all patients was 24.14 degrees.

Data from which the graph in Fig. 10 is constructed.

Source: Fabry G, MacEwen GD, Shands AR Jr. Torsion of the femur. *J Bone Joint Surg (Am)* 1973;55:1726–38.

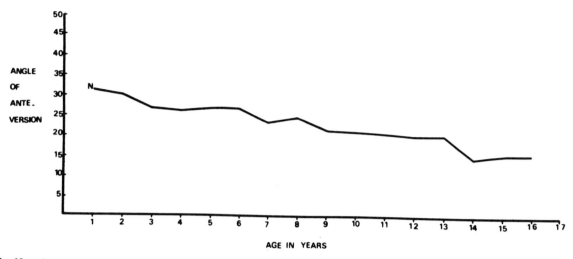

FIG. 10. Angle of anteversion versus age in 432 normal children.

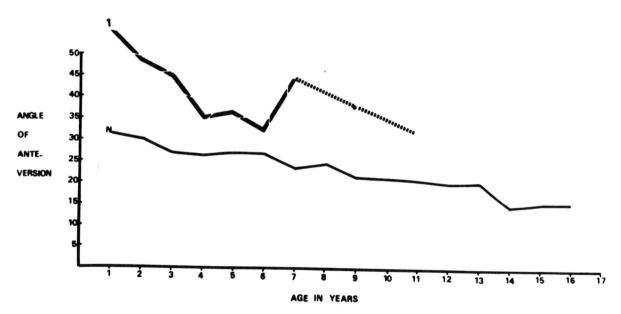

FIG. 11. Femoral anteversion in 151 studies of 93 patients with congenital dislocation of the hip plotted against the normal curve.

The curve was not extended beyond the age of 11 years because of the small number of hips examined in children older than 11. Curve 1 represents the children with dislocated hips. Curve N represents the normals.

Source: Fabry G, MacEwen GD, Shands AR Jr. Torsion of the femur. *J Bone Joint Surg (Am)* 1973;55:1726–38.

TABLE 7. *Anteversion in 93 patients with congenital dislocation of the hip*

Age (Yrs.)	No. of Studies	Average Anteversion (Degrees)	Standard Deviation (Degrees)	P Value
1	3	55.33	1.155	
2	21	48.15	5.393	0.001
3	38	44.62	7.286	0
4	21	34.67	8.898	0.007
5	20	35.73	9.743	0.007
6	13	31.80	8.672	0
7	12	43.67	8.214	0
8	0	0	0	
9	6	38.00	5.228	0
10	0	0	0	
11	7	31.50	2.121	0
12	3	36.00	9.899	0.001
13	2	32.50	8.257	0
14	4	27.00	7.213	0.005
15	1	30.00	0	
16	0	0	0	

These are the data from which the graph in Fig. 11 was constructed.

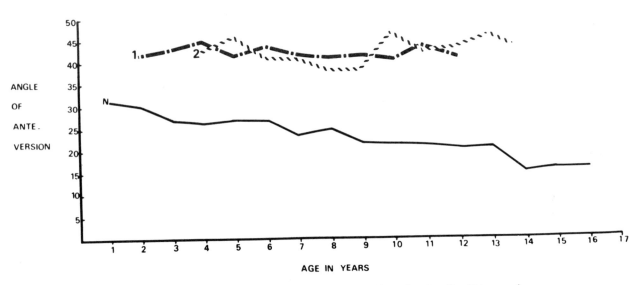

FIG. 12. Comparison of femoral torsion in 154 hips of 77 patients with toeing in after 5½ years' follow-up. Curve 1 represents the first study, curve 2 represents those with toeing in, and curve N represents the normals.

Source: Fabry G, MacEwen GD, Shands AR Jr. Torsion of the femur. *J Bone Joint Surg (Am)* 1973;55:1726–38.

TABLE 8. *Anteversion in 77 patients with toeing-in gait after an average 5½ years' follow-up*

Age (Yrs.)	No. of Hips	Average Anteversion (Degrees)	Standard Deviation (Degrees)	P Value
1	0	0	0	
2	0	0	0	
3	4	35.75	10.971	0.056
4	4	42.00	5.598	0.035
5	18	44.89	8.595	0.001
6	24	40.21	7.271	0
7	28	40.20	9.002	0.012
8	10	37.50	8.303	0.003
9	22	37.65	8.676	0
10	10	45.83	10.057	0
11	10	41.80	6.877	0
12	8	42.33	2.944	0
13	8	45.00	3.543	0.001
14	6	43.00	10.728	0.002
15	0	0	0	
16	2	32.50	6.364	0

These are the data from which the graph in Fig. 12 was constructed.

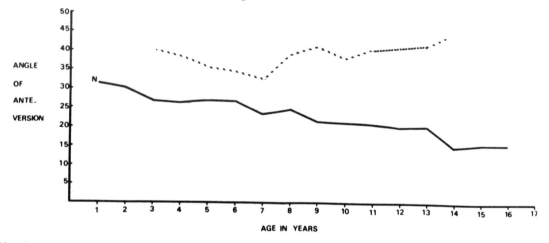

FIG. 13. Increased anteversion in 180 hips of patients with cerebral palsy. N = normal.

TABLE 9. *Anteversion in 91 patients with cerebral palsy*

Age (Yrs.)	No. of Hips	Average Anteversion (Degrees)	Standard Deviation (Degrees)	P Value
1	0	0	0	
2	0	0	0	
3	6	40.00	8.025	0
4	20	38.10	4.506	0.001
5	4	35.25	7.805	0.008
6	38	34.11	9.226	0.007
7	22	32.10	10.279	0.009
8	32	38.74	6.967	0.001
9	10	40.43	6.241	0
10	12	37.50	10.210	0.001
11	8	40.27	7.994	0
12	2	40.00	5.657	0
13	12	41.00	6.723	0
14	10	43.67	5.132	0.002
15	0	0	0	
16	4	48.00	6.321	0

These are the data from which the graph in Fig. 13 was constructed.

Femoral Head Diameter

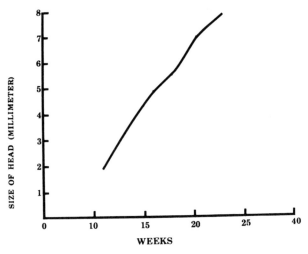

FIG. 14. Femoral head diameter vs weeks of gestation.

This was a study of 144 embryos and fetuses representing a total of 288 hip joints.

***

Source: Watanabe RS. Embryology of the human hip. *Clin Orthop* 1974;98:8–26.

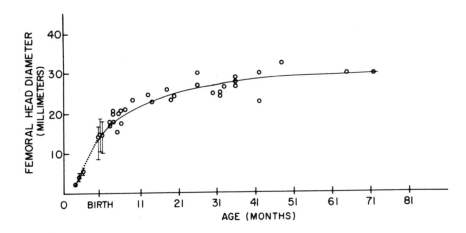

FIG. 15. Femoral head diameter vs age.

The data in Fig. 15 were derived from 129 femoral heads measured with a micrometer. There were 51 specimens from fetuses with an estimated age of 2.8 to 4.8 months, and 78 specimens from children (52 boys and 26 girls) ranging in age from birth to 16 years 10 months. Newborns weighing less than 2.5 kg and patients with connective tissue abnormalities were excluded.

***

Source: Chung SMK. *Hip disorders in infants and children.* Philadelphia: Lea & Febiger, 1981.

Derivation of Quotients

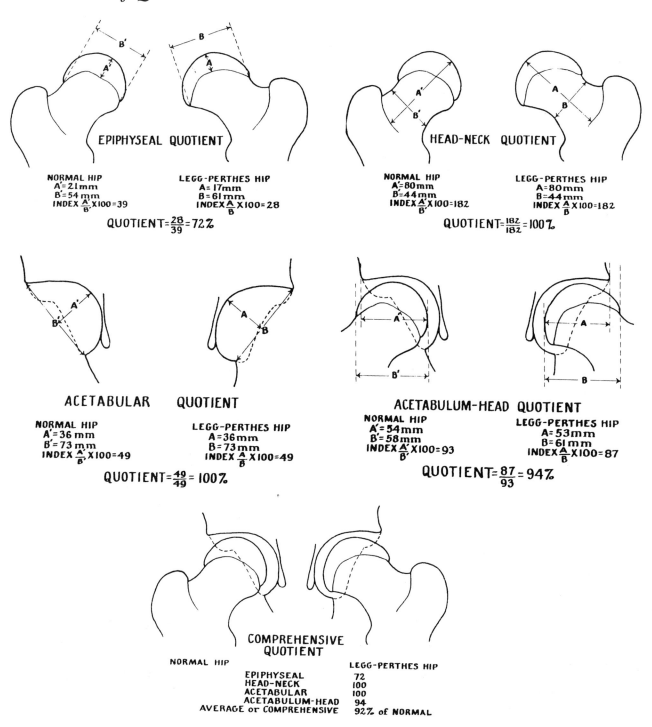

FIG. 16. Measurement system proposed by Heyman and Herndon for the more precise appraisal of roentgenographic results and for comparative statistical studies. The diagrams illustrate the method of measurement, comparing the normal hip **(left)** and a hip with Legg-Perthes disease **(right)**.

Source: Heyman CH, Herndon CH. Legg-Perthes disease, a method for the measurement of the roentgenographic result. *J Bone Joint Surg (Am)* 1950;32:767–78.

Heyman-Herndon Measurements

Ten normal children between the ages of 5 and 13 were examined radiologically in the following manner: Supine and prone anteroposterior roentgenograms of the pelvis were obtained with the pelvis flat and the hips in a neutral attitude. Keeping the tube in the same position, a supine anterior roentgenogram with a 1-cm elevation under the left buttock was then obtained with both hips in a neutral position, followed by bilateral internal and external rotation exposures as well as a lateral exposure. The epiphyseal Heyman-Herndon measurements were then determined. The epiphyseal (EQ), head and neck (HNQ), acetabular (AQ), and acetabular head (AHQ) quotients were measured with the hips in a neutral position and the pelvis flat and elevated by 1 cm on the left side. A modified comprehensive quotient (CQ) was created by leaving the HNQ out in the compilation of the standard CQ.

TABLE 10. *Changes in the Heyman-Herndon quotients caused by a 1-cm pelvic tilt along the longitudinal axis in 10 normal children*

	EQ		HNQ		AQ		AHQ		CQ	
	Flat	Tilt	Flat	Tilt	Flat	Tilt	Flat	Tilt	Flat	Tilt
Average (%)	100	100	98	97	98	94	96	100	99	98
Range (%)	All 100	All 100	94–100	89–100	90–100	86–100	87–100	97–100	98–100	96–100

Values were recorded for the other side.

TABLE 11. *Changes in the HNQ and AH indices caused by hip rotation in 10 normal children*

	H.N.Q.			A.H.I.		
	Internal rotation	Neutral	External rotation	Internal rotation	Neutral	External rotation
Average (%)	99	97	66	92	90	85
Range (%)	90–100	89–100	56–86	85–100	83–100	72–92

Values were recorded for the rotated side.

Source: Schiller MG. Legg-Calve-Perthes syndrome (L.C.P.S.): a critical analysis of roentgenographic measurements. *Clin Orthop* 1972;86:34–42.

Medial Joint Space Measurements

The teardrop distance or Waldenstroms interval is the distance between the metaphysis margin of the medial proximal femur and the lateral pelvic teardrop margin.

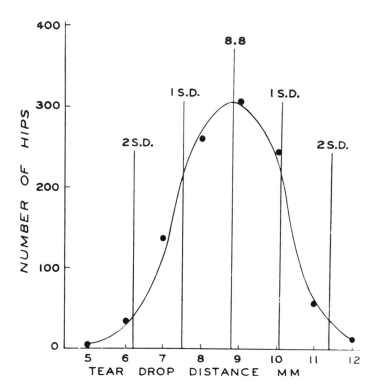

FIG. 17. Graph illustrating the distribution of the teardrop distance in 1,070 hips with no known hip joint disease.

TABLE 12. *Data from which Fig. 17 was constructed*

Study	Age (yrs)	No. of hips	Average MJS (mm)	Range (mm)
Eyring et al.[a]	6 mo–11	1,070	8.8	5–12
Schiller & Axer[b]	5–13	20	7.0	5–10

[a]Eyring EJ, Bjornson DR, Peterson CA. Early diagnostic and prognostic signs in Legg-Calve-Perthes disease. *AJR* 1965;93:382.

[b]Schiller MD, Axer A. Legg-Calve-Perthes syndrome (L.C.P.S.): a critical analysis of roentgenographic measurements. *Clin Orthop* 1972;86:34–42.

MJS = medial joint space.

Source: Eyring EJ, Bjornson DR, Peterson CA. Early diagnostic and prognostic signs in Legg-Calve-Perthes disease. *AJR* 1965;93:382.

Acetabular Depth

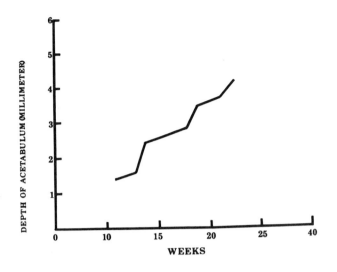

FIG. 18. Depth of the acetabulum vs weeks' gestation.

Source: Watanabe RS. Embryology of the human hip. *Clin Orthop* 1974;98:8–26.

Depth of Acetabulum and Size of Femoral Head

Roentgenograms with dye injected into the hip were measured. The measurements indicated that both dimensions increase with advancing age. The size of the femoral head increased slightly more than the depth of the acetabulum.

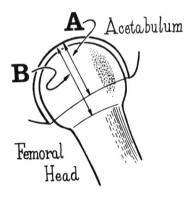

FIG. 19. Measurement of the depth of the acetabulum **(A)** and the size of the femoral head **(B)**.

TABLE 13. *Depth of the acetabulum and length of the femoral head in 10 hips of otherwise normal fetuses*

Crown-to-Rump Length (*Millimeters*)	Specimen No.	Age (*Weeks*)	Acetabulum (*Millimeters*)	Femoral Head (*Millimeters*)
90	9	14	2.30	2.70
110	7	15	2.40	3.00
128	22	16	3.30	3.40
135	21	18	3.20	3.60
155	27	19	4.00	4.00
175	25	21	3.60	3.60
185	15	23	5.00	6.60
210	16	25	6.00	5.90
300	94	34	8.5	11.00
	33	Term	8.5	10.00

Source: Laurenson RD. Development of the acetabular roof in the fetal hip. *J Bone Joint Surg (Am)* 1965;47:975–83.

Acetabular Measurements

Forty-four hip joints were studied in 15 fetuses and 29 children. The diameter and depth of the acetabulum were determined, as well as the diameter and height of the femoral head.

Acetabulum diameter: The greatest width of the cavity a^1 was measured with calipers. Depth: This was measured by using two wires. One was placed across the greatest diameter of the mouth of the cavity lying on the fibrocartilaginous labrum; the second wire, at right angles to the first marked the distance a^2 between this "bridge" and the deepest part of the socket.

Femoral head diameter: The greatest diameter h^1 was measured with calipers. Height: This dimension (h^2), at right angles to the above and representing the distance from the greatest convexity of the head to the articular margin, was also measured with calipers.

Cover of the femoral head: The head was returned to the acetabulum in that position in which it was most completely covered, i.e., when the axis of the cavity and that of the femoral neck were identical. The line of the acetabular margin was then marked out on the head either by drawing with a fine felt-tipped pen or by marking it with a line of pins. The distance between this line and the convexity of the head was then measured (h^3) so that the proportion of the total height of the head covered by the acetabulum could be calculated (h^3/h^2).

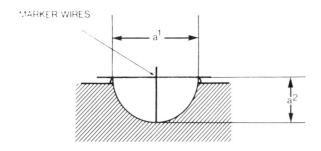

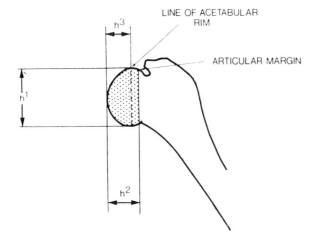

FIG. 20. Methods of measuring the acetabulum.

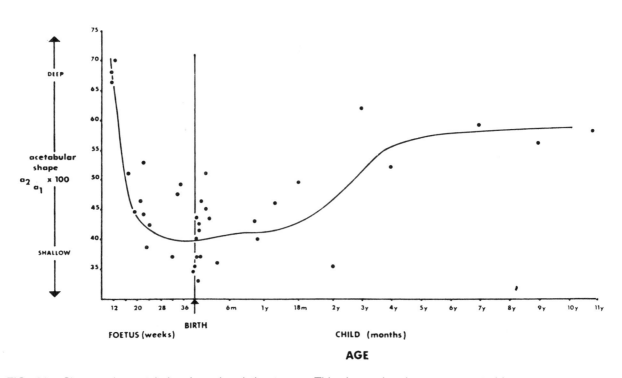

FIG. 21. Changes in acetabular shape in relation to age. This change has been represented by expressing the depth (a_2) as a percentage of the width (a_1), so that if the cavity is deep and represents more than a complete hemisphere the ratio will be greater than 50%.

In the embryo the femoral head is quite globular, representing as much as 80% of the complete sphere, but as birth approaches it becomes closer to a hemisphere. After birth the globular appearance returns to some extent, although the head never again attains the sphericity seen in the embryo.

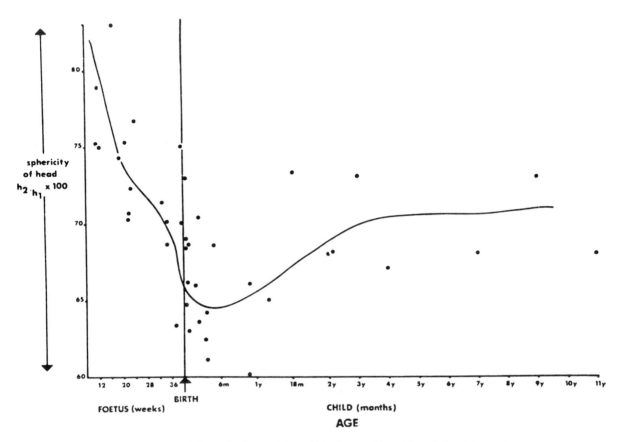

FIG. 22. Changes in the shape of the articular position of the femoral head in relation to age. h_2 represents height and h_1 the width.

Source: Ralis Z, McKibbin B. Changes in shape of the human hip joint during its development and their relation to its stability. *J Bone Joint Surg (Br)* 1973;55:780–5.

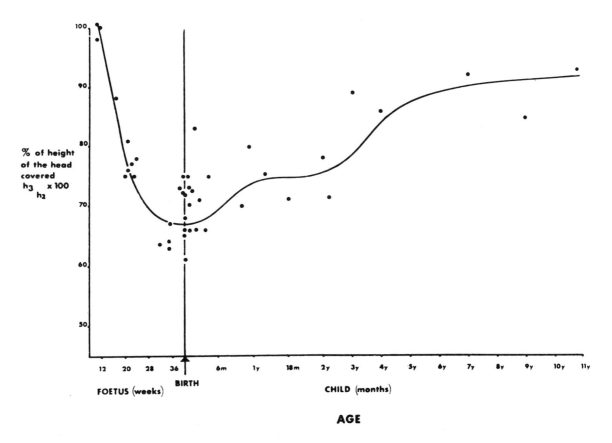

FIG. 23. Changes in proportion of the femoral head covered by the acetabulum in relation to age. This figure demonstrates that the proportion of the head contained within the acetabulum gradually diminishes as the fetus grows, reaching a minimum at the time of birth.

Source: Ralis Z, McKibbin B. Changes in shape of the human hip joint during its development and their relation to its stability. *J Bone Joint Surg (Br)* 1973;55:780–5.

Sagittal Acetabular Inclination

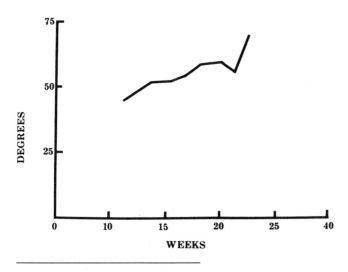

FIG. 24. Sagittal acetabular inclination versus weeks of gestation.

Source: Watanabe RS. Embryology of the human hip. *Clin Orthop* 1974;98:8–20.

Symphysis/Os Ischium Angle

When the acetabular index (Hilgenreiner) is measured, twisting the pelvis can be controlled by dividing the diameter of the right foramen obturatum by that on the left side. In a neutral position this index would be 1. By turning to the right side the diameter of the right foramen gets smaller and the left one larger. Therefore the index shows values below 1 when the pelvis is turned to the right and above 1 when turned to the left.

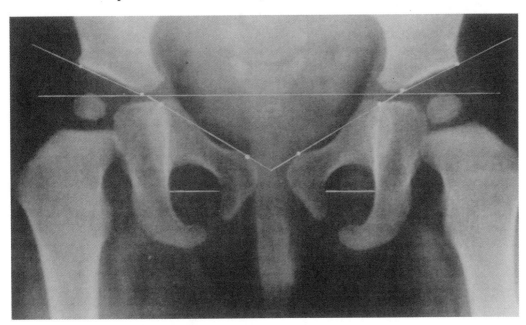

FIG. 25. Method for evaluating twisting of pelvis.

The angle was measured, and the material was used to prepare a normal distribution curve. A mean distribution for each age group in which most of the cases are included has been determined and is shown in Table 14.

TABLE 14. *Symphysis/os ischium angle measured on 1,582 X-rays (3,164 normal hip joints)*

Age (months)	Symphysis/os ischium angle (°)
1–2	98–130
3–4	100–135
5–6	98–128
7–12	96–126
13–18	90–127
19–24	92–128
25–36	90–124
37–60	85–115

Source: Tonnis D. Normal values of the hip joint for the evaluation of X-rays in children and adults. *Clin Orthop* 1976;119:39–48.

Acetabular Angle

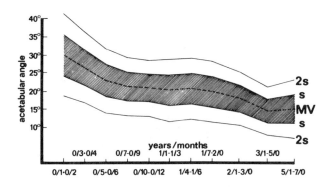

FIG. 26. Acetabular angle plotted against age. A total of 2,294 acetabular angles, mean values, and one (s) and two (2s) standard deviations were evaluated. Patients with no other diseases and apparently normal hip joints were included, as were those in whom there were doubts as to the normalcy of hip joints.

Source: Tonnis D. Normal values of the hip joint for the evaluation of X-rays in children and adults. *Clin Orthop* 1976;119:39–48.

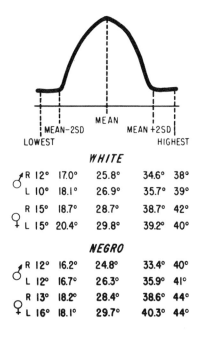

FIG. 27. Acetabular angle.

WHITE

♂ R	12°	17.0°	25.8°	34.6°	38°
L	10°	18.1°	26.9°	35.7°	39°
♀ R	15°	18.7°	28.7°	38.7°	42°
L	15°	20.4°	29.8°	39.2°	40°

NEGRO

♂ R	12°	16.2°	24.8°	33.4°	40°
L	12°	16.7°	26.3°	35.9°	41°
♀ R	13°	18.2°	28.4°	38.6°	44°
L	16°	18.1°	29.7°	40.3°	44°

Roentgenograms were studied for evidence of displacement in 1,000 normal infants. X-rays were obtained at birth and the acetabular angle measured.

Source: Ryder CT, Mellin GW, Caffey J. The infant's hip—normal or dysplastic? *Clin Orthop* 1962;22:7–15.

Acetabular Angle—Mean and Range Newborn, 6 Months and 1 Year

This was a study of 627 infants examined during the first week of life for clinical signs of predislocation and for the acetabular angle by the Hilgenreiner method radiologically. The same infants were later examined in the same way at 6 and 12 months of age. Examined were 627 newborns of whom 551 were later reexamined at 6 months, and 527 at 12 months. Data are further broken down into white (344:197 males and 147 females), and black (283:134 males and 149 females).

TABLE 15. *Acetabular angle in 627 infants (males and females)*

	White male (right)		White male (left)		White female (right)		White female (left)		Black male (right)		Black male (left)		Black female (right)		Black female (left)	
	Mean	Range	Mean	Range	Mean	Range	Mean	Range	Mean	Range	Mean	Range	Mean	Range	Mean	Range
Newborn	25.8	34–17	27.0	37–17	28.3	38–18	29.4	39–20	24.8	34–15	26.0	36–16	27.7	38–18	29.4	39–19
6 mo.	19.4	26–12	20.9	28–13	22.1	30–14	23.4	32–15	21.4	31–12	23.0	32–14	23.9	32–16	25.4	33–18
12 mo.	19.1	26–12	20.6	28–13	20.5	28–13	21.9	20–14	20.5	29–12	21.9	30–14	22.5	30–15	24.4	32–16

Range = 2 SD.

Source: Caffey J, Ames R, Silverman W, Ryder CT, Hough G. Contradiction of the congenital dysplasia-predislocation of the hip through a study of the normal variation in acetabular angles at successive periods in infancy. *Pediatrics* 1956;17:632–41.

Center Edge (CE) Angle

TABLE 16. *Size of the CE angle in 200 normal hips in children 6 to 17 years old*

AGE	SEX	15°	16°	17°	18°	19°	20°	21°	22°	23°	24°	25°	26°	27°	28°	29°	30°	31°	32°	33°	34°	35°	36°	37°	38°	39°	40°	41°	42°	43°	44°	45°	46°	Total
17	♀	—	—	—	—	—	—	—	—	—	—	—	—	—	—	—	—	—	—	—	1	—	—	—	1	—	—	—	—	—	—	—	—	2
	♂	—	—	—	—	—	—	—	—	—	—	—	—	—	—	—	—	—	—	—	—	—	—	—	—	—	—	—	—	—	—	—	—	..
16	♀	—	—	—	—	—	—	—	—	—	1	—	—	—	—	—	1	1	2	—	1	1	—	3	1	—	2	1	—	—	—	—	—	14
	♂	—	—	—	—	—	—	—	—	—	—	—	—	—	—	—	—	—	—	1	1	—	—	—	—	—	—	—	—	—	—	—	—	2
15	♀	—	—	—	—	—	—	—	—	—	—	—	—	—	1	1	—	—	3	—	1	3	—	—	—	2	1	—	1	1	—	1	1	16
	♂	—	—	—	—	—	—	1	—	1	—	1	—	—	—	1	—	3	—	3	—	—	—	—	—	—	—	—	—	—	—	—	—	10
14	♀	—	—	—	—	—	—	—	—	—	—	—	—	—	1	—	—	5	—	—	2	—	—	—	—	1	1	—	—	—	—	—	—	10
	♂	—	—	—	—	—	—	—	—	—	1	—	1	1	—	—	—	3	1	—	1	—	—	—	1	1	—	—	—	—	—	—	—	10
13	♀	—	—	—	—	—	—	—	—	1	2	1	—	—	—	—	—	2	3	2	—	2	1	—	—	—	—	—	—	—	—	—	—	14
	♂	—	—	—	—	—	—	—	—	—	—	—	—	—	—	—	—	3	—	1	1	1	—	—	—	—	—	—	—	—	—	—	—	6
12	♀	—	—	—	—	—	1	1	—	—	1	1	1	—	—	—	—	—	1	—	—	1	1	—	—	—	—	—	—	—	—	—	—	8
	♂	—	—	—	—	—	1	—	1	1	3	1	—	1	—	2	—	—	—	—	—	—	—	—	—	—	—	—	—	—	—	—	—	10
11	♀	—	—	—	—	—	—	—	—	—	—	—	—	—	—	—	—	1	2	—	1	3	—	1	—	—	—	—	—	—	—	—	—	8
	♂	—	—	—	1	1	—	—	—	—	—	—	1	1	2	—	—	—	2	—	—	2	—	—	—	—	—	—	—	—	—	—	—	10
10	♀	—	—	—	—	—	—	—	—	—	—	—	—	—	—	—	—	—	—	—	1	1	—	—	—	—	—	—	—	—	—	—	—	2
	♂	—	—	—	—	—	1	—	—	—	—	—	—	—	—	1	—	—	1	1	—	1	1	—	—	—	—	—	—	—	—	—	—	6
9	♀	—	—	—	1	1	—	—	—	—	—	—	—	—	—	—	—	—	1	—	—	1	—	—	—	—	—	—	—	—	—	—	—	4
	♂	—	—	—	—	—	—	1	1	—	3	—	—	—	—	—	—	1	—	—	—	—	—	—	—	—	—	—	—	—	—	—	—	6
8	♀	—	1	—	—	—	2	—	—	2	—	—	—	—	1	1	—	1	—	1	—	—	—	1	—	—	—	—	—	—	—	—	—	10
	♂	—	—	—	—	—	—	—	—	—	1	—	—	1	—	1	1	1	2	—	1	—	—	—	—	—	—	—	—	—	—	—	—	8
7	♀	1	—	1	—	2	1	—	—	1	2	2	1	—	—	—	—	—	1	—	—	—	—	—	—	—	—	—	—	—	—	—	—	12
	♂	—	—	—	—	1	1	—	1	1	3	—	—	—	1	1	—	2	2	—	—	—	—	—	—	—	—	—	—	—	—	—	—	12
6	♀	—	—	—	—	—	—	—	—	—	—	—	—	—	—	—	2	—	—	—	—	2	—	—	—	—	—	—	—	—	—	—	—	4
	♂	—	—	—	—	3	—	—	—	—	2	3	1	—	—	2	3	—	—	—	—	2	—	—	—	—	—	—	—	—	—	—	—	16
Total		**1**	**—**	**1**	**1**	**—**	**8**	**5**	**6**	**7**	**11**	**13**	**11**	**6**	**10**	**8**	**23**	**16**	**15**	**10**	**15**	**6**	**6**	**4**	**4**	**3**	**4**	**1**	**2**	**1**	**—**	**1**	**1**	

TABLE 17. *Size of the CE angle in 400 normal hips in persons 6 to 35 years of age*

	Age in years					
CE angle	6—13		14—17		20—25	
	Number of hips	%	Number of hips	%	Number of hips	%
15° . . .	1		—		—	
16° . . .	—		—		—	
17° . . .	1	2 %	—		—	
18° . . .	1		—		—	
19° . . .	—		—		—	
20° . . .	8		—		1	
21° . . .	5		—		2	
22° . . .	6	34½ %	—	4½ %	4	9 %
23° . . .	7		—		5	
24° . . .	9		2		6	
25° . . .	12		1			
26—30° . . .	42	31 %	16	25 %	54	27 %
31—35° . . .	38	28 %	24	37½ %	66	33 %
36—40° . . .	6	4½ %	15	23½ %	44	22 %
41—45° . . .	—	—	5	8 %	15	7½ %
46°— . . .	—	—	1	1½ %	3	1½ %
	136	**100 %**	**64**	**100 %**	**200**	**100 %**

(Wiberg's series)

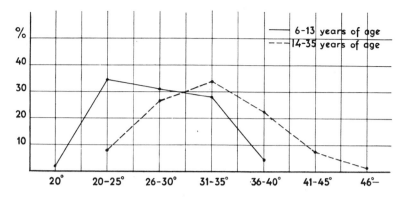

FIG. 28. Relative frequency of different CE angles in different age groups (400 hips).

Source: Severin E. Congenital dislocation of the hip joint. *Acta Chir Scand* 1941;84(Suppl 63):93–142.

Visibility of Femoral Capital Epiphysis

There were 247 apparently normal infants, ages 6 to 7 months in this study. All infants were white and predominantly of northern European descent. The frequency and presence of the ossification center of the femoral capital epiphysis at the two age levels is recorded.

TABLE 18. *Visibility of the femoral capital epiphysis in 247 infants*

Age (months)	Males			Females			Total		
		Visible			Visible		Both sexes	Visible	
	Total	Number	Per cent	Total	Number	Per cent		Number	Per cent
6	61	41	67.2	81	72	88.9	142	113	79.6
7	58	49	84.5	47	46	97.9	105	95	90.5
Total	119	90	75.6	128	118	92.2	247	208	84.2

Source: Harris LE, Lipscomb PR, Hodgson JR. Hilgenreiner measurement of the hip roentgenograms in 247 normal infants 6 and 7 months of age. *Pediatrics* 1960;56:478–84.

Hilgenreiner's Measurements

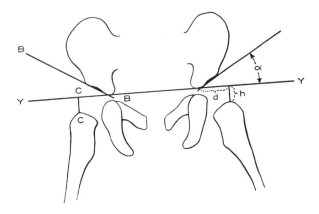

FIG. 29. Hilgenreiner's measurements. Lines *(YY)* are drawn through the acetabulum so as to touch the visible tips of the ilia. *BB* is the line drawn tangentially to the visible acetabular face and through the medial and lateral bony edges of the acetabular face. (This line is difficult to draw accurately in the newborn infant because of the insufficient roentgenographic definition at this age.) *CC* is a line drawn perpendicularly from most cephalic portion of the point of the femoral diaphysis to the YY line. Alpha (α) is the angle between the BB line and the YY line, known as the acetabular angle. *d* Is the distance between the point of transection of the YY line by the CC line, generally referred to as the d line of Hilgenreiner. *h* Is the distance between the most cephalic point of the femoral diaphysis and the point where the CC line transects the YY line.

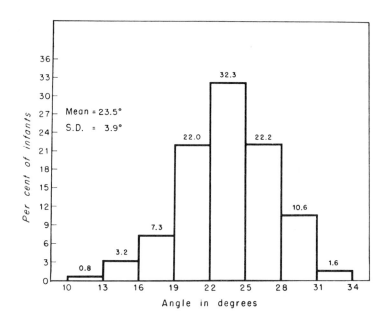

FIG. 30. Acetabular angle (α of Hilgenreiner). This figure shows the distribution (percentages) of 247 normal infants, 6 to 7 months of age, according to the magnitude of the acetabular angle (α of Hilgenreiner).

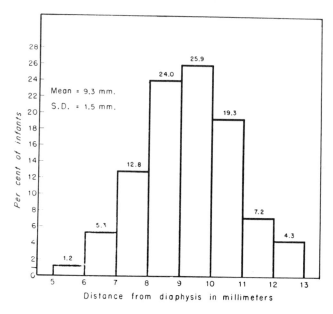

FIG. 31. Distance from diaphysis to Y line (h of Hilgenreiner). This figure shows the distribution (percentages) of infants according to the distance from the diaphysis to the Y line (h of Hilgenreiner).

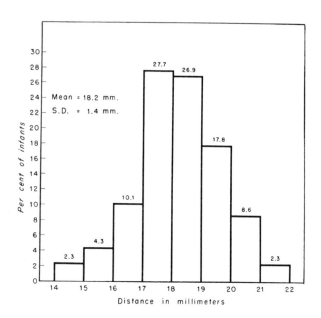

FIG. 32. Distance from diaphysis to acetabulum (d of Hilgenreiner). This figure shows the distribution (percentages) of infants according to the distance from the diaphysis to the acetabulum (d of Hilgenreiner).

Source: Harris LE, Lipscomb PR, Hodgson JR. Hilgenreiner measurement of the hip roentgenograms in 247 normal infants 6 and 7 months of age. *Pediatrics* 1960;56:478–84.

Time of Appearance of Pelvic Ossification Centers

Roentgenograms of 640 fetuses whose crown-rump lengths ranged from 32 to 472 mm were examined to determine the status of ossification of the pelvis. Table 19 shows the length of the fetus at the onset of ossification of the various portions of the pelvis and lumbosacral spine. In every case the length is that at which 50% of the specimens in the group displayed ossification of the center under study. Male fetuses tend to initiate ossification a little later than female fetuses of the same size in the groups 160 mm and over; in fetuses less than 160 mm there was no obvious difference between the two sexes. There was no evidence of any variation of the onset of ossification due to race.

TABLE 19. *Appearance of pelvic ossification centers*

Center	Crown-Rump Length
Ilium	60 mm.
Ischium	130–140 mm.
Pubis	160 mm.
Upper three sacral centra	80–90 mm.
Fourth sacral centrum	160 mm.
Fifth sacral centrum	200 mm.
Transverse processes of sacral vertebrae	Soon after respective centra
First lateral sacral center	210 mm.
Second lateral sacral center	280 mm.
Third lateral sacral center	340 mm.
First coccygeal center	Birth

Source: Francis CC. Appearance of centers of ossification in the human pelvis before birth. *AJR* 1951;65:778–83.

Ossification of Pubic Bones at Birth

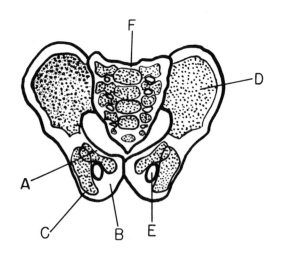

FIG. 33. Study of roentgenograms of the pelvis in 1,286 randomly selected newborn infants. *A:* Location of ossification centers in the pelvic cartilage at birth. The ossification centers of the bones which are visible in roentgenograms are stippled. *B:* Ossified superior ramus of pubic bone. *C:* Nonossified inferior ramus. *D:* Ilium. *E:* Obturator foramen. *F:* Sacrum.

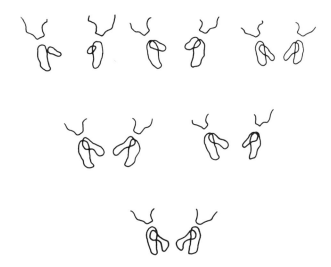

FIG. 34. Different types of ossification centers in pubic bones. Type A **(top row)**, a single bony mass is limited to the superior ramus. Ossification does not extend as far medially as the junction of the superior and inferior rami, so that the medial end of the ossification center is not enlarged. Type B **(middle row)**, a single bony mass shaped like a dumbbell, produces an opaque strip in the superior ramus with globular expansions laterally in the body of the pubis and medially at the junction of the horizontal and descending rami. Ossification does not extend into the descending ramus. Type C **(bottom row)** ossification center is shaped like a hook owing to the extension of ossification beyond the junction of the rami into the descending ramus. Type D includes all cases in which there were two or more ossification centers in one or both pubic bones.

TABLE 20. *Types of ossification centers and their incidence*

Type	Premature	Fullterm	All cases
A	12 (14.3%)	92 (7.6%)	104 (8.1%)
B	52 (61.9%)	637 (52.9%)	689 (53.6%)
C	19 (22.6%)	454 (37.7%)	473 (36.8%)
D	1 (1.2%)	19 (1.6%)	20 (1.6%)
Total	84	1,202	1,286

Source: Caffey J, Madell SH. Ossification of the pubic bones at birth. *Radiology* 1956;67:346–50.

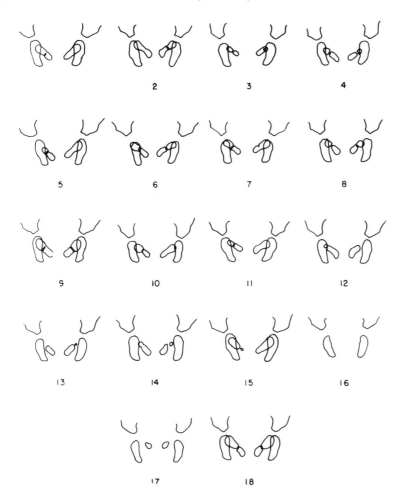

FIG. 35. Eighteen varieties of double ossification centers in the pubic rami.

FIG. 36. Progressive changes in pubic bones with double ossification centers. **A:** Premature infant with no pubic ossification centers at birth. **B:** Fullterm infant with double ossification centers in each pubic bone at birth. At 9 weeks the radiolucent strip is still present, but the marginal bone has become sclerotic. At 5 months the pubic bones are normal. **C:** A single small center in each pubic bone at the junction of the two rami on the 11th day of life. At 7 weeks there are three pubic ossification centers in the right side of the pelvis and two on the left side. At 6 months there is a single transverse radiolucent strip with marginal sclerosis in each superior ramus.

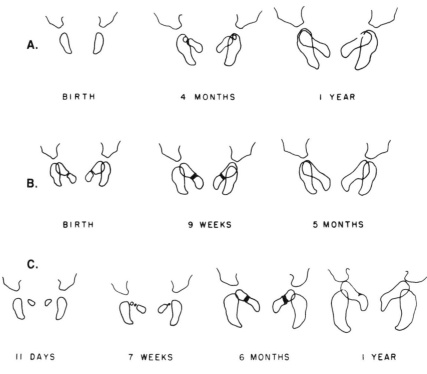

Source: Caffey J, Madell SH. Ossification of the pubic bones at birth. *Radiology* 1956;67:348–50.

Roentgenographic Studies of the Pelvic Girdle

A group of 46 boys and 49 girls had 467 sets of roentgenograms taken during the first postnatal year. Subjects were white babies born in southwestern and central Ohio, all participants in an intensive and long-term study on growth and development conducted by the S. Fels Research Institute. The infants were X-rayed at birth and at 1, 3, 6, 9, and 12 months of age. Careful tracings were made of the shadows of the bony ilium, ischium, and pubis on both sides at birth and at 1 month. At the upper age levels the left side only was traced. The study is confined to conclusions derived from measurements taken on these tracings.

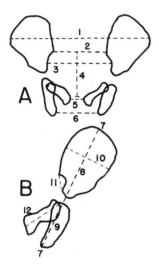

FIG. 37. Measurements taken from a pelvic tracing **(A)** and a hip tracing **(B)**. *(1)* Pelvis breadth. *(2)* Interiliac breadth. *(3)* Inlet breadth. *(4)* Sagittal inlet diameter. *(5)* Interpubic breadth. *(6)* Bi-ischium breadth. *(7)* Pelvis height. *(8)* Ilium length. *(9)* Ischium length. *(10)* Ilium breadth. *(11)* Breadth of sciatic notch. *(12)* Pubis length.

Source: Reynolds EL. The bony pelvic girdle in early infancy. *Am J Phys Anthropol* 1945;3:321–54.

TABLE 21. *Data from eight pelvic items from birth to 1 year*

Age	n	Boys Mean	S.D.	C.V.	n	Girls Mean	S.D.	C.V.
Pelvis height (mm)								
Birth	46	56.1	3.3	5.9	49	55.7	3.2	5.7
1 month	37	61.8	3.4	5.5	38	61.1	3.0	4.9
3 months	36	72.9	3.2	4.4	40	70.8	3.9	5.5
6 months	36	82.8	3.5	4.2	37	80.5	3.8	4.7
9 months	28	89.9	3.5	3.9	31	87.6	4.1	4.7
12 months	29	94.9	3.9	4.1	30	92.7	4.0	4.3
Inter-pubic breadth (mm)								
Birth	46	7.2	1.6	22.2	48	7.7	1.8	23.3
1 month	37	7.6	1.3	17.0	39	8.2	1.1	13.5
3 months	34	8.5	1.3	15.3	40	8.4	1.4	16.6
6 months	32	8.6	1.6	18.6	36	8.1	1.7	21.0
9 months	30	8.3	1.2	14.5	24	8.1	1.4	17.2
12 months	24	7.8	1.7	21.7	23	7.6	1.6	21.0
Ilium length (mm)								
Birth	46	32.4	2.4	7.4	49	32.9	2.1	6.4
1 month	39	36.0	1.9	5.3	39	36.1	2.0	5.5
3 months	36	41.3	1.9	4.6	41	40.7	2.4	5.9
6 months	36	47.2	2.3	4.9	38	46.4	2.7	5.8
9 months	28	51.9	2.3	4.4	31	51.6	2.9	5.6
12 months	29	54.5	2.8	5.1	30	54.3	2.6	4.8
Ilium breadth (mm)								
Birth	46	22.4	3.6	16.0	49	22.6	3.8	16.8
1 month	39	26.4	3.1	11.8	39	25.1	3.5	13.9
3 months	36	29.2	3.6	12.3	42	27.1	4.4	16.2
6 months	36	33.1	4.2	12.7	39	31.1	5.2	16.7
9 months	29	35.8	4.8	13.4	32	33.3	6.3	18.9
12 months	30	38.0	5.1	13.4	31	36.1	6.7	18.6
Ischium length (mm)								
Birth	46	19.6	1.5	7.6	49	19.7	1.6	8.1
1 month	37	22.0	1.9	8.6	38	22.3	1.5	6.7
3 months	37	26.8	1.8	6.7	41	26.7	2.1	7.9
6 months	38	30.8	2.0	6.5	38	31.0	2.0	5.8
9 months	31	34.2	2.2	6.4	36	34.4	2.0	5.8
12 months	33	36.7	1.9	5.2	34	36.6	1.7	4.6
Pubis length (mm)								
Birth	39	15.6	1.8	11.5	44	16.7	2.0	12.0
1 month	37	18.6	1.6	8.6	39	18.8	1.3	6.9
3 months	37	22.0	1.7	7.7	42	22.0	1.4	6.3
6 months	38	25.6	2.0	7.8	41	25.8	1.7	6.6
9 months	30	28.7	2.4	8.4	34	28.6	1.9	6.6
12 months	32	30.6	1.9	6.2	31	30.4	1.9	6.3
Breadth of greater sciatic notch (mm)								
Birth	46	9.0	1.6	17.8	48	10.0	1.9	19.3
1 month	39	10.6	2.0	18.5	39	11.2	1.8	16.2
3 months	37	9.8	1.8	18.1	42	10.7	2.4	22.3
6 months	38	11.3	2.2	19.6	42	11.4	2.9	25.4
9 months	31	13.5	2.7	19.7	35	14.1	3.0	21.6
12 months	31	14.0	2.9	20.9	32	14.7	2.3	15.9
Iliac index								
Birth	46	69.3	10.7	15.4	49	68.8	11.3	16.4
1 month	39	72.7	8.0	11.0	39	69.5	8.2	11.8
3 months	36	70.7	8.3	11.7	41	66.8	10.0	15.0
6 months	36	70.3	9.2	13.1	38	66.7	10.5	15.7
9 months	28	69.1	9.2	13.3	31	65.2	11.0	16.9
12 months	29	70.0	9.3	13.3	30	67.4	12.0	17.8

TABLE 22. *Data for 10 pelvic items at birth and 1 month (boys and girls)*

| ITEM | | BOYS | | | | | | |
| | | Birth | | | | 1 month | | |
	n	Mean	S.D.	C.V.	n	Mean	S.D.	C.V.
Pelvis breadth	45	75.8 mm.	4.9	6.5	38	83.6 mm.	4.5	5.4
Inlet, sagittal	44	22.3 mm.	3.2	14.3	36	25.1 mm.	2.5	10.0
Inlet breadth	45	37.0 mm.	2.4	6.5	38	40.4 mm.	2.5	6.2
Inter-iliac br.	45	27.6 mm.	2.9	10.5	38	30.4 mm.	2.4	7.9
Bi-ischial br.	46	21.9 mm.	2.4	10.8	36	22.3 mm.	2.1	9.6
Pelvic index	45	74.3%	2.8	3.8	36	74.0%	2.4	3.2
Inlet index	44	60.2%	7.2	12.0	36	62.4%	6.4	10.3
Sacral index	45	36.4%	3.1	8.5	38	36.4%	2.8	7.7
Relative inlet br.	45	48.9%	1.7	3.5	38	48.4%	1.9	3.9
Anterior segm. ix.	44	125.4%	10.0	8.0	36	124.2%	6.6	5.3

| ITEM | | GIRLS | | | | | | |
	n	Mean	S.D.	C.V.	n	Mean	S.D.	C.V.
Pelvis breadth	49	74.4 mm.	4.7	6.3	39	81.6 mm.	4.7	5.8
Sagittal inlet	47	23.0 mm.	2.9	12.6	39	25.2 mm.	3.0	11.9
Inlet breadth	48	36.8 mm.	2.5	6.8	39	40.2 mm.	2.2	5.5
Inter-iliac br.	49	26.9 mm.	2.6	9.7	39	30.0 mm.	1.7	5.7
Bi-ischial br.	49	23.1 mm.	2.8	12.3	37	23.5 mm.	2.9	12.5
Pelvic index	49	74.9%	3.6	4.8	38	74.9%	2.9	3.9
Inlet index	47	62.9%	7.8	12.4	39	62.8%	7.6	12.1
Sacral index	49	36.1%	2.8	7.8	39	36.9%	2.1	5.7
Relative inlet br.	48	49.6%	2.0	4.0	39	49.2%	1.6	3.2
Anterior segm. ix.	47	127.3%	8.2	6.4	39	130.0%	11.4	8.8

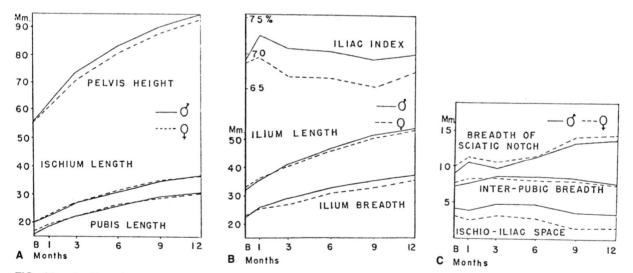

FIG. 38. A: Growth curves for pelvic height, ischium length, and pubis length. **B:** Growth curves for iliac index, ilium length, and ilium breadth. **C:** Growth curves for breadth of sciatic notch, interpubic breadth, and ischioiliac space. Boys = solid line; girls = dotted line.

This article represents the continuation of Reynolds' longitudinal study and contains similar data on 14 males and 16 females 9 to 18 years of age. The original text should be consulted as it represents a great deal of data which cannot be satisfactorily condensed.

Source: Reynolds EL. The bony pelvic girdle in early infancy. *Am J Phys Anthropol* 1945;3:321–54.

Related reference: Coleman WH. Sex differences in the growth of the human bony pelvis. *Am J Phys Anthropol* 1969;31:125–52.

Ischiopubic Synchondrosis Incidence of Fusion and Swelling

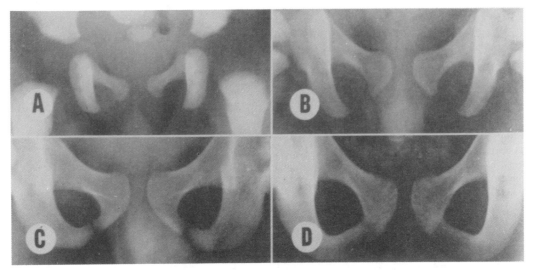

FIG. 39. Normal ischiopubic synchondrosis studied in 549 roentgenograms of the pelvises of children 2 to 12 years of age. **A:** Two-day-old infant. **B:** At 12 months. **C:** At 2½ years. **D:** At 6½ years after completed fusion of the ischial and pubic rami.

Because of the wide range, there is no average age at which fusion occurs, especially since the annual increment of bilaterally completed fusions does not exceed 20% in any year and is well below the figure in most years. Similarly, the existence of unilateral fusion indicates that the fusion does not occur simultaneously on both sides. Fusion on the second side usually follows fusion on the first side within 1 year.

TABLE 23. *Fusions*

No. of Cases	Age (years)	Boys				Girls				Entire Group				
		Right Side	Left Side	Total Uni-lateral	Bilateral	Right Side	Left Side	Total Uni-lateral	Bilateral	Right Side	Left Side	Total Uni-lateral	Bilateral	Per Cent of New Fusions
50	4								3(10%)				3(6%)	6
60	5	3	1	4	3(9%)	2	—	2	2(7%)	5	1	6	5(8%)	2
60	6	1	1	2	4(19%)	3	—	3	5(13%)	4	1	5	9(15%)	7
60	7	2	1	3	9(29%)	—	1	1	7(24%)	2	2	4	16(27%)	12
66	8	2	3	5	9(31%)	1	—	1	17(46%)	3	3	6	26(39%)	12
58	9	2	4	6	12(46%)	3	1	4	21(65%)	5	5	10	33(57%)	18
57	10	2	1	3	17(55%)	2	1	3	15(58%)	4	2	6	32(56%)	—
25	11	1	1	2	11(78%)	1	—	1	8(73%)	2	1	3	19(76%)	19
23	12	—	—	—	10(83%)	—	—	—	9(82%)	—	—	—	19(83%)	7

Source: Caffey J, Ross SE. The ischiopubic synchondrosis in healthy children: some normal roentgenologic findings. *AJR* 1956;76:488–94.

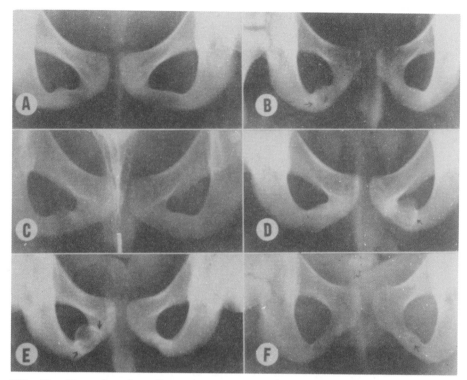

FIG. 40. Examples of swelling with and without uneven mineralization at the ischiopubic synchondrosis in healthy children. **A:** Swelling in a child 7 years of age. Mineralization is even. **B–E:** Swelling with uneven mineralization; children aged 4 years, 9 years, 7½ years, and 7 years, respectively. **F:** Child with only slight swelling.

Swelling and uneven mineralization is a finding between the fifth and tenth years. Statistical evaluation suggests that swelling with or without mineralization is present at some time in almost all children, and that it precedes fusion by 3 years or more on the average and lasts until fusion occurs.

TABLE 24. *Swelling and uneven mineralization*

No. of Cases	Age (years)	Boys Uni-lateral	Boys Bi-lateral	Girls Uni-lateral	Girls Bi-lateral	Entire Group Right Side	Left Side	Total	Bi-lateral	Total
40	2	—	—	—	2	—	—	—	2	2(5%)
50	3	1	1	—	4	1	—	1	5	6(12%)
50	4	1	5	4	2	2	3	5	7	12(24%)
60	5	8	9	5	7	4	9	13	16	29(48%)
60	6	4	7	13	19	2	15	17	26	43(72%)
60	7	6	14	5	14	2	9	11	28	39(65%)
66	8	7	13	5	16	5	7	12	29	41(62%)
58	9	8	5	12	7	11	9	20	12	32(55%)
57	10	6	12	5	6	6	5	11	18	29(51%)
25	11	1	2	1	4	1	1	2	6	8(32%)
23	12	1	1	—	3	1	—	1	4	5(22%)

Source: Caffey J, Ross SE. The ischiopubic synchondrosis in healthy children: some normal roentgenologic findings. *AJR* 1956;76:488–94.

GAIT

Earliest Photographic Studies of Gait in Childhood

Eadweard Muybridge was a transplanted Englishman who worked as a photographer on the Pacific Coast of the United States. During the 1870s he was sponsored by Lehman Stanford, the builder of the Central Pacific Railroad, former governor of California, and benefactor of Stanford University. Muybridge developed a successful method for photographing animals in motion, particularly Mr. Stanford's horses. Later, under the sponsorship of the University of Pennsylvania, he developed a more sophisticated system and completed his larger work at the University of Pennsylvania from 1884 to 1885, *The Human Figure in Motion*, which was published in 1887. This original work was reprinted by Dover Publications in 1955.

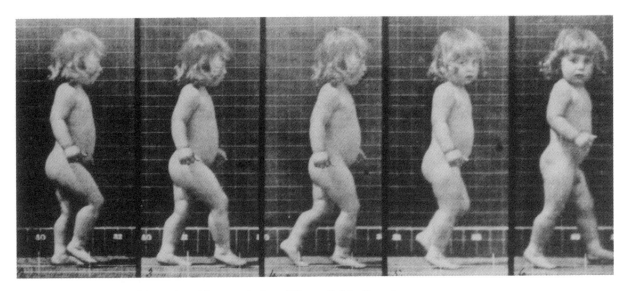

FIG. 1.   Boy walking. (Reproduced by permission of Dover Publications.)

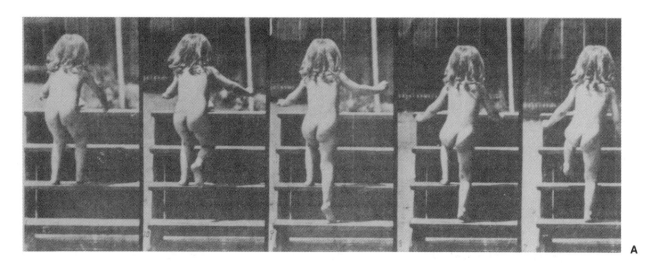

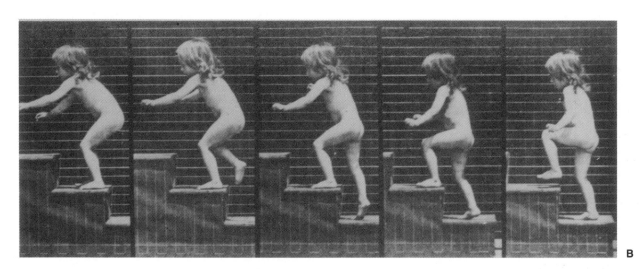

FIG. 2.   Girl walking upstairs. **A:** Posterior–anterior. **B.** Left lateral.

Source: Muybridge E. *Human Figure in Motion*. New York, Dover Publications, 1955, plates 183 and 190.

Step and Stride Length

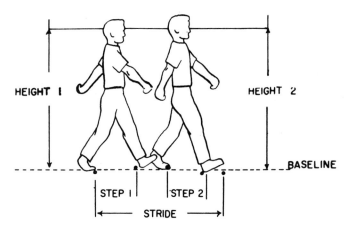

FIG. 3. Method used to calculate step and stride length as a percentage of height.

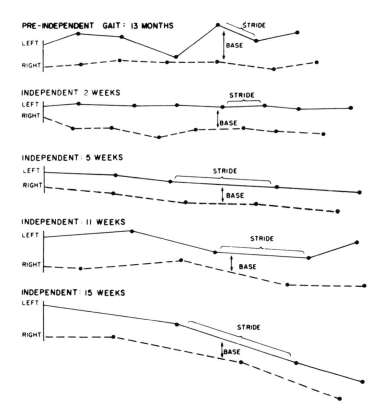

FIG. 4. Length of stride measured from photographic film of five children who were followed for periodic intervals from the onset of independent gait to 19–27 months of age. Stride length is recorded in percentage of body height. Chart demonstrates an increasing stride length and a narrowing of base.

TABLE 1. *Stride length recorded in percentage of body height*

Subject	Sex	Weeks independent gait																		
		2	3	4	6	8	10	12	14	16	18	20–25	26–30	31–35	36–40	41–45	46–50	51–55	56–60	61–70
1	M		23·4		37·3	57·3	58·9	61·8		45·7	55·2	64·6	65·9	57·6		55·7			63·3	62·8
2	M		30·3		30·3		44·2		62·2		51·2	65·9	54·2	71·6	75·3	76·3			65·9	63·3
3	M	30·6		34·8		54·1							50·7	56·7						
4	M	50·9		44·8			84·5		74·7									72·8		
5	F		67·4				67·3			50·7		55·7	69·4	73·7		80·2	88·1		54·3	71·9
6	F	25·7		28·3	42·6	37·2		43·6		54·1		25·6	26·6	38·2	27·8					
7	F	32·0		27·6			48·2			44·6			42·1	6·28						

Data for subjects 1–5 obtained from films. Data for subjects 6 and 7 obtained from paper record. Note the long stride taken by subjects 4 and 5 at two and three weeks respectively.

Source: Burnett CN, Johnson EW. Development of gait in childhood. Part I. Method. *Dev Med Child Neurol* 1971;13:196–206.

Transitional Stage from Supported Walking to Independent Walking

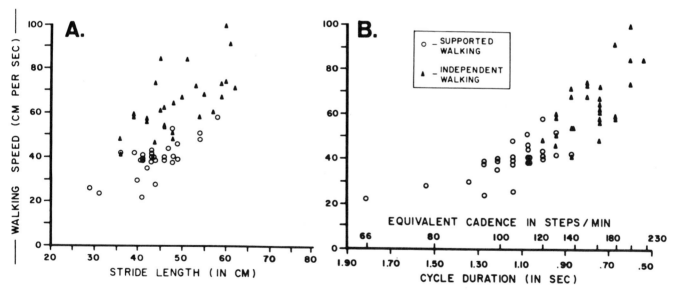

FIG. 5. Relationships between walking speeds and stride lengths **(A)** and between walking speed and walking cycle durations **(B)** of the same seven normal children studied photographically. Four measurements (of two successive left and two successive right walking cycles) were made for each child during supported walking and during independent walking.

Source: Statham L, Murray MP. Early walking patterns of normal children. *Clin Orthop* 1971;79:11–24.

Displacement Patterns of Lower Limb While Walking

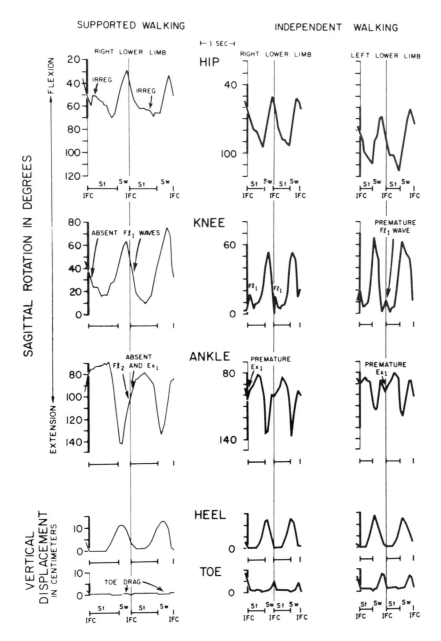

FIG. 6.   Left: Displacement patterns of the right lower limb during supported walking of a normal child. **Right:** Displacement patterns of the lower limbs during independent walking of the same child. Patterns were measured at 0.067-sec intervals throughout two successive walking cycles. Walking cycles begin and end at instants of initial floor contact (IFC) and are comprised of one period of distance (St bar) and one period of swing (Sw). For sagittal rotation patterns, upward deflections on the ordinate represent flexion (fl) and downward deflections represent extension (Ex). Flexion of the ankle equals dorsiflexion; extension of the ankle equals plantar flexion. For heel and toe patterns, ordinate values indicate distance of the heel target from the floor (zero on ordinate scale).

Source: Statham L, Murray MP. Early walking patterns of normal children. *Clin Orthop* 1971;79:11–24.

Muscle Phasic Activity

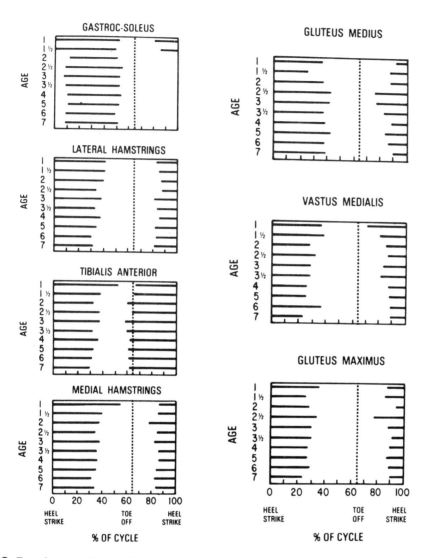

FIG. 7. Average timing of the phasic activities of the muscles and muscle groups investigated in each of 10 age groups. Data were obtained using surface electrodes. *Broken vertical lines* represent the average time of toe off for all age groups.

Source: Sutherland DH, Olshen R, Cooper L, Woo S. The development of mature gait. *J Bone Joint Surg (Am)* 1980;62:336–53.

Factors Influencing Gait

Hip rotation (not shown) was measured with the subjects prone, the hip in extension, and the knees flexed. Both internal and external hip rotation were measured with a gravity goniometer. Total excursion of hip motion was calculated.

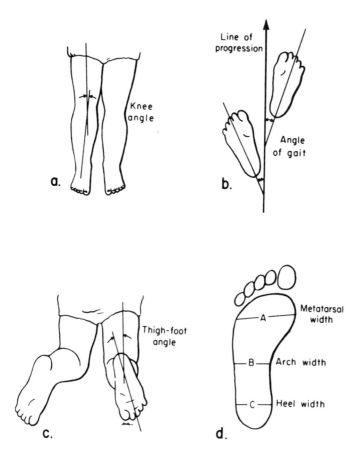

FIG. 8.   Methods of measurement with definition of terms. **a.** The knee angle is the angle formed by the midlongitudinal axis of the thigh and tibia and assesses genu valgum or varum. **b.** The angle of gait is the degree of in-toeing and out-toeing, and is measured photographically, utilizing a glass gait ramp over an inclined mirror. **c.** The thigh–foot axis is the angle between the long axis of the foot in its neutral position and the thigh. **d.** Arch development is assessed utilizing footprint tracings in which the widest forefoot length is called the metatarsal width, and the midfoot width is called the arch width. Data were derived from a study of 160 normal infants and children.

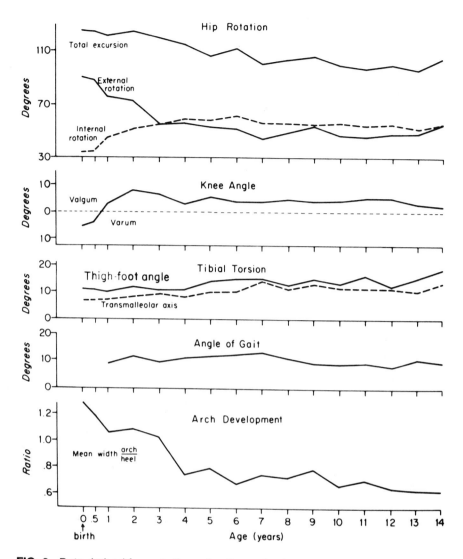

FIG. 9. Data derived from studies using the methods outlined in Fig. 7.

Source: Engel G, Staheli LT. The natural history of torsion and other factors influencing gait in childhood. *Clin Orthop* 1974;99:13.

Development of Mature Gait

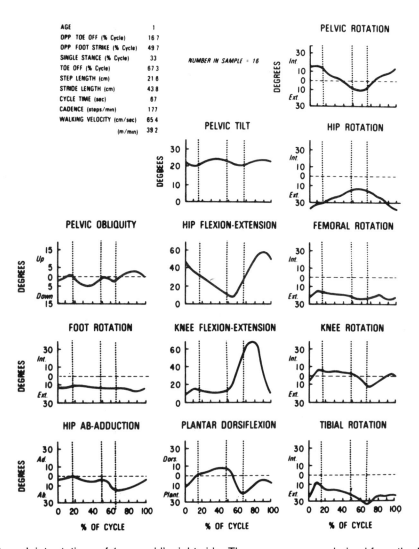

FIG. 10.   Joint rotations of 1-year-old's right side. These curves were derived from the Fourier trigonometric model by least squares using values obtained from 16 one-year-old subjects. *Broken vertical lines* from left to right indicate left toe off, left foot strike, and right toe off.

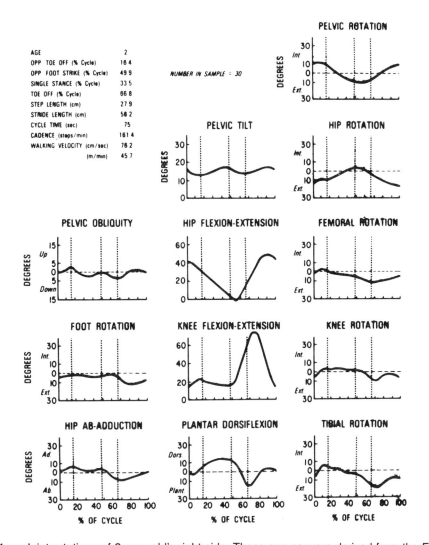

AGE   2
OPP TOE OFF (% Cycle)   16.4
OPP FOOT STRIKE (% Cycle)   49.9
SINGLE STANCE (% Cycle)   33.5
TOE OFF (% Cycle)   66.8
STEP LENGTH (cm)   27.9
STRIDE LENGTH (cm)   56.2
CYCLE TIME (sec)   .75
CADENCE (steps/min)   161.4
WALKING VELOCITY (cm/sec)   78.2
                (m/min)   45.7

NUMBER IN SAMPLE = 30

FIG. 11.   Joint rotations of 2-year-old's right side. These curves were derived from the Fourier trigonometric model by least squares, from 30 two-year-old subjects. *Broken vertical lines* from left to right indicate left toe off, left foot strike, and right toe off.

Source: Sutherland DH, Olshen R, Cooper L, Woo S. The development of mature gait. *J Bone Joint Surg (Am)* 1980;62:336–53.

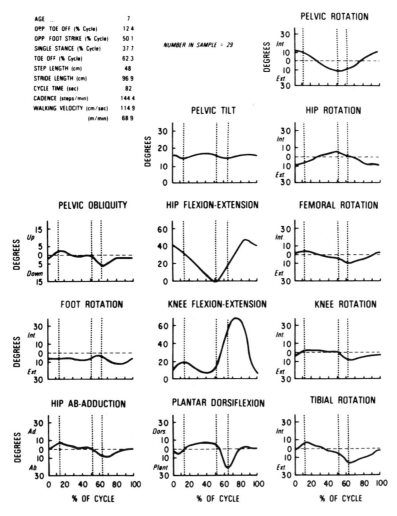

FIG. 12. Joint rotations of 7-year-old's right side. The curves were derived from the Fourier trigonometric model by least squares, using data from 29 seven-year-old subjects. *Broken vertical lines from left to right indicate left toe off, left foot strike, and right toe off.*

Source: Sutherland DH, Olshen R, Cooper L, Woo S. The development of mature gait. *J Bone Joint Surg (Am)* 1980;62:336–53.

Analysis of Normal Gait

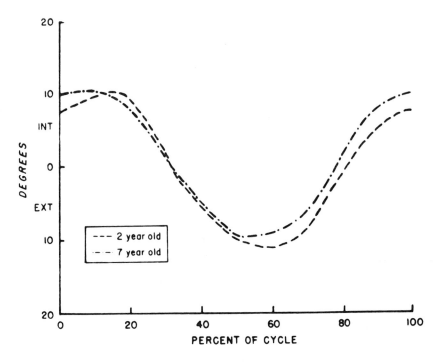

FIG. 13. Pelvic rotation curves derived from the Fourier trigonometric model by least squares. One curve is a composite of 20 two-year-olds, and the other is a composite of 20 seven-year-olds.

Source: Sutherland DH, Olshen R, Cooper L, Woo S. The development of mature gait. *J Bone Joint Surg (Am)* 1980;62:336–53.

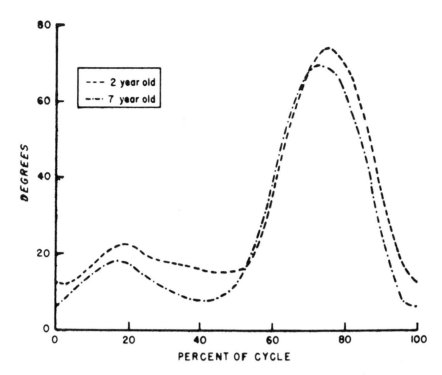

FIG. 14. Knee flexion–extension. These curves were derived from the Fourier trigonometric model by least squares. One curve is a composite of 20 two-year-olds, and the other is a composite of 20 seven-year-olds.

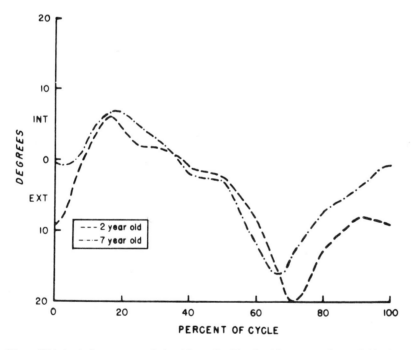

FIG. 15. Tibial rotation curves derived from the Fourier trigonometric model by least squares. One curve is a composite of 20 two-year-olds, and the other is a composite of 20 seven-year-olds.

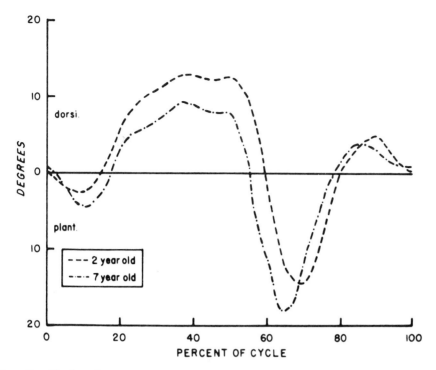

FIG. 16.   Dorsiflexion-plantar flexion curves derived from the Fourier trigonometric model by least squares. One curve is a composite of 20 two-year-olds, and the other is a composite of 20 seven-year-olds.

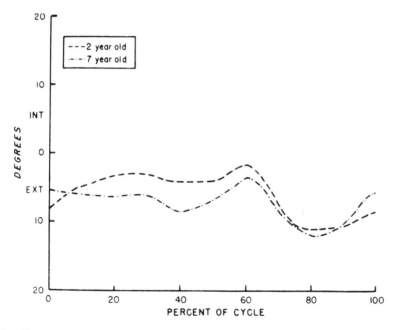

FIG. 17.   Foot rotation curves derived from the Fourier trigonometric model by least squares. One curve is a composite of 20 two-year-olds, and the other is a composite of 20 seven-year-olds.

Source: Sutherland DH, Olshen R, Cooper L, Woo S. The development of mature gait. *J Bone Joint Surg (Am)* 1980;62:336–53.

Single Limb Stance

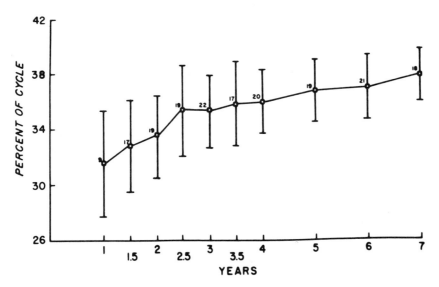

FIG. 18.   Duration of single limb stance versus age. The numbers at each point on the curve refer to numbers of children and respective ages. *Vertical lines* are ±1 SD.

Source: Sutherland DH, Olshen R, Cooper L, Woo S. The development of mature gait. *J Bone Joint Surg (Am)* 1980;62:336–53.

Determinants of Gait

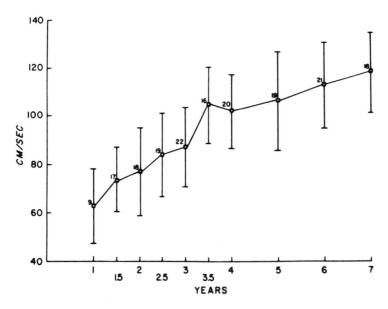

FIG. 19.   Velocity versus age. The numbers at the different points on the curve refer to the numbers of subjects and their corresponding age groups. *Vertical bars* are ±1 SD.

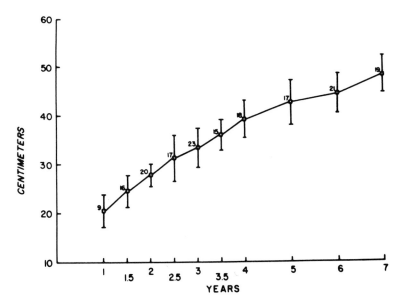

FIG. 20.   Step length versus age. The numbers at each point on the curve refer to the numbers of subjects and corresponding age groups. *Vertical bars* are ±1 SD.

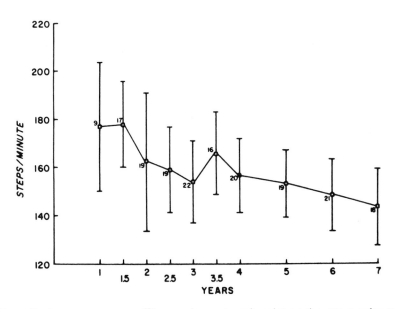

FIG. 21.   Cadence versus age. The numbers at each point on the curve refer to the numbers of subjects and their corresponding age groups. *Vertical bars* are ±1 SD.

Source: Sutherland DH, Olshen R, Cooper L, Woo S. The development of mature gait. *J Bone Joint Surg (Am)* 1980;62:336–53.

Development of Pelvic Span/Ankle Spread

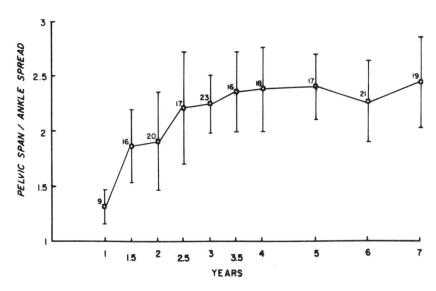

FIG. 22. Pelvic span is the body width at the level of the anterior–superior iliac spines. Ankle spread is the distance between the left and right ankle centers during double-limb support time. The value for each subject was averaged from five separate measurements. *Vertical bars* are equal to ± 1 SD from the mean.

Source: Sutherland DH, Olshen R, Cooper L, Woo S. The development of mature gait. *J Bone Joint Surg (Am)* 1980;62:336–53.

Gait Velocity

Foot switches were placed under the heel and at the metatarsal joints of 230 normal children aged 3 to 16 years, and a recording was made and evaluated by computer. All subjects were videotaped. Subjects were instructed to walk at three different velocities. Both start and stop were made at a few meters from the beginning and end of a 10-meter walkway. Velocities were freely chosen by the subjects themselves with the instruction that they should correspond to (a) ordinary, (b) very slow, and (c) very fast.

Source: Norlin R. Gait development in the normal child. *J Pediatr Orthop* 1981;1:261–6.

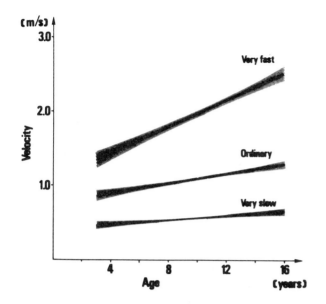

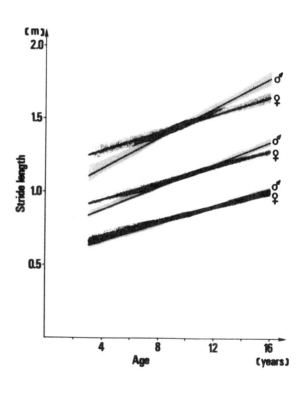

FIG. 23. Relationship between age and gait velocity m/sec for the whole group at the requested velocities. The 5% confidence intervals are marked. Velocity presented at each requested speed increases with increasing age according to the following equations: Very slow: V = 0.42 + 0.014 × age. Ordinary: V = 0.77 + 0.031 × age. Very fast: V = 1.09 + 0.087 × age.

FIG. 24. Stride length versus age for boys and girls at three requested velocities: very fast **(top)**, ordinary **(center)**, and very slow **(bottom)**. The 5% confidence intervals are marked. Stride length is correlated to both age and sex according to the following equations: Very slow: L = 0.59 + 0.026 × age. Ordinary: L = 0.84 + 0.028 × age (female); L = 0.73 + 0.039 × age (male). Very fast: L = 1.16 + 0.31 × age (female); L = 0.96 + 0.052 × age (male).

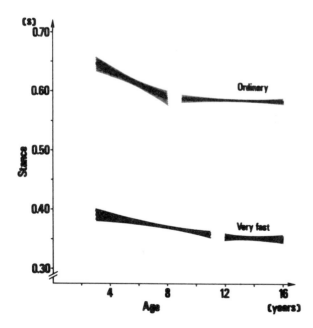

FIG. 25. Stance versus age for the whole group at ordinary and very fast gaits. The 5% confidence levels are marked.

Duchenne's Muscular Dystrophy

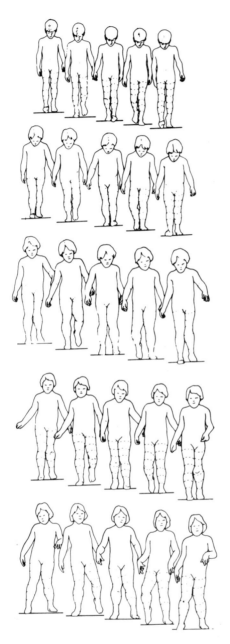

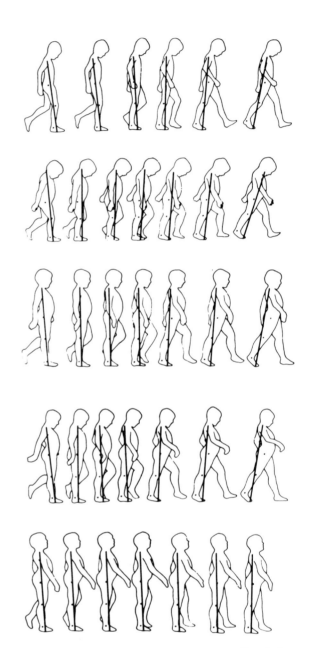

FIG. 26. Pathomechanics of gait in Duchenne's muscular dystrophy. Tracings taken directly from camera film of five standard gait cycle events. Four studies of patient R.C. are compared with those of a 7-year-old normal boy **(top)**. Note the arm position, increased lateral trunk sway, and widening of the support base. **Top to bottom:** normal 7-year-old boy; then patient R.C. at 5 years, 7 years 6 months, 7 years 11 months, and 8 years 2 months. Gait cycle (left to right) is the right foot strike, left toe off, left foot strike, right toe off, right foot strike.

FIG. 27. Tracings taken from side camera film during single-limb support. Heavy black line is the result of the vertical force and fore-aft shear vectors. Note the position of the force vector in relation to the hip, knee, and ankle joint centers for a normal 7-year-old boy **(top)**, and for patient R.C. as his disease progresses at 5 years, 7 years 6 months, 7 years 11 months, and 8 years 2 months.

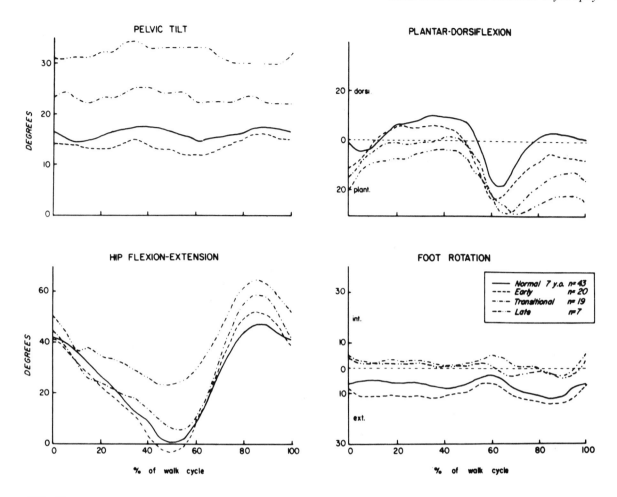

FIG. 28. Mean joint angle curves for the degree of involvement and stage of the illness (early, transitional, and late groups) compared with a normal 7-year-old. Initiation of the swing phase for each group is difference and is as follows: normal 7-year-old (62%), early group (63%), transitional group (64%), and late group (68%).

Source: Sutherland DH, Olshen R, Cooper L, Watt MD, Leach J, Mubarak S, Schultz PP. The pathomechanics of gait in Duchenne muscular dystrophy. *Dev Med Child Neurol* 1981;23:2–22.

BIOMECHANICS

Relationship of Radial Fractures and Epiphyseal Displacement and Growth

The data are from 119 patients with epiphyseal displacement types I and II (Salter–Harris classification) and 100 consecutive cases of simple fracture of the radial shaft. All patients were below the age of 19 years, and all were analyzed in the same manner.

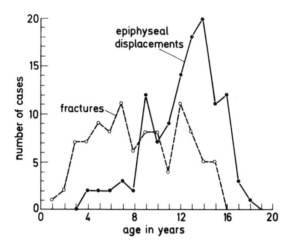

FIG. 1. Age distribution of radial fractures and epiphyseal displacement (sexes combined).

TABLE 1. *Mean ages of patients with radial fractures and epiphyseal displacements*

Sex	Epiphyseal displacement		Shaft fracture		Significance of difference
Male and female	12.4	(*N* = 119)	8.5	(*N* = 100)	*p* = 0.001
Male	11.9	(*N* = 88)	8.8	(*N* = 64)	
Female	10.9	(*N* = 34)	7.8	(*N* = 36)	
Male/female ratio	2.8:1		1.8:1		NS

Source: Alexander CG. Effect of growth rate on the strength of the growth plate–shaft junction. *Skeletal Radiol* 1976;1:67–76.

Relationship of Epiphyseal Displacement and Age

Dr. Alexander believed that statistical data were not satisfactory from New Zealand and as a consequence used data from Belgium (Quetelet. *Of Growth and Form*. Washington, D.C.: Thompson, 1959:97).

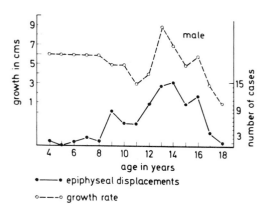

FIG. 2. Incidence of traumatic epiphyseal displacement of the radius in New Zealand boys compared with the growth rate in Belgian boys.

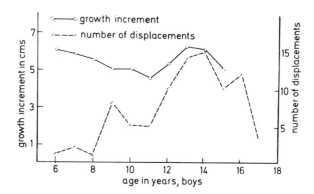

FIG. 3. Incidence of traumatic epiphyseal displacement compared with the cross-sectional growth rate for New Zealand males, by age.

Source: Alexander CG. Effect of growth rate on the strength of the growth plate–shaft junction. *Skeletal Radiol* 1976;1:67–76.

Relationship of Radial Metaphyseal Band Width to Stature Velocity

Thirty-five boys and 32 girls were surveyed in a longitudinal growth study. The boys were in the study for an average of 10 years, the girls for an average of 10.3 years. These children underwent roentgenograms of the wrists, stature measurements, and other anthropometric measurements at 6-month intervals. During the period of adolescent growth and the interval between, measurements were reduced to 3 months. (A total of 657 roentgenograms for boys and 673 for girls were examined.) Stature velocity at any age was calculated by determining the velocity over the shortest period of time at which there was an age center equivalent to the age for which the roentgenogram was made. The radial metaphyseal band width was measured to the nearest 0.1 mm with a precision caliper and a magnifying glass.

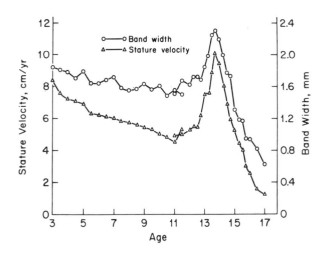

FIG. 4. Relationship between stature velocity and band width in normal boys.

TABLE 2. *Boys' preadolescent and adolescent growth and band data used to construct Fig. 4*

Preadolescent

Age, yr	Sample Size	Band Width, mm (Mean ± SD)	Height Velocity,* cm/yr (Mean ± SD)
3.0	17	1.84 ± .12	8.40 ± 1.25
3.5	23	1.81 ± .17	7.61 ± 1.16
4.0	24	1.78 ± .22	7.19 ± 0.94
4.5	24	1.70 ± .20	7.14 ± 0.78
5.0	23	1.79 ± .20	6.88 ± 1.09
5.5	24	1.64 ± .26	6.31 ± 0.88
6.0	24	1.64 ± .23	6.23 ± 0.76
6.5	25	1.68 ± .22	6.14 ± 0.74
7.0	23	1.71 ± .20	6.00 ± 0.68
7.5	23	1.58 ± .30	5.82 ± 0.65
8.0	24	1.55 ± .31	5.70 ± 0.69
8.5	24	1.57 ± .27	5.57 ± 0.43
9.0	25	1.63 ± .30	5.42 ± 0.46
9.5	23	1.57 ± .35	5.26 ± 0.61
10.0	25	1.61 ± .31	5.04 ± 0.80
10.5	24	1.49 ± .41	4.82 ± 0.68
11.0	24	1.55 ± .30	4.48 ± 0.69
11.5	20	1.50 ± .25	5.24 ± 0.77

Adolescent

Age, yr	Sample Size	Band Width, mm (Mean ± SD)	Height Velocity,* cm/yr (Mean ± SD)
11.00	15	1.51 ± .20	4.87 ± 0.78
11.50	17	1.67 ± .31	4.95 ± 0.66
12.00	22	1.62 ± .19	5.24 ± 1.01
12.25	16	1.72 ± .29	5.50 ± 1.09
12.50	23	1.72 ± .33	5.42 ± 1.24
12.75	20	1.68 ± .29	6.23 ± 1.36
13.00	24	1.84 ± .36	7.48 ± 1.38
13.25	24	1.98 ± .32	7.55 ± 1.36
13.50	25	2.24 ± .38	8.86 ± 1.45
13.75	25	2.30 ± .32	10.05 ± 1.53
14.00	21	2.19 ± .28	9.41 ± 1.34
14.25	20	1.99 ± .34	8.04 ± 1.21
14.50	16	1.77 ± .33	6.94 ± 1.29
14.75	19	1.74 ± .43	5.95 ± 1.57
15.00	16	1.31 ± .42	5.24 ± 1.05
15.25	13	1.18 ± .20	4.43 ± 0.96
15.50	10	1.17 ± .37	4.00 ± 1.17
15.75	10	0.95 ± .26	3.03 ± 0.82
16.00	11	0.94 ± .28	2.56 ± 0.61
16.50	5	0.82 ± .19	1.62 ± 0.28
17.00	6	0.63 ± .09	1.28 ± 0.18

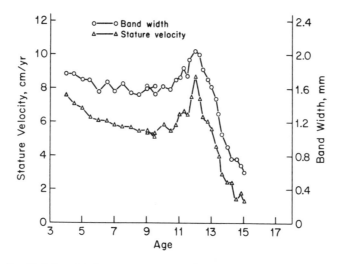

FIG. 5. Relationship between stature velocity and band width in normal girls.

TABLE 3. *Girls' preadolescent and adolescent growth and band data used to construct Fig. 5*

Preadolescent

Age, yr	Sample Size	Band Width, mm (Mean ± SD)	Height Velocity,* cm/yr (Mean ± SD)
4.0	22	1.78 ± .23	7.60 ± 0.94
4.5	25	1.77 ± .21	7.10 ± 0.84
5.0	23	1.70 ± .26	6.78 ± 0.72
5.5	22	1.69 ± .21	6.30 ± 0.89
6.0	22	1.56 ± .23	6.08 ± 1.08
6.5	22	1.66 ± .22	6.04 ± 0.90
7.0	22	1.58 ± .24	5.95 ± 0.82
7.5	22	1.63 ± .24	5.69 ± 0.78
8.0	23	1.54 ± .21	5.67 ± 0.66
8.5	22	1.52 ± .28	5.54 ± 0.64
9.0	19	1.59 ± .27	5.51 ± 0.66
9.5	18	1.62 ± .22	5.13 ± 0.52

Adolescent

Age, yr	Sample Size	Band Width, mm (Mean ± SD)	Height Velocity,* cm/yr (Mean ± SD)
9.00	16	1.62 ± .10	5.42 ± 0.58
9.50	14	1.53 ± .31	5.38 ± 0.78
10.00	16	1.62 ± .27	5.86 ± 0.92
10.50	18	1.59 ± .30	5.52 ± 1.14
10.75	10	1.70 ± .45	5.87 ± 1.36
11.00	20	1.73 ± .32	6.46 ± 0.87
11.25	17	1.84 ± .29	6.66 ± 0.94
11.50	26	1.75 ± .24	6.42 ± 0.90
11.75	21	1.94 ± .25	7.53 ± 0.97
12.00	26	2.04 ± .34	8.73 ± 1.06
12.25	23	2.00 ± .26	7.75 ± 0.87
12.50	22	1.82 ± .30	6.28 ± 1.12
12.75	22	1.71 ± .32	5.94 ± 1.37
13.00	22	1.61 ± .36	5.56 ± 1.30
13.25	21	1.48 ± .34	4.61 ± 1.10
13.50	23	1.31 ± .35	3.99 ± 1.45
13.75	20	1.05 ± .34	2.90 ± 1.17
14.00	23	0.90 ± .22	2.43 ± 1.07
14.25	14	0.76 ± .29	2.39 ± 1.28
14.50	19	0.76 ± .16	1.53 ± 0.86
14.75	8	0.69 ± .15	1.86 ± 1.14
15.00	14	0.61 ± .22	1.32 ± 0.73

Source: Edlin JC. Relationship of radial metaphyseal bandwidth to stature velocity. *Am J Dis Child* 1976;130:160–3.

Shear Strength of the Human Femoral Capital Epiphyseal Plate

Twenty-five pairs of femurs from children whose ages ranged from newborn to 15 years were obtained at autopsy. Specimens were then tested to failure for shear strength in the anterior-posterior plane, cut in half with a band saw after testing, and photographed again. One specimen of each pair was tested after removal of the perichondral fibrocartilaginous complex; the other was tested with the perichondral complex undisturbed and served as a control. The forces necessary to cause failure between the secondary center of ossification and the metaphysis were recorded by an Instron testing machine and by a CGS/Lawrence Instron machine at a loading ram speed of 2 mm/min.

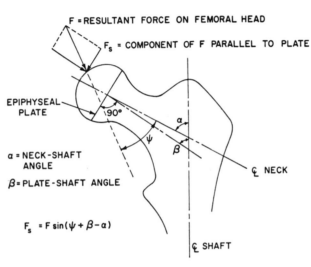

FIG. 6. Proximal end of the femur (anterior view) showing the forces acting on the femoral head.

Source: Chung et al. Shear strength of the human femoral capital epiphyseal plate. *J Bone Joint Surg (Am)* 1976;58:98–103.

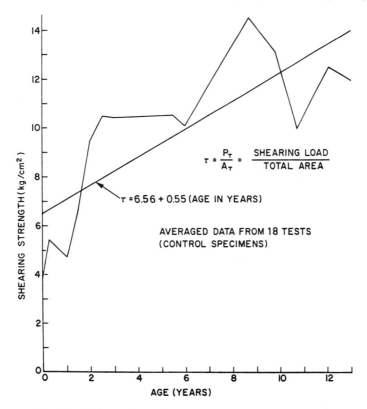

FIG. 7. Shear stress versus age for 18 control specimens. The straight line represents a least squares fit of the data.

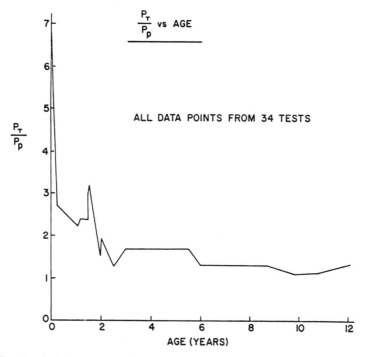

FIG. 8. Ratio of the failure load of the control to that of the experimental specimen versus age for seventeen pairs of specimens. In the younger children the perichondral complex is a major contributor to the shear resistance of the perichondral complex-epiphyseal plate combination. P_T = Failure load of the control. P_p = failure load of the specimen.

Source: Chung et al. Shear strength of the human femoral capital epiphyseal plate. *J Bone Joint Surg (Am)* 1976;58:98–103.

Incidence of Schmorl's Nodes by Age

This was a survey of good quality but otherwise unselected dorsal and lumbar spine films of 1,107 radiologically apparent Schmorl's nodes. A node was defined as a localized or incongruous depression of the endplate exceeding 3 mm in diameter. The incidence of nodes was determined by age group.

TABLE 4. *Age incidence of 1,107 radiological Schmorl's nodes*

Age (years)	Lumbar spine No. of patients	Per-centage with nodes	Dorsal spine No. of patients	Per-centage with nodes	Mean inci-dence (%)
10–14	26	31	20	30	30.5
15–19	46	46	33	58	52
20–24	55	36	38	63	49.5
25–29	50	38	23	69	53.5
30–39	161	30	60	65	47.5
40–49	160	28	59	59	43.5
50–59	100	19	33	60	39.5

Source: Alexander CJ. Effect of growth rate on the strength of the growth plate shaft junction. *Skeletal Radiol* 1976;1:67–76.

Sequential Changes in Weight Density and Percentage Ash Weight of Human Skeletons from an Early Fetal Period Through Old Age

The weight density and percentage ash weight of dry, fat-free osseous human skeletons were examined from 16 weeks' gestation to 100 years of age. Data were drawn from 426 skeletons of American whites and blacks of both sexes.

TABLE 5. *Mean weights of four skeletal divisions and the total according to race, sex, and age*

	Fetal Age in weeks				Young Age in years				Adult Age in years		
	16–20	21–28	29–36	37–44	B–0.5	> 0.5–3.0	> 3.0–13.0	> 13.0	25–44	45–64	≧ 65
White male											
	(1)	(11)	(13)	(4)	(7)	(5)	(7)	(9)	(1)	(11)	(18)
Mean age	16.0	24.5	32.1	40.8	0.26	1.5	7.2	18.8	34.0	54.9	69.2
Skull	1.2	8.3	18.8	43.9	48.2	133.4	365.6	697.3	978.0	611.6	554.0
Postcranial	0.7	4.4	10.4	26.0	19.3	71.8	192.0	756.2	1013.1	596.6	544.4
Superior limb	0.7	3.1	6.4	14.8	11.5	36.3	127.8	703.6	936.1	672.1	600.6
Inferior limb	0.8	4.3	9.0	23.6	16.7	74.9	247.2	1847.3	2488.0	1658.2	1485.7
Total	3.4	20.1	44.6	108.3	95.8	315.8	932.6	4004.4	5415.2	3538.4	3184.7
White female											
	(2)	(6)	(8)	(15)	(3)	(4)	(10)	(3)	(2)	(13)	(15)
Mean age	19.0	23.8	33.1	39.0	0.26	2.0	8.2	17.7	34.5	56.0	77.8
Skull	2.8	8.7	29.4	35.7	30.1	129.3	312.0	524.0	514.7	505.2	519.4
Postcranial	1.7	4.3	15.0	20.1	16.9	62.2	250.4	559.0	602.3	406.0	378.6
Superior limb	1.4	2.6	8.8	11.4	10.1	27.5	160.9	468.3	527.8	391.6	338.9
Inferior limb	1.7	3.8	13.9	17.9	13.9	49.4	409.1	1173.0	1439.6	1033.4	894.0
Total	7.7	19.5	67.1	85.1	71.0	268.4	1132.4	2724.3	3084.4	2336.2	2130.0
Negro male											
	(2)	(9)	(13)	(9)	(4)	(13)	(9)	(29)	(2)	(15)	(13)
Mean age	18.5	24.3	32.2	39.6	0.22	1.3	7.8	18.2	34.5	53.9	71.7
Skull	3.7	8.4	22.8	35.2	48.7	125.9	438.9	690.1	575.4	685.4	701.9
Postcranial	1.9	4.5	13.2	18.9	25.2	56.0	262.8	772.7	706.6	702.4	697.0
Superior limb	1.6	3.1	8.4	11.6	14.5	30.0	209.7	824.7	761.6	788.8	737.1
Inferior limb	2.1	4.4	12.2	16.9	21.7	48.4	545.2	1941.0	1866.5	1796.6	1716.5
Total	9.3	20.4	56.6	82.5	110.0	260.2	1456.6	4228.5	3910.1	3973.2	3852.4
Negro female											
	(1)	(4)	(8)	(11)	(4)	(7)	(11)	(19)	(9)	(7)	(14)
Mean age	16.0	24.8	33.4	40.5	0.11	1.9	8.2	18.1	37.4	57.3	78.0
Skull	3.1	9.0	25.4	37.7	45.4	182.4	379.5	629.8	729.3	626.5	594.8
Postcranial	1.6	4.9	14.1	20.6	24.6	75.7	241.0	632.0	576.6	536.1	464.8
Superior limb	1.3	3.6	9.1	12.5	12.9	44.2	182.2	549.3	523.8	508.0	457.7
Inferior limb	1.5	5.0	13.2	18.6	19.5	80.1	502.9	1445.1	1297.4	1334.6	1103.2
Total	7.6	22.5	61.7	89.3	102.3	382.3	1305.6	3256.2	3127.2	3005.2	2620.5

TABLE 6. *Means of percentages of the total weight of the skeleton contributed by four divisions according to race, sex, and age.*

	Fetal Age in weeks				Young Age in years				Adult Age in years		
	16–20	21–28	29–36	37–44	B–0.5	> 0.5–3.0	> 3.0–13.0	> 13.0	25–44	45–64	≧ 65
White male											
	(1)	(11)	(13)	(4)	(7)	(5)	(7)	(9)	(1)	(11)	(18)
Skull	36	41	43	41	50	46	41	19	18	17	17
Postcranial	21	22	23	24	20	23	21	19	19	17	17
Sup. limb	21	16	14	14	12	11	13	17	17	17	17
Inf. limb	23	21	20	22	18	20	25	45	46	47	47
White female											
	(2)	(6)	(8)	(15)	(3)	(4)	(10)	(3)	(2)	(13)	(15)
Skull	37	43	44	42	42	46	33	19	17	22	24
Postcranial	22	22	22	23	23	26	22	21	19	17	18
Sup. limb	18	14	13	13	14	10	14	17	17	17	16
Inf. limb	22	20	21	21	21	18	31	43	47	44	42
Negro male											
	(2)	(9)	(13)	(9)	(4)	(13)	(9)	(29)	(2)	(15)	(13)
Skull	39	41	41	43	45	48	34	17	15	17	18
Postcranial	21	22	23	23	22	22	18	18	18	18	18
Sup. limb	17	16	15	14	14	12	14	19	19	20	19
Inf. limb	23	22	21	20	19	18	34	46	48	45	45
Negro female											
	(1)	(4)	(8)	(11)	(4)	(7)	(11)	(19)	(9)	(7)	(14)
Skull	41	39	41	42	44	48	30	20	23	21	23
Postcranial	21	21	23	23	24	21	19	19	18	18	18
Sup. limb	17	17	15	14	13	11	14	17	17	17	17
Inf. limb	20	22	22	21	19	20	37	44	41	44	42

Source: Trotter M, Hixon BB. Sequential changes in weight density and percentage ash weight of human skeletons from an early fetal period through old age. *Anat Rec* 1976;179:1–18.

TABLE 7. *Mean percentage ash weights of the individual bones, bone sets, and total skeleton of white males according to age*

	Fetal Age in weeks 16–44	Young Age in years				Adult Age in years 30–85
		B–0.5	> 0.5–3.0	> 3.0–13.0	> 13.0–22	
	(29)	(4)	(4)	(12)	(9)	(30)
Cranium	65.3	66.0	66.3	66.8	67.2	67.3
Mandible	63.8	64.9	70.2	72.0	71.1	69.5
Cervical v.	67.2	63.2	64.1	63.2	64.3	65.4
Thoracic v.	68.2	63.9	61.9	60.7	62.8	63.6
Lumbar v.	68.0	63.0	61.6	59.2	62.4	63.9
Sacrum	67.2	60.0	59.6	57.6	61.9	63.0
Sternum	66.7	62.4	58.8	56.2	59.7	64.8
Ribs	65.5	63.9	63.9	63.7	64.4	65.8
Scapula	65.2	63.1	62.3	62.9	64.1	66.3
Clavicle	64.6	63.3	64.4	63.6	65.2	67.0
Humerus	65.7	63.2	60.7	64.4	66.4	67.7
Radius	65.2	63.1	60.9	63.5	66.5	67.8
Ulna	65.6	62.3	63.0	63.0	66.0	66.5
Hand bones	63.9	58.3	51.7	58.3	60.8	64.8
Hip	65.1	62.8	60.8	60.2	62.8	67.0
Femur	66.1	64.0	59.3	63.4	66.0	67.2
Tibia	65.4	63.4	56.2	62.6	65.6	67.8
Fibula	64.5	62.9	58.0	64.0	66.3	66.2
Foot bones	63.4	59.4	49.9	55.0	60.3	66.4
Total	65.6	64.6	63.3	64.0	65.1	

TABLE 8. *Rank orders of bones or bone sets according to decreasing mean percentage ash weight in fetal, young, and adult skeletons*

	Fetal	Young B–0.5	> 0.5–3.0	> 3.0–13.0	> 13.0–22.0	Adult	Fetal	B–0.5	> 0.5–3.0	> 3.0–13.0	> 13.0–22.0	Adult
	White male						*White female*					
	(29)	(4)	(4)	(12)	(9)	(30)	(31)	(2)	(5)	(5)	(2)	(30)
Cranium	11	1	2	2	2	5	7	1	2	2	2	5
Mandible	18	2	1	1	1	1	17	2	1	1	1	1
Cervical v.	4	8	4	9	11	13	4	4	4	12	4	13
Thoracic v.	1	4	8	13	14	18	1	5	12	15	13	17
Lumbar v.	2	12	9	15	15	16	2	6	17	17	17	16
Sacrum	3	17	13	17	16	17	3	3	15	18	19	18
Sternum	5	15	15	18	19	19	5	15	19	19	16	19
Ribs	9	5	5	5	10	14.5	11	10	5	7	8	14
Scapula	13	10.5	7	11	12	12	9	8	13	11	9	12
Clavicle	15	7	3	6	9	10	13	7	3	10	3	11
Humerus	7	9	12	3	4	7	12	11	9	5	12	6
Radius	12	10.5	10	7	5	4	15	17	6	9	5	4
Ulna	8	16	6	10	6	2	10	14	8	8	6	2
Hand bones	17	19	18	16	17	9	18	19	14	16	11	9
Hip	14	14	11	14	13	14.5	8	13	16	14	18	15
Femur	6	3	14	8	7	8	6	12	11	4	10	8
Tibia	10	6	17	12	8	6	16	16	10	6	15	7
Fibula	16	13	16	4	3	3	14	9	7	3	7	3
Foot bones	19	18	19	19	18	11	19	18	18	13	14	10
	Negro male						*Negro female*					
	(36)	(3)	(6)	(2)	(0)	(30)	(27)	(4)	(4)	(1)	(1)	(30)
Cranium	7	7	2	2		6	10	3	3	2	10	6
Mandible	17	1	1	1		1	16	1	1	1	1	1
Cervical v.	4	2	3	4		13	4	7.5	10	5.5	11	15
Thoracic v.	1	4	11	10		19	2	11	14	13	16	18
Lumbar v.	2	3	13	9		17	1	15	5	15	17	17
Sacrum	3	14	14	15		16	3	18	2	18	19	16
Sternum	5	15	17	17		18	5	14	15	17	14	19
Ribs	10	6	5	6		14	9	5	4	8	9	13
Scapula	9	9	7	5		12	8	10	13	9	12	11
Clavicle	16	8	4	3		11	12	9	6	7	7	10
Humerus	8	12	6	8		7	11	2	11	14	4	5
Radius	15	10	12	13		2	17	6	17	12	6	3
Ulna	11	5	8	16		4	14	4	16	10	8	2
Hand bones	18	18	19	18		9	18	17	19	19	15	7
Hip	12	11	15	7		15	6	16	12	16	18	14
Femur	6	16	10	12		8	7	7.5	7	4	5	9
Tibia	13	17	16	14		5	15	12	9	3	3	8
Fibula	14	13	9	11		3	13	13	8	5.5	2	4
Foot bones	19	19	18	19		10	19	19	18	11	13	12

Source: Trotter M, Hixon BB. Sequential changes in weight density and percentage ash weight of human skeletons from an early fetal period through old age. *Anat Rec* 1976;179:1–18.

Ash Weight of Bones by Race, Sex, and Age

A total of 66 skeletons, unequally divided among American whites and blacks of both sexes and unevenly spread over an age range from birth to 23 years, were ashed. The weight of the ash was determined as a percentage of the weight of dry, fat-free bone of 19 bones or one group for each skeleton (excluding unfused epiphyses), and for the total skeleton. The methods used in earlier studies of fetal and adult skeletons were followed in an effort to describe the pattern of development of percentage ash weight in the intervening age span.

TABLE 9. *Mean percentage ash weights for each race-sex group by age*

	White male (29)				White female (14)			
	B-0.5 (4)	>0.5-3 (4)	>3-13 (12)	>13-22 (9)	B-0.5 (2)	>0.5-3 (5)	>3-13 (5)	>13-22 (2)
Mandible	64.92	70.15	71.96	71.11	67.94	70.58	71.70	66;89
Cranium	66.02	66.26	66.84	67.19	69.32	64.77	66.31	64.60
Humeri	63.16	60.68	64.38	66.30	64.62	62.00	63.98	59.09
Radii	63.09	60.88	63.52	66.28	62.60	62.76	63.26	61.74
Ulnae	62.34	62.99	63.03	66.04	63.58	62.47	63.47	61.46
Femora	63.97	59.32	63.41	65.96	64.48	60.63	64.17	59.81
Tibiae	63.40	56.15	62.61	65.63	63.04	61.27	63.72	57.34
Fibulae	62.88	58.01	63.96	66.60	65.44	62.54	64.19	61.30
Clavicles	63.30	64.38	63.58	65.16	66.02	63.17	63.10	62.17
Scapulae	63.09	62.32	62.94	64.14	65.90	60.45	62.82	60.40
Ribs	63.87	63.91	63.74	64.38	64.98	62.84	63.67	60.44
Hip bones	62.84	60.81	60.20	62.84	64.02	58.58	60.40	54.48
CV	63.17	64.06	63.23	64.32	67.16	62.86	62.26	61.80
TV	63.88	61.91	60.74	62.75	66.99	60.46	60.29	58.75
LV	62.98	61.59	59.18	62.39	66.66	58.54	59.70	54.55
Sacrum	60.01	59.58	57.59	61.93	67.82	59.56	59.20	53.24
Sternum	62.39	58.80	56.20	59.72	63.41	56.04	56.35	54.64
Hand bones	58.26	51.74	58.28	60.80	57.68	60.03	59.95	59.76
Foot bones	59.44	49.90	55.03	60.33	58.72	57.08	60.81	58.34
Total Skeleton	64.57	63.28	64.04	65.09	66.92	62.79	64.18	60.45

Source: Trotter M. Percentage of ash weight of young human skeletons. *Growth* 1973;37:153–63.

TABLE 10. *Rank order according to decreasing percentage ash weights of bones or bone groups in the four age periods within each race-sex group*

Age (years)	B—0.5				>0.5—3				>3—13				>13—23			
Race-Sex	WM	WF	NM	NF	WM	WF	NM	NF	WM	WF	NM	NF	WM	WF	NM	NF
N	(4)	(2)	(3)	(4)	(4)	(5)	(6)	(4)	(12)	(5)	(2)	(1)	(9)	(2)	(0)	(1)
Mandible	2	2	1	1	1	1	1	1	1	1	1	1	1	1		1
Cranium	1	1	7	3	2	2	2	3	2	2	2	2	2	2		10
Humeri	9	11	12	2	12	9	6	11	3	5	8	14	4	12		4
Radii	10.5	17	10	6	10	6	12	17	7	9	13	12	5	5		6
Ulnae	16	14	5	4	6	8	8	16	10	8	16	10	6	6		8
Femora	3	12	16	7.5	14	11	10	7	8	4	12	4	7	10		5
Tibiae	6	16	17	12	17	10	16	9	12	6	14	3	8	15		3
Fibulae	13	9	13	13	16	7	9	8	4	3	11	5.5	3	7		2
Clavicles	7	7	8	9	3	3	4	6	6	10	3	7	9	3		7
Scapulae	10.5	8	9	10	7	13	7	13	11	11	5	9	12	9		12
Ribs	5	10	6	5	5	5	5	4	5	7	6	8	10	8		9
Hip bones	14	13	11	16	11	16	15	12	14	14	7	16	13	18		18
CV	8	4	2	7.5	4	4	3	10	9	12	4	5.5	11	4		11
TV	4	5	4	11	8	12	11	14	13	15	10	13	14	13		16
LV	12	6	3	15	9	17	13	5	15	17	9	15	15	17		17
Sacrum	17	3	14	18	13	15	14	2	17	18	15	18	16	19		19
Sternum	15	15	15	14	15	19	17	15	18	19	17	17	19	16		14
Hand bones	19	19	18	17	18	14	19	19	16	16	18	19	17	11		15
Foot bones	18	18	19	19	19	18	18	18	19	13	19	11	18	14		13

See explanation for Table 9.

Source: Trotter M. Percentage of ash weight of young human skeletons. *Growth* 1973;37:153–63.

Bone Mineral Content in Children as Determined by Radiographic Techniques

The direct photon absorption method was used to measure the bone mineral content of 322 white schoolage children (6 to 14 years) from Middleton, WI. Linear scans were made with a ^{125}I source at the distal third of the radius and across the midhumerus of all children and at the distal third of the ulna in 128 subjects. Bone width and the mineral width ratio were derived from the absorptiometric scans.

Radiographic morphometry was done with Helios calipers on standard radiographs (36 in. focal film distance). The thickness of the total bone and the medullary canal diameter were measured at the absorption scan site on the radius, thereby permitting direct comparisons of the two methods. Compact bone thickness was derived, and the total cross-sectional area and the area of the compact bone were calculated assuming a circular model. The commonly used ratios of compact bone/total bone thickness and area were also calculated. The skeletal age was determined using the standards of Gruelich WW, Pyle SI. *Radiographic atlas of skeletal development of the hand and wrist.* 2nd ed. Stanford: Stanford University Press, 1959.

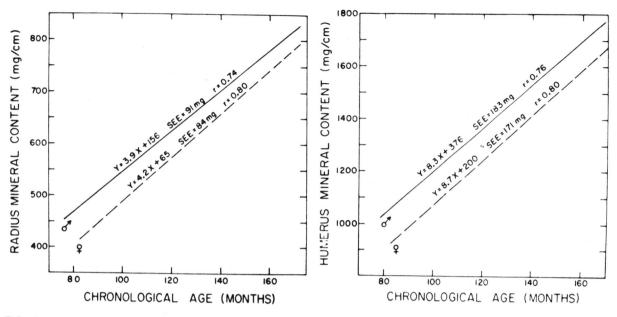

FIG. 9. Bone mineral content in children 6 to 14 years of age.

TABLE 11. *Means and coefficients of variation for bone mineral measurements of schoolchildren*

Age	Radius						Humerus						Ulna					
	Mineral		Width		M/W		Mineral		Width		M/W		Mineral		Width		M/W	
	F	**M**	**F**	**M**	**F**	**M**	**F**	**M**	**F**	**M**	**F**	**M**	**F**	**M**	**F**	**M**	**F**	**M**
Means																		
6	436	466	9.1	9.5	47.5	48.6	943	1018	13.7	14.4	69.2	70.9	354	343	7.6	8.1	46.6	42.1
7	457	510	9.1	10.0	49.9	50.9	1001	1109	14.3	14.7	69.8	75.7	374	411	8.2	8.6	45.9	48.2
8	490	557	9.4	10.2	52.2	54.3	1106	1249	14.9	15.6	74.2	80.2	413	480	8.8	9.1	47.2	52.7
9	542	584	9.7	10.5	55.6	55.4	1216	1276	15.7	15.9	77.3	79.9	481	475	8.4	9.2	57.5	51.6
10	565	633	9.9	11.1	56.6	57.3	1226	1442	15.8	16.8	77.4	85.7	473	554	8.6	9.5	54.6	58.6
11	645	691	10.8	11.3	59.6	61.0	1354	1478	16.5	17.2	81.7	85.9	540	567	9.6	9.8	55.0	58.0
12	716	763	11.3	12.0	63.1	62.9	1533	1662	17.3	19.0	88.1	87.1	—	595	—	10.4	—	57.0
13	742	781	11.5	12.6	64.0	61.6	1627	1624	18.2	18.0	89.4	90.6	—	—	—	—	—	—
14	878	792	12.1	11.9	71.9	66.0	1875	1855	19.1	19.8	98.1	93.2	—	—	—	—	—	—
Coefficients of Variation																		
6	18	11	12	9	10	8	11	12	13	12	10	8	16	10	7	7	15	8
7	12	14	10	8	8	8	11	15	8	14	7	7	14	12	9	13	12	9
8	12	15	9	10	9	9	14	12	9	11	8	7	17	12	9	11	17	11
9	13	12	10	10	6	7	11	13	9	8	7	9	9	15	13	10	7	12
10	17	13	11	10	9	13	12	14	9	10	8	9	16	14	12	7	9	12
11	18	16	11	12	12	8	18	10	11	8	12	8	26	10	12	11	16	9
12	12	16	10	11	8	9	16	13	12	9	9	8	—	10	—	7	—	8
13	13	17	10	12	8	8	12	14	9	11	9	13	—	—	—	—	—	—
14	14	18	14	12	2	10	6	19	6	12	5	12	—	—	—	—	—	—

These data were used to construct Fig. 9.

Source: Mazess RB. Growth of bone in schoolchildren: comparison of radiographic morphometry and photon absorptiometry. *Growth* 1972;36:77–92.

TABLE 12. *Means and coefficients of variation for radiographic morphometry of the radial shaft in schoolchildren*

	Thickness (mm)						Area (mm²)				Compact/Total (%)			
	Total		Medullary		Compact		Total		Compact		Thickness		Area	
Age	F	M	F	M	F	M	F	M	F	M	F	M	F	M
Means														
6	9.4	10.0	4.4	4.6	5.0	5.4	70	79	54	62	54	54	78	79
7	9.7	10.3	4.4	4.8	5.2	5.5	75	84	58	65	54	54	79	78
8	9.6	10.6	4.2	4.9	5.4	5.7	73	89	59	69	56	54	81	78
9	9.9	10.8	4.4	5.2	5.5	5.6	78	93	62	71	56	52	80	77
10	10.3	11.2	4.6	5.0	5.7	6.2	84	101	67	80	56	55	80	80
11	11.2	11.4	4.8	5.2	6.3	6.2	99	103	80	81	56	55	81	79
12	11.5	12.0	5.2	5.7	6.3	6.3	105	113	82	87	55	53	79	77
13	11.6	12.2	4.9	5.5	6.7	6.6	107	117	87	92	58	55	82	79
14	11.7	12.3	4.8	5.5	7.0	6.8	109	120	91	95	60	56	84	80
Coefficients of Variation														
6	12	10	24	20	15	13	25	20	23	20	15	12	10	7
7	12	8	20	17	10	10	23	15	20	14	9	10	6	7
8	8	10	18	20	12	13	16	20	16	19	11	12	7	8
9	12	9	28	16	9	11	23	18	17	17	14	10	9	6
10	12	11	21	20	12	13	24	22	22	21	11	11	7	7
11	10	9	19	21	15	10	20	19	22	16	12	12	7	7
12	9	9	28	16	11	11	18	17	11	17	17	10	11	6
13	10	9	22	21	12	14	19	18	18	18	12	14	7	9
14	11	13	18	23	7	14	22	26	19	25	6	13	3	8

Source: Mazess RB. Growth of bone in schoolchildren: comparison of radiographic morphometry and photon absorptiometry. *Growth* 1972;36:77–92.

Bone Mineral Content in the Os Calcis

Bone mineral content (BMC) was measured in 66 boys aged 3 to 16 years and in 71 girls aged 3 to 20 years. These were children of the hospital staff and others who were examined in the course of a field study of chronic lead incorporation. The investigations were carried out by a method developed by the authors following principles of photon absorptiometry. The BMC is expressed in grams per centimeter length unit and in grams per cubic centimeter bone volume, indicating the bone density. The figure demonstrates the normal values of bone mineral (length and volume) content, expressed as a percentage of the standard for normal adults (male and female).

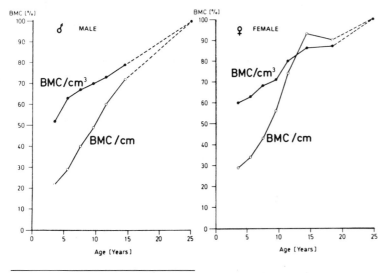

FIG. 10. Graph of bone mineral content in the os calcis.

Source: Klemm DH, Banzer U, Schneider. Bone mineral content of the growing skeleton. *AJR* 1976;126:1283–4.

TABLE 13. *Bone mineral content of the os calcis in children*

AGE |YEARS| ♂	n	BMC		C−WIDTH	C−THICKNESS	HEIGHT	WEIGHT
		M ± SD |mg/cm³|	M ± SD |g/cm|	M ± SD |mm|	M ± SD |mm|	M ± SD |cm|	M ± SD |kg|
3 − 4	6	145 ± 24	0.82 ± 0.23	32.0 ± 1.8	24.8 ± 1.9	108 ± 4.0	16.8 ± 2.1
5 − 6	10	176 ± 36	1.07 ± 0.21	35.5 ± 1.6	25.6 ± 4.0	117 ± 8.2	21.3 ± 2.5
7 − 8	17	188 ± 20	1.48 ± 0.26	39.3 ± 2.8	29.2 ± 2.5	132 ± 5.9	27.0 ± 4.2
9 − 10	13	195 ± 28	1.83 ± 0.39	43.6 ± 5.3	32.0 ± 3.3	139 ± 9.2	34.4 ± 7.1
11 − 12	8	206 ± 26	2.23 ± 0.38	47.3 ± 4.3	33.9 ± 2.6	152 ± 5.6	42.3 ± 5.9
13 − 16	12	222 ± 31	2.68 ± 0.40	49.8 ± 2.6	36.3 ± 2.7	161 ± 9.6	51.0 ± 9.1

AGE |YEARS| ♀	n	BMC		C−WIDTH	C−THICKNESS	HEIGHT	WEIGHT
		M ± SD |mg/cm³|	M ± SD |g/cm|	M ± SD |mm|	M ± SD |mm|	|cm|	|kg|
3 − 4	6	165 ± 34	0.90 ± 0.18	33.0 ± 4.1	24.0 ± 3.7	108 ± 5.4	17.7 ± 1.0
5 − 6	17	172 ± 37	1.05 ± 0.25	34.3 ± 4.0	26.2 ± 3.3	118 ± 7.0	21.4 ± 3.7
7 − 8	12	186 ± 26	1.33 ± 0.28	37.1 ± 3.6	27.9 ± 2.6	129 ± 6.6	26.9 ± 4.1
9 − 10	11	195 ± 24	1.74 ± 0.32	43.1 ± 3.1	30.8 ± 1.9	142 ± 6.5	32.6 ± 4.1
11 − 12	6	221 ± 36	2.29 ± 0.42	45.7 ± 4.1	33.5 ± 1.8	149 ± 12.5	37.5 ± 6.0
13 − 16	6	236 ± 34	2.88 ± 0.50	49.3 ± 1.2	36.3 ± 2.7	165 ± 8.3	50.3 ± 8.0
17 − 20	13	239 ± 35	2.80 ± 0.38	48.7 ± 3.4	35.7 ± 1.8	165 ± 7.5	53.2 ± 6.7

The subjects were males aged 3 to 16 years and females aged 3 to 20 years. The data here were used to construct Fig. 10. The results are given as the mean ± SD.

Related data for bone mineral content in the radius and ulna may be found in Mazess RB, Cameron JR. Bone mineral content in normal U.S. Whites. In: *International Conference on Bone Mineral Measurement, Chicago, 1973*. DHEW publication No. (NIH)75–68, pp. 228–37.

Source: Schuster W, Reiss KH, Kromer K. Quantitatif mineralsalzbestimmung am kindlichen skelett. *Dtsch Med Wochenschr* 1969;94:183–7.

Bone Mineral Content of Full-Term Infants Measured by Direct Photon Absorptiometry

Sixty-two full-term (38 to 42 weeks' gestation) infants were studied during the first 3 days of life. Measurements were performed in the left ulna and radius at one-third and one-tenth from the distal end of both bones. Gestational age was categorized from the first day of the last menstrual period according to the history obtained from the mother and was verified by clinical assessment of physical and neuromuscular maturity.

TABLE 14. *Normal values for bone mineral content in full-term infants, appropriate for gestational age*

					RADIUS				ULNA			
					1/3		1/10		1/3		1/10	
				MATERN								
BLACK MALE	WT	LENGTH	H C	AGE	BMC	BW	BMC	BW	BMC	BW	BMC	BW
n=12												
X̄	3211	49.47	34.1	22.92	.0964	.484	.1144	.720	.0833	.475	.0797	.552
SE	96.43	.515	.375	1.124	.0083	.027	.0114	.065	.0074	.040	.0092	.045
SD	373.46	1.995	1.454	4.051	.0248	.082	.0302	.172	.0210	.114	.0245	.119
WHITE MALE												
n=18												
X̄	3311	50.14	34.17	24.231	.1006	.497	.1178	.707	.0857	.482	.0752	.643
SE	83.84	.387	.256	1.602	.0056	.024	.0071	.038	.0034	.023	.0067	.040
SD	365.44	1.643	1.085	5.776	.0239	.105	.0274	.148	.0137	.093	.0201	.122
BLACK FEMALE												
n=20												
X̄	3067	49.75	33.61	21.08	.1069	.574	.1088	.652	.0804	.443	.0690	.548
SE	60.12	.37	.2	1.059	.0097	.063	.0178	.085	.0045	.023	.0055	.041
SD	275.52	1.737	.938	3.818	.0432	.284	.0617	.296	.0190	.099	.0182	.137
WHITE FEMALE												
n=12												
X̄	3313	51.35	33.95	26.2	.1081	.502	.1230	.815	.0953	.416	.1010	.581
SE	89.12	.236	.311	1.772	.0071	.045	.0151	.118	.0038	.018	.0205	.077
SD	282.1	.747	.985	3.962	.0202	.129	.0369	.291	.0100	.049	.0410	.155

WT = weight in grams; LENGTH in centimeters; HC = head circumference in centimeters; BW = bone width in centimeters; BMC = bone mineral content in grams/centimeters.

Source: Steicher JJ, Kaplan B, Edwards N, Tsang RD. Conference on bone mineral measurement. *AJR* 1976;126:1284–5.

Variation of Roentgenographic Density of the Os Calcis and Phalanx by Sex and Age

Roentgenograms of the left os calcis and phalanx (fifth finger, second bone) were taken of 738 male and 746 female subjects from various geographic locations. These were compared with measurements of a standard wedge.

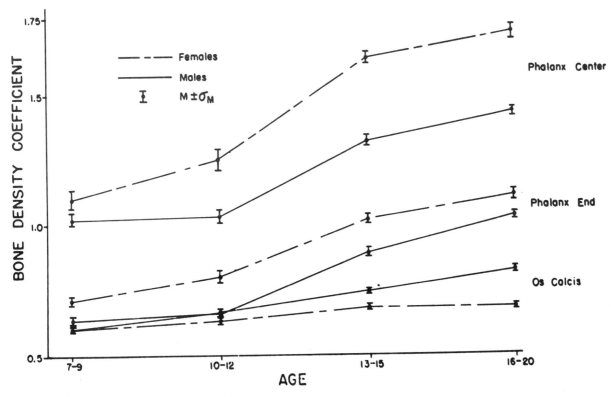

FIG. 11. Variation in bone density coefficients of the os calcis and phalanx trace paths, by sex and age.

TABLE 15. *Mean density coefficients of the os calcis and phalanx of subjects aged 7 to 20 years*

AGE GROUP	OS CALCIS						PHALANX END						PHALANX CENTER					
	MALES			FEMALES			MALES			FEMALES			MALES			FEMALES		
	MEAN	SD	NO.	MEAN	SD	NO.	MEAN	SD	NO.	MEAN	SD	NO.	MEAN	SD	NO.	MEAN	SD	NO.
7-9	0.60	0.09	138	0.60	0.09	139	0.64	0.11	77	0.71	0.16	97	1.02	0.23	77	1.10	0.21	97
10-12	0.67	0.10	183	0.63	0.08	138	0.66	0.16	101	0.80	0.18	56	1.03	0.28	101	1.25	0.30	56
13-15	0.74	0.10	254	0.68	0.10	296	0.89	0.21	225	1.02	0.18	135	1.32	0.30	225	1.64	0.22	135
16-20	0.82	0.05	163	0.68	0.09	173	1.03	0.19	221	1.11	0.18	107	1.43	0.24	221	1.74	0.31	107

Source: Scharer H. Variation in the roentgenographic density of the os calcis and phalanx with sex and age. *J Pediatr* 1968;52:416–23.

Measurement of the Second Metacarpal at Its Midshaft

Standard values for medullary width, cortical width, cortical area, and percent cortical area are based on findings in more than 2,000 well-nourished clinically healthy Ohio subjects.

TABLE 16. *Standards for metacarpal width, cortical thickness, cortical area, and percent cortical area*

Age (yr)	Total width Mean	SD	Medullary width Mean	SD	Cortical width Mean	SD	Cortical area Mean	SD	Cortical area (%) Mean	SD
Males										
1	4.50	0.34	3.04	0.45	1.46	0.30	8.63	1.65	54.22	9.40
2	5.11	0.44	3.24	0.62	1.85	0.39	12.09	2.35	59.28	10.85
4	5.53	0.49	3.04	0.62	2.48	0.37	16.65	2.54	69.49	8.47
6	6.05	0.53	3.06	0.66	2.98	0.44	21.26	3.51	73.94	8.53
8	6.57	0.54	3.13	0.66	3.43	0.45	26.08	3.90	76.88	7.29
10	7.16	0.59	3.28	0.66	3.88	0.49	31.81	4.97	78.72	6.52
12	7.73	0.65	3.43	0.72	4.29	0.60	37.66	6.37	79.87	6.67
14	8.52	0.77	3.63	0.72	4.89	0.68	46.83	8.52	81.45	5.85
16	9.11	0.72	3.81	0.75	5.29	0.51	53.82	7.53	82.29	5.14
18	9.31	0.68	3.56	0.90	5.75	0.66	57.94	7.55	84.91	6.04
30	9.36	0.68	3.41	0.81	5.94	0.43	59.59	6.62	86.49	4.67
40	9.35	0.50	3.72	0.83	5.63	0.60	57.59	5.29	83.77	5.97
50	9.65	0.88	3.84	0.93	5.81	0.63	61.54	9.64	83.85	5.67
60	9.69	0.62	4.44	0.84	5.24	0.62	58.03	6.82	78.67	6.43
70	9.38	0.58	4.61	1.05	4.76	0.73	52.99	5.28	76.25	6.23
80	9.07	0.51	4.23	0.62	4.89	0.56	50.10	5.30	76.00	5.23
Females										
1	4.35	0.36	2.87	0.38	1.47	0.31	8.40	1.94	56.04	8.36
2	4.91	0.47	3.12	0.53	1.79	0.36	11.29	2.41	59.32	9.36
4	5.37	0.49	3.04	0.49	2.32	0.35	15.39	2.79	67.68	7.12
6	5.76	0.53	3.01	0.51	2.76	0.43	18.98	3.41	72.41	6.28
8	6.26	0.58	3.05	0.58	3.20	0.41	23.51	4.01	76.04	6.25
10	6.80	0.63	3.26	0.64	3.53	0.48	28.01	4.95	76.70	6.71
12	7.40	0.68	3.25	0.74	4.14	0.57	34.72	6.09	80.22	6.70
14	7.77	0.62	2.94	0.68	4.83	0.57	40.64	6.20	85.25	5.53
16	7.79	0.61	2.71	0.71	5.08	0.60	41.91	6.15	87.43	5.33
18	7.90	0.64	2.71	0.72	5.18	0.68	43.22	6.94	87.63	5.03
30	7.94	0.55	2.61	0.80	5.33	0.69	43.96	5.85	88.49	5.82
40	8.08	0.65	2.59	0.89	5.45	0.81	45.79	7.06	88.85	6.13
50	7.79	0.66	2.27	0.71	5.52	0.75	43.67	7.13	90.89	4.98
60	8.12	0.43	3.26	0.88	4.85	0.68	43.02	4.03	83.20	7.59
70	8.34	0.70	4.38	0.88	3.99	0.63	38.65	4.15	70.93	7.00
80	8.29	0.61	5.00	0.64	3.30	0.51	34.47	4.15	63.38	6.70

Source: Garn SM, Poznanski AK, Nagy JM. Bone measurement in the differential diagnosis of osteopenia and osteoporosis. *Radiology* 1971;100:509–19.

REMODELING

Remodeling After Distal Forearm Fractures in Children

The effect of residual fracture angulation on the distal radial and ulnar epiphyseal plates was studied in children aged 1 to 15 years. Thirty-eight fractures located in the distal fifth of the forearm bones were observed for 1 to 25 months after the fractures had healed. Forearms were examined radiographically on 2 to 5 occasions, and the inclinations of the epiphyseal plates in relation to the long axis of the proximal fragments were measured.

The results demonstrated that an abnormal inclination of the epiphyseal plate after healing of a distal forearm fracture induced an alteration of growth in the epiphyseal plate. The redistribution of growth tended to correct the abnormal inclination. The rate of correction followed an exponential course. The age of the child at the time of the fracture and the distance from the fracture to the epiphyseal plate did not influence the capacity for correction.

TABLE 1. *Capacity for correction of the epiphyseal line inclination expressed in degrees/ month. Means and standard deviations are given*

	Radius		Ulna
	Doroso-volar plane	Radio-ulnar plane	Doroso-volar plane
All observations	0.91 ± 0.57	0.80 ± 0.31	0.82 ± 0.43
Primary angulation 0°–14°	0.25 ± 0.28	—	—
Primary angulation 5°–14°	0.75 ± 0.56	0.74 ± 0.28	0.68 ± 0.37
Primary angulation ≥15°	1.18 ± 0.47	1.08 ± 0.29	1.36 ± 0.08

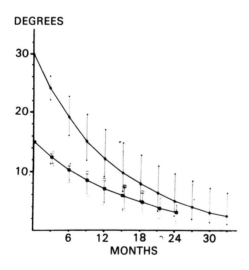

FIG. 1. Normalization of the epiphyseal plate. This graph represents two hypothetical patients, one with a primary angulation of 15° *(lower line)* and a second with angulation of 30° *(upper line)*. The mean value of B (individual correction factor) found in the lateral view of the radius has been used. (B = 0.074 + 1 × SD = 0.029). The mean constant percentage correction was 6.1%.

Source: Friberg KSI. Remodeling after distal forearm fractures in children. I. The effect of residual angulation on the spatial orientation of the epiphyseal plates. *Acta Orthop Scand* 1979;50:537–46.

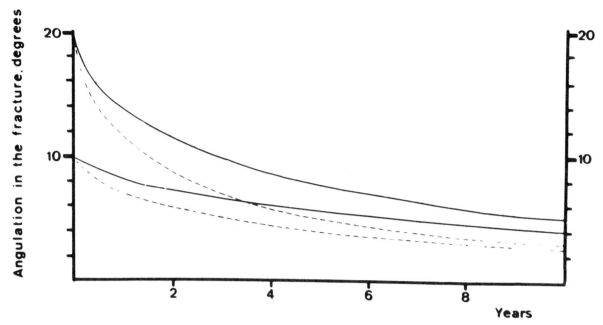

FIG. 2. The correction of angulation of distal forearm fractures. The outcome of residual angulation of the radius after 38 distal forearm fractures in children was investigated. The period of observation ranged from 4 months to 10 years, 8 months. The graph indicates four hypothetical patients. Remodeling was calculated using the formula:

$$\tan \beta = \frac{\sin \alpha \times D}{G + (\cos \alpha \times D)}$$

where G = the longitudinal growth produced by the epiphyseal plate. D = distance from the fracture to the epiphyseal plate. $A = \sin \alpha \times D$ = adaxial displacement of the epiphyseal plate. α = angulation of the fracture at the time of healing. β = residual angulation of the fracture. The unbroken line equals 10 mm of adaxial displacement of the distal epiphyseal plate. The broken line equals 5 mm of adaxial displacement of the distal epiphyseal plate.

Correction of the residual angulation after fracture was shown to be governed by three factors: (1) an increase in the time between the healing of the fracture and completed growth at the epiphyseal plates resulted in a more complete correction; (2) a larger adaxial dislocation of the epiphyseal plate at the time of healing of the fracture, reflecting a larger primary fracture angulation and a greater distance from the fracture to the epiphyseal plate, resulted in less complete correction; and (3) a more complete correction or overcorrection of the distal epiphyseal plate increased the correction of the angulation of the fracture. These findings indicate the process of correction of a residual angulation after a healed fracture can be explained in terms of the combined effects of the direction and amount of longitudinal growth at the epiphyseal plate. A trigonometric equation based on this theory predicted the residual angulations of fractures at follow-up with an error of less than 1°.

Source: Friberg KSI. Remodeling after distal forearm fractures in children. III. Correction of residual angulation in fractures of the radius. *Acta Orthop Scand* 1979;50:741–9.

Incidence of Double Contour, Cupping, and Spurring in Long Bones of Infants

Roentgenograms of the long bones, wrists and ankles were obtained routinely at monthly intervals up to the eighth month of life from 100 consecutive prematurely born babies. A total of approximately 800 roentgenograms were viewed.

The author defines cupping and spurring as the elongated appearance of the edges of the epiphyseal plate when concave or convex. These findings resemble the spurring, lipping, and cupping seen in scurvy or rickets.

TABLE 2. *Month of first visibility of "double contour" by individual bone and of "cupping" and/or "spurring" of the epiphyseal line*

Month of first visibility of "double contour" (100 infants)

Bone	1st	2nd	3rd	4th	5th	6th	7th	8th	Total
Ulna	1	9	15	19	11	18	2	3	78
Radius	1	3	15	23	10	15	5	4	76
Tibia	1	4	19	12	6	6			49
Fibula			5	8	4	5	5	1	28

Month of first visibility of "cupping" and/or "spurring" (100 infants)

Bone	1st	2nd	3rd	4th	5th	6th	7th	8th	Total
Ulna		3	25	20	13	8	1	3	73
Radius			8	18	12	4	1	3	46
Tibia			2	3	1	3			9
Fibula			1	3		2			6

Note: Each asterisk indicates a case which showed the "double contour," "cupping," or "spurring" for the first time during the respective month.

Source: Glaser K. Double contour, cupping and spurring in roentgenograms of long bones in infants. *AJR* 1949;61:482–92.

TABLE 3. *Month of disappearance of "double contour," "cupping," and/or "spurring"*

Month of disappearance of "double contour" (100 infants)

Bone:	1st	2nd	3rd	4th	5th	6th	7th	8th	Total
Ulna			* 1		** 2	*** 3	****** 6	******** ******** **** 20	32
Radius			* 1			****** 6	**** 4	******** ******** 16	27
Tibia				* 1		****** 6	**** 4	******** ***** 13	24
Fibula						** 2	* 1	***** 5	8

Month of disappearance of "cupping" and/or "spurring" (100 infants)

Bone:	1st	2nd	3rd	4th	5th	6th	7th	8th	Total
Ulna					* 1	**** 4	******** ******** 16	******** ******** ******** ****** 30	51
Radius				* 1	* 1	**** 4	******* 7	******** ******** *** 19	32
Tibia						** 2	* 1	****** 6	9
Fibula								***** 5	5

Note: Each asterisk indicates a case which for the first time during the respective month *failed to show* the previously visible "double contour," "cupping" or "spurring."

Source: Glaser K. Double contour, cupping and spurring in roentgenograms of long bones in infants. *AJR* 1949;61:482–92.

Incidence of Double Contour Effect

One-hundred and seventeen infants of whom the majority were premature (97 during life and 20 after death) were studied. A double contour effect was noted on the radiographs of the long bones as a single continuous linear shadow running adjacent to the diaphysis on its outer side, and separated from it by a radiolucent strip about 1 mm in width. This thin pencilled line, which was never laminated, was limited to the diaphyseal portion of the bone and never extended beyond the metaphyseal region, at which point it merged with the outline of the diaphysis.

TABLE 4. *Incidence of the double contour effect in individual bones*

Bone	No. of infants showing double contour	Percentage
Tibia	15	22
Ulna	14	20
Fibula	9	12
Femur	7	10
Radius	7	10
Humerus	2	3

TABLE 5. *Incidence of double contour effect in combinations of bones in the same patients*

Combination of bones	No. of infants showing double contour	Percentage
Radius and ulna	8	11
Tibia and fibula	6	8
Tibia, fibula, radius, and ulna	2	3

TABLE 6. *Incidence of double contour effect at different birth weights*

Birth weight	No. of infants showing double contour	Percentage
Under 3 lb	5	80
3 lb–3 lb 15 oz.	26	42
4 lb–4 lb 15 oz.	27	26
5 lb–5 lb 7 oz.	5	20
5 lb 8 oz.–5 lb 15 oz.	3	None
6 lb and over	7	None

Source: Hancox NM, Hay JD, Holden WS, Moss PD, Whitehead AS. The radiologic "double contour" effect in the long bones of newlyborn infants. *Arch Dis Child* 1961;26:543–8.

Acetabular Development After Reduction in Congenital Dislocation of the Hip

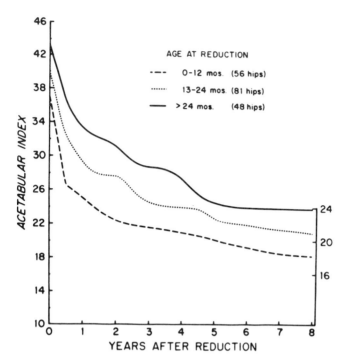

FIG. 3. Acetabular index related to age at reduction and years after reduction. Roentgenograms were made at approximately 6-month intervals for the first 5 years and yearly thereafter.

TABLE 7. *Acetabular indices from age at reduction to 7 years after reduction*

Age at Reduction	Years after Reduction														
	0	½	1	1½	2	2½	3	3½	4	4½	5	5½	6	6½	7
0-12 mos.	38.3	26.5	25.5	23.3	23.1	21.7	23.0	21.5	20.8	21.2	20.0	19.3	20.9	17.2	18.7
(56 hips)	±7.3	±5.6	±5.8	±4.7	±4.8	±5.1	±4.5	±4.7	±4.2	±3.4	±4.5	±4.3	±2.7	±3.7	±5.2
13-24 mos.	40.3	32.4	29.8	28.0	28.2	25.5	24.7	24.3	24.1	24.4	22.0	23.1	22.1	21.6	22.0
(81 hips)	±7.5	±6.8	±5.8	±5.1	±5.0	±6.1	±5.4	±4.2	±5.1	±5.7	±5.7	±7.0	±6.1	±6.3	±7.1
> 24 mos.	44.5	36.2	33.1	32.1	31.8	28.5	28.6	29.2	26.6	27.5	22.5	24.9	23.1	25.8	22.2
(48 hips)	±8	±4.8	±5.2	±5.3	±5.7	±5.2	±5.5	±4.8	±6.0	±5.2	±5.7	±6.6	±6.8	±5.5	±5.8

Data from which the graph in Fig. 3 was constructed.

Source: Lindstrom JR, Ponseti IV, Wenger DR. Acetabular development after reduction in congenital dislocation of the hip. *J Bone Joint Surg (Am)* 1979;61:112–18.

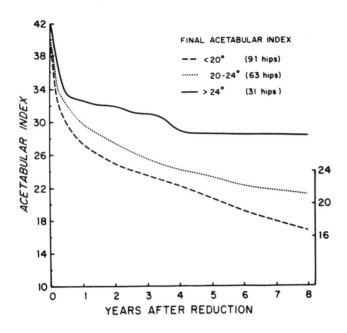

FIG. 4. Acetabular development related to final acetabular index and years after reduction.

TABLE 8. *Acetabular development related to final acetabular index and years after reduction*

Final acetabular index	Years after reduction														
	0	½	1	1½	2	2½	3	3½	4	4½	5	5½	6	6½	7
20 (91 hips)	39.8	29.4	28.5	25.1	25.5	22.3	23.4	22.8	22.0	22.9	19.4	18.7	19.7	17.9	18.1
	± 7.1	± 7.5	± 6.5	± 5.6	± 5.6	± 4.9	± 5.2	± 4.4	± 5.3	± 4.5	± 4.7	± 3.6	± 5.0	± 4.7	± 4.0
20–24 (63 hips)	41.3	31.7	29.6	28.3	29.3	26.4	25.0	25.1	24.0	24.2	21.7	23.5	21.4	23.7	21.5
	± 7.7	± 6.5	± 5.8	± 5.7	± 5.6	± 5.9	± 4.7	± 4.1	± 4.6	± 5.2	± 4.2	±7.2	± 3.7	± 4.3	± 6.1
24 (31 hips)	42.8	33.3	32.8	32.2	32.1	31.1	31.1	30.9	28.5	28.5	29.0	29.2	27.8	29.0	28.7
	± 9.9	± 5.8	± 6.0	± 4.6	± 5.2	± 4.8	± 4.3	± 5.5	± 5.2	± 5.9	± 5.1	± 4.1	± 4.5	± 5.4	± 6.5

Data from which the graph in Fig. 4 was constructed.

Source: Lindstrom JR, Ponseti IV, Wenger DR. Acetabular development after reduction in congenital dislocation of the hip. *J Bone Joint Surg (Am)* 1979;61:112–18.

Development of Center Edge (CE) Angle Following Reduction in Congenital Dislocation of the Hip

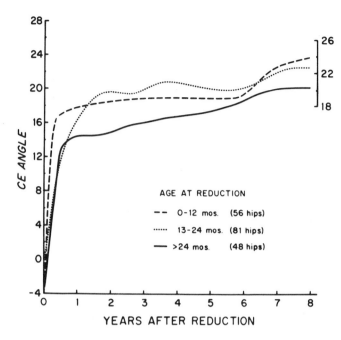

FIG. 5. Center-edge angle related to age at reduction and years after reduction.

Source: Lindstrom JR, Ponseti IV, Wenger DR. Acetabular development after reduction in congenital dislocation of the hip. *J Bone Joint Surg (Am)* 1979;61:112–18.

Femoral Head and Final Acetabular Index Following Reduction in Congenital Dislocation of the Hip

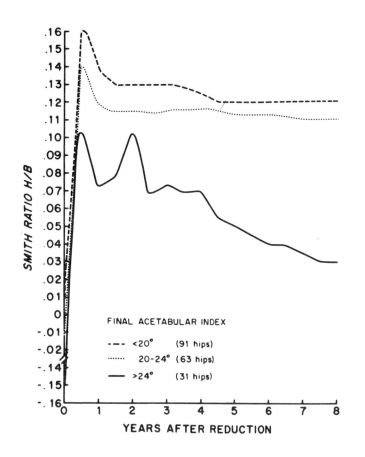

FIG. 6. Location of the femoral head relative to the final acetabular index and years after reduction.

TABLE 9. *Acetabular indices from age at reduction to seven years after reduction*

Final acetabular index	Years after reduction						
	0	½	1	1½	2	2½	3
20 (91 hips)	0.009	0.155	0.138	0.134	0.137	0.132	0.131
	± 0.164	± 0.057	± 0.047	± 0.039	± 0.038	± 0.054	± 0.076
20–24 (63 hips)	− 0.009	0.140	0.118	0.115	0.115	0.114	0.115
	± 0.159	± 0.043	± 0.050	± 0.0.42	± 0.045	± 0.050	± 0.042
24 (31 hips)	− 0.147	0.103	0.073	0.077	0.102	0.069	0.073
	± 0.164	± 0.046	± 0.074	± 0.045	± 0.090	± 0.067	± 0.075

Data from which Fig. 6 was constructed.

Source: Akeson J, Staheli LT. The radiographic appearance of the normal forearm in pronation and supination. *J Pediatr Orthop (in preparation.)*

Normal Forearm in Pronation and Supination

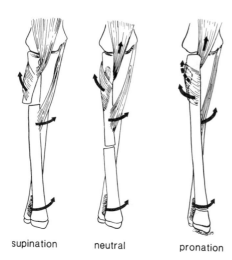

supination   neutral   pronation

FIG. 7. Rotation of the proximal radial fragment as determined by the muscle forces acting at each level.

Source: Akeson J, Staheli LT. The radiographic appearance of the normal forearm in pronation and supination. *J Pediatr Orthop (In preparation.)*

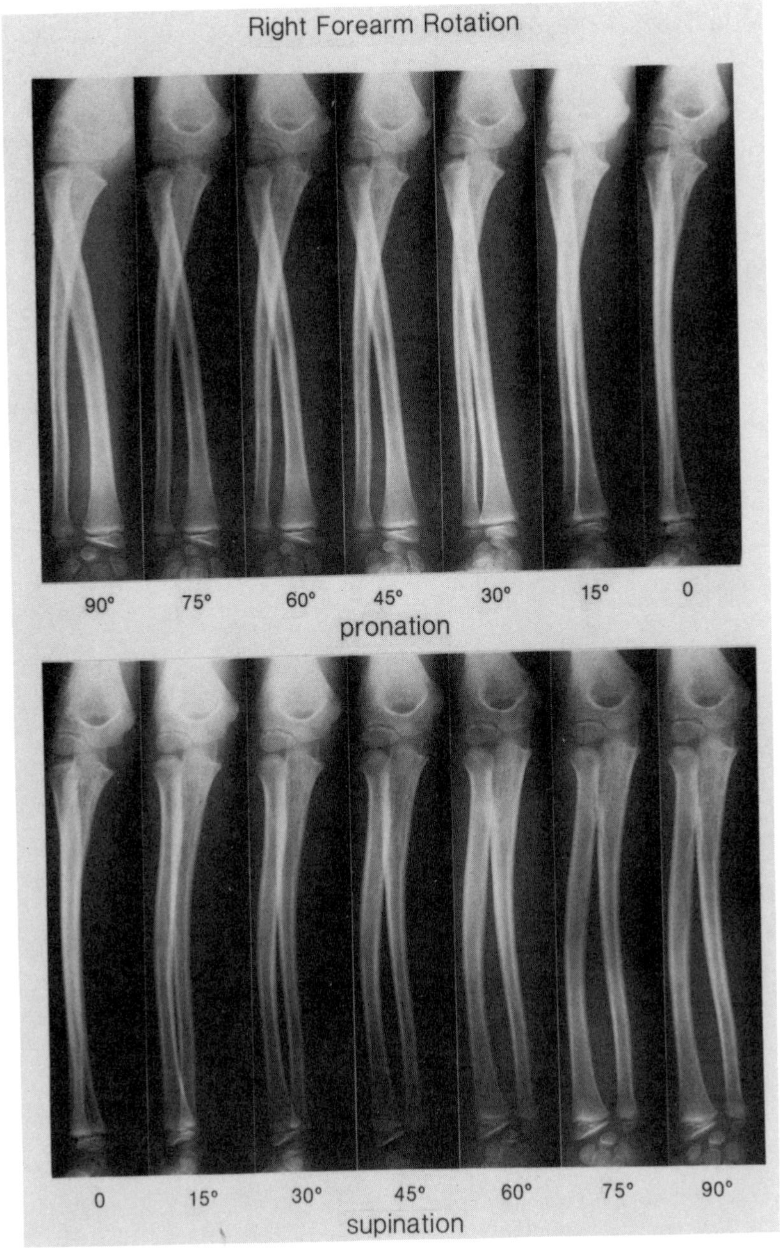

FIG. 8.   Top: Radiographs of the right forearm as it moves from 90° pronation to neutral. **Bottom:** Radiographs of the right forearm as it moves from neutral to 90° supination.

Source: Akeson J, Staheli LT. The radiographic appearance of the normal forearm in pronation and supination. *J Pediatr Orthop (In preparation.)*

UPPER EXTREMITY

Time Schedule for the Appearance of Primary Ossification Centers in the Shafts of Long Bones and the Hand During Fetal Life

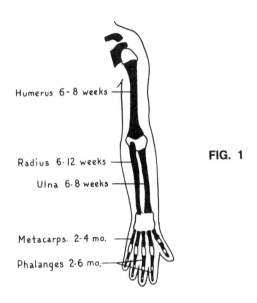

Humerus 6-8 weeks

Radius 6-12 weeks

Ulna 6-8 weeks

Metacarps. 2-4 mo.

Phalanges 2-6 mo.

FIG. 1

Source: Reproduced with permission from Caffey J, Silverman FN, Baker DH, Berdon WE, Dorst JP, Girdany BR, Lee FA, Shopfner CE. *Pediatric x-ray diagnosis.* 7th ed. Chicago: Yearbook Medical Publishers, 1978.

Time of Ossification of Bones of the Upper Extremity

TABLE 1. *Giving the time of the ossification of the bones of the arm*

No.	E	168	53	D	263,b	42	271	C	263,c	333	56	B	202	274	263,b,2
Length	15	15	15	16	16	18	18	18	19	—	24	29	30	31	32
Age	39	39	39	40	40	42	42	42	44	—	49	54	55	56	56
Clavicle	?	*	*	*	*	*	*	*	*	*	*	*	*	*	*
Humerus	—	—	—	—	—	—	—	*	*	*	*	*	*	*	*
Radius	—	—	—	—	—	⌐	—	—	*	*	*	*	*	*	*
Ulna	—	—	—	—	—	—	—	—	*	*	*	*	*	*	*
Scapula	—	—	—	—	—	—	—	—	—	—	—	—	*	*	*
Metacarpal 1	—	—	—	—	—	—	—	—	—	—	—	—	—	—	—
Metacarpal 2	—	—	—	—	—	—	—	—	—	—	—	—	—	—	—
Metacarpal 3	—	—	—	—	—	—	—	—	—	—	—	—	—	—	—
Metacarpal 4	—	—	—	—	—	—	—	—	—	—	—	—	—	—	—
Metacarpal 5	—	—	—	—	—	—	—	—	—	—	—	—	—	—	—
Phalanges I 1	—	—	—	—	—	—	—	—	—	—	—	—	—	—	—
Phalanges I 2	—	—	—	—	—	—	—	—	—	—	—	—	—	—	—
Phalanges I 3	—	—	—	—	—	—	—	—	—	—	—	—	—	—	—
Phalanges I 4	—	—	—	—	—	—	—	—	—	—	—	—	—	—	—
Phalanges I 5	—	—	—	—	—	—	—	—	—	—	—	—	—	—	—
Phalanges II 2	—	—	—	—	—	—	—	—	—	—	—	—	—	—	—
Phalanges II 3	—	—	—	—	—	—	—	—	—	—	—	—	—	—	—
Phalanges II 4	—	—	—	—	—	—	—	—	—	—	—	—	—	—	—
Phalanges II 5	—	—	—	—	—	—	—	—	—	—	—	—	—	—	—
Phalanges III 1	—	—	—	—	—	—	—	—	—	—	—	—	—	*	*
Phalanges III 2	—	—	—	—	—	—	—	—	—	—	—	—	—	—	*
Phalanges III 3	—	—	—	—	—	—	—	—	—	—	—	—	—	—	*
Phalanges III 4	—	—	—	—	—	—	—	—	—	—	—	—	—	—	*
Phalanges III 5	—	—	—	—	—	—	—	—	—	—	—	—	—	—	*

No.	266	263,b,1	272	J	I	282	K	L	284	288,b	M	N	300	O	S	306,c	Q	306,b	P	R
Length	33	34	34	36	41	42	53	54	54	57	69	70	73	73	75	75	81		105	110
Age	57	58	58	60	64	65	72	73	73	75	83	83	85	85	87	87	90	105	105	110
Clavicle	*	*	*	*	*	*	*	*	*	*	*	*	*	*	*		*	*	*	*
Humerus	*	*	*	*	*	*	*	*	*	*	•	*	*	*	*	*	*	*	*	*
Radius	*	*	*	*	*	*	*	*	*	*	*	*	*	*	*	*	*	*	*	*
Ulna	*	*	*	*	*	*	*	*	*	*	*	*	*	*	*	*	*	*	*	*
Scapula	*	*	*	*	*	*	*	*	*	*	*	*	*	*	*	*	*	*	*	*
Metacarpal 1	—	—	*	*	*	*	*	*	*	*	*	*	*	*	*	*	*	*	*	*
Metacarpal 2	*	*	*	*	*	*	*	*	*	*	*	*	*	*	*	*	*	*	*	*
Metacarpal 3	*	*	*	*	*	*	*	*	*	*	*	*	*	*	*	*	*	*	*	*
Metacarpal 4	—	*	*	*	*	*	*	*	*	*	*	*	*	*	*	*	*	*	*	*
Metacarpal 5	—	*	*	0	*	*	*	*	*	*	*	*	*	*	*	*	*	*	*	*
Phalanges I 1	—	—	*	—	*	*	*	*	*	*	*	*	*	*	*	*	*	*	*	*
Phalanges I 2	—	—	*	—	*	*	*	*	*	*	*	*	*	*	*	*	*	*	*	*
Phalanges I 3	—	—	—	—	*	*	*	*	*	*	*	*	*	*	*	*	*	*	*	*
Phalanges I 4	—	—	—	—	*	*	*	*	*	*	*	*	*	*	*	*	*	*	*	*
Phalanges I 5	—	—	—	—	*	*	*	*	*	*	*	*	*	*	*	*	*	*	*	*
Phalanges II 2	—	—	—	—	—	*	*	*	*	*	*	*	*	*	*	*	*	*	*	*
Phalanges II 3	—	—	—	—	—	—	*	*	*	*	*	*	*	*	*	*	*	*	*	*
Phalanges II 4	—	—	—	—	—	—	—	—	*	*	*	*	*	*	*	*	*	*	*	*
Phalanges II 5	—	—	—	—	—	—	—	—	*	*	*	*	*	*	*	*	*	*	*	*
Phalanges III 1	*	*	*	*	*	*	*	*	*	*	*	*	*	*	*	*	*	*	*	*
Phalanges III 2	*	*	*	*	*	*	*	0	*	*	*	*	*	*	*	*	*	*	*	*
Phalanges III 3	*	*	*	*	*	*	*	0	*	*	*	*	*	*	*	*	*	*	*	*
Phalanges III 4	*	*	*	0	*	*	*	·0	*	*	*	*	*	*	*	*	*	*	*	*
Phalanges III 5	*	*	*	0	*	*	*	0	*	*	*	*	*	*	*	*	*	*	*	*

Notes: The first line is the designation of each specimen, the second line the crown/rump length in millimeters, and the third line the probable age in days. An asterisk indicates that the bone given in the first column is ossified. The question mark indicates that the ossification is uncertain, and zero indicates that the specimen is injured.

Source: Mall FP. On ossification centers in human embryos less than one hundred days old. *Am J Anat* 1906;5:433–58.

Humeral Head and Coracoid Ossification in the Newborn (<35 to 44 Weeks' Gestation)

This table represents the authors' review of the literature on humeral head ossification and gestational age. They noted that prenatal ossification of the humeral head in black infants probably occurs at a more rapid rate than in whites. In order to adapt the material from Christie, gestational age was calculated from birth weight assuming each black newborn was within 1 standard deviation of the mean weight according to Cassady's standards and assuming that each white newborn was within 1 standard deviation of the mean birth weight according to the standard of Usher and McLean.

TABLE 2. *Humeral head ossification and gestational age*

	Race, sex	<35	35	36	37	38	39	40	41	42	43	44
Present study			0%(31)	5%(20)		15%(20)		40%(20)	50%		82%(11)	
Garn												
Stampfel & Tscherne	WM							18%(39)			58%(11)	
	WF							26.5%(41)			70%(18)	
Menes & Holly	WM							46%(122)				
	WF							47%(112)				
Lempberg & Liliequist	WM		8%(24)	11%(9)		12.5%(8)		37%(32)		67%(3)		66%(3)
	WF		0%(19)	3.7%(8)		50%(4)		61%(23)		67%(9)		0%(2)
Christie	WM	0%(24)		7.7%(23)		7.7%(29)				41%(135)		
	WF	0%(22)		12.5%(116)		5.6%(31)				56%(125)		
	BM	0%(11)						28.8%(184)				
	BF	0%(13)						37.3(97)				

The data are compiled from several sources. (1) 102 white singleton newborns of both sexes from the C. S. Mott Children's Hospital: each was examined within 4 days of birth by the method of Dubowitz, and, for those infants who were post-mature, by maternal history. Results are not separated according to sex, because previous authors were not able to find any difference in humeral head ossification between newborn males and females. (2) 92 infants delivered over a 1-year interval and who had had chest radiographs within the first 24 hours of life at the Wayne County General Hospital. (3) 115 unselected newborns with respiratory distress syndrome of prematurity seen over the past 1.5 years. (4) Finally, there were newborns seen for serious congenital heart disease.

Related References:

Cassady G. Body composition in intrauterine growth retardation. *Pediat Clin N Am* 1970;17:79–99.

Christie A. Prevalence and distribution of ossification centers in the newborn infant. *Am J Dis Child* 1949;77:355–61.

Dubowitz LM, Dubowitz V, Goldberg C. Clinical assessment of gestational age in the newborn infant. *J Pediat* 1970;77:1–10.

Garn SM, Rohmann CG, Silverman FN. Radiographic standards for postnatal ossification and tooth calcification. *Med Radiogr Photogr* 1967;43:45–66.

Lemperg R, Liliequist B. Appearance of the ossification centre in the proximal humeral epiphysis of newborn children. *Acta Radiol (diagn)* 1972;12:76–80.

Menees TO, Holly LE. The ossification in the extremities of the new-born. *Am J Roentgenol* 1932;28:389–90.

Stampfel K, Tscherne E. Die Rontgendiagnose der ubertragenen Frucht. *Z Geburtsch Gynaek* 1939;119:31–44.

Usher R, McLean F. Intrauterine growth of live-born Caucasian infants at sea level: standards obtained from measurements in 7 dimensions of infants born between 25 and 44 weeks of gestation. *J Pediat* 1969;74:901–10.

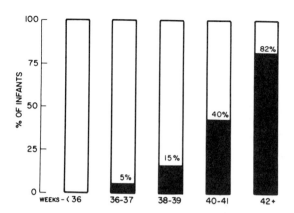

FIG. 2. The ossification of the humeral head of 102 infants is shown in relation to gestational age, as determined by a verified maternal history.

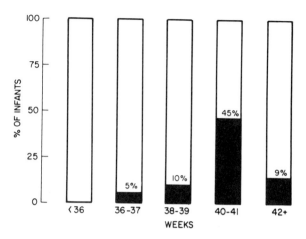

FIG. 3. Coracoid ossification relative to gestational age in the same 102 white newborns shown in Fig. 2. Note the low incidence of coracoid visualization in the postmature infant.

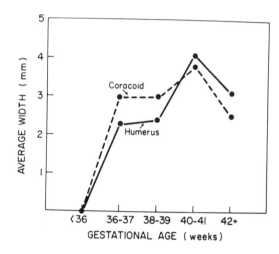

FIG. 4. The sizes of the shoulder epiphysis, coracoid, and humerus are shown in relation to gestational age in 102 newborns.

Note that the epiphyses are smaller in the postmature infants than in term newborns. The authors concluded that it is more reliable to determine ossification of the humeral head on chest roentgenograms in the newborn than of the coracoid epiphysis when assessing gestational age.

Source: Kuhns LR, Sherman MP, Poznanski AK, Holt JF. Humeral-head and coracoid ossification in the newborn. *Radiology* 1973;107:145–9.

Time of Appearance of the Primary Ossification Centers of the Upper Extremity in the First Five Prenatal Months

The data are from 136 human embryos ranging in crown/rump length from 14 to 235 mm. The chart notes: column 1, the bone; column 2, the smallest specimen with an ossification center present (the main entry in this column refers to the crown/rump length in millimeters; when there was more than one specimen at that crown/rump length which also had the ossification present, their lengths are indicated in parentheses); column 3, specimen of a crown/rump length in which the ossification center was always observed; column 4, specimens between those listed in columns 2 and 3, with the bone ossified; and column 5, reviews of the previous literature pertaining to those specific bones.

TABLE 3. *Appearance of ossification centers during the first five prenatal months*

1 Centers	2 Smallest specimen(s) with center present (mm CR)	3 Specimen(s) of a CR length after which center always observed	4 Specimens between those listed in columns 2 and 3 with the bone ossified	5 Data in literature in mm CR
Clavicle	20(4)	24(2,3)	23	15(M),17(F)
Scapula	29(2)	35(2,4)	31,34(2)	30(M)
Humerus	23	30(2)	24(1,2),27,28(3),29(1,2)	18(M)
Radius	24(2)	35(2,3)	28(3),29(1,2),31,32,34(1,2)	19(M)
Ulna	24(2,3)	35(2,3,4)	28(3),29(1,2),31,32,34(1,2)	24(M)
Metacarpal 1	45(1,4)	56(1,2)	49,50,52	34(M)
Metacarpal 2	37	44(1,2)	38(1,4),39,40(1,3,4),42	33(M)
Metacarpal 3	37	45(1,2,3,4)	38(4),39,40(1,3,4),44(1,2)	33(M)
Metacarpal 4	38(4)	45(1,2,4)	40(3,4),44(1,2)	34(M)
Metacarpal 5	38(4)	49	40(3),44(1),45(1,4),48(1)	34(M)
Prox. phalanges 1	52	60(1,2)	56(1),57	41(M)
Prox. phalanges 2	50	60(1,2)	51,52,56(1,2),57	34–41(M)
Prox. phalanges 3	50	60(1,2)	51,52,53,56(1,2),57,59	34–41(M)
Prox. phalanges 4	52	60(1,2)	56(1,2),57	41(M)
Prox. phalanges 5	60(1,2)	60(1,2)		41(M)
Middle phalanges 2	60(2)	72	61(1),65(1,3),67,69(1,2),70	57(M)
Middle phalanges 3	60(2)	70	61(1),65(1,3),67,69(1,2)	57(M)
Middle phalanges 4	60(2)	70	61(1),65(1,3),67,69(1,2)	57(M)
Middle phalanges 5	69(1)	102(2)	76,78,83(2),84(2),88,89, 91,94,97(1,2,3)	70(M)
Distal phalanges 1	29(2)	35(2,4)	34(2)	31(M)
Distal phalanges 2–5	29(2)	35(2,4)	34(2)	32(M)

Notes: (F), Fawcett E. The development and ossification of the human clavicle. *J Anat Physiol* 1913;45:378–405. (M), Mall FP. On ossification centers in human embryos less than one hundred days old. *Am J Anat* 1906;5:433–58.

Source: Noback CR, Robertson GG. Sequences of appearance of ossification centers in the human skeleton during the first five prenatal months. *Am J Anat* 1951;89:15.

Postnatal Skeletal Development of the Proximal Humerus

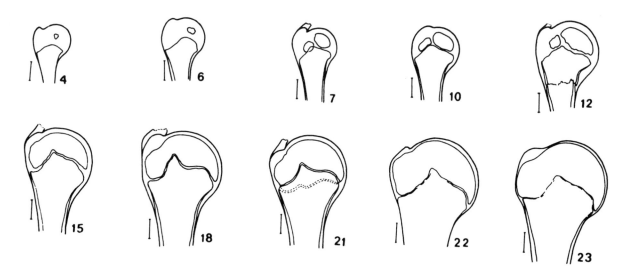

FIG. 5. Twenty-three pairs of proximal humeri obtained from human cadavers ranging in age from full-term stillborns to 14 years were studied morphologically and radiologically. The figure depicts the development of the proximal humeral epiphysis and metaphysis based on the findings in the cadaver specimens. The reference line to the left of each figure represents 1 cm. The number represents the specimen used for the drawing: 4, a 2-month-old; 6, a 3-month-old; 7, a 7-month-old; 10, a 2-year old; 12, a 3-year old; 15, a 7-year-old; 18, a 9-year-old; 21, a 10-year-old; 22, a 13-year-old; and 23, a 14-year-old. At 5 to 7 years of age the specimens demonstrated complete fusion of the two major ossification centers.

Source: Ogden JA, Conlogue CJ, Jensen P. Radiology of postnatal skeletal development: the proximal humerus. *Skeletal Radiol* 1978;2:153–60.

Time Schedule for Appearance of Secondary Epiphyseal Ossification Centers in the Upper Extremity

For a more detailed review of time of ossification, the reader is referred to the chapter on growth and maturation.

BOYS

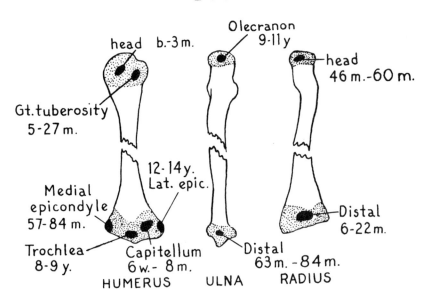

GIRLS

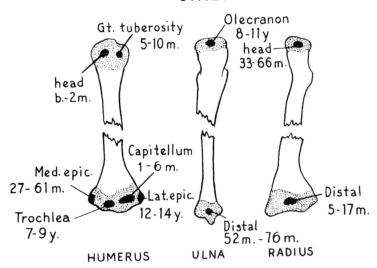

m. = months   y. = years   b. = birth.

FIG. 6. Time schedule for ossification centers, boys and girls.

Source: Reproduced with permission from Caffey et al., 1978 (see Fig. 1 of this chapter). Modified from Vogt EC, Vickers VS. Osseous growth and development. *Radiology* 1938;31:441–4.

Normal Secondary Epiphyseal Ossification Centers at the Elbow

For the exact timed appearance of these ossification centers, the reader is referred to the chapter on growth and maturation.

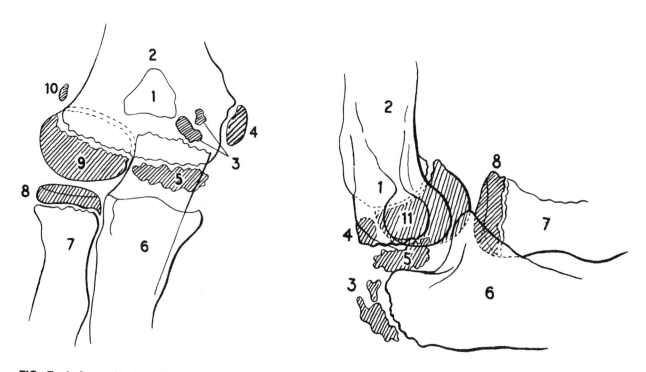

FIG. 7. Left panel is frontal view; right panel is lateral view. Key: (1) Olecranon fossa. (2) Shaft of the humerus. (3) Centers of the olecranon process. (4) Medial epicondyle. (5) Trochlea. (6) Shaft of the ulna. (7) Shaft of the radius. (8) Capitellum of the radius. (9) Capitellum of the humerus. (10) Lateral epicondyle. (11) Lateral projection of the diaphyseal end.

Source: Reproduced with permission from Caffey et al., 1978 (see Fig. 6 of this chapter).

Linear Growth of Long Bones of the Upper Extremity

The data are compiled from several groups. The first 55 children whose bone lengths were measured were 2 months through 3 to 4 years of age. The second group (59 children) were 3 to 4 years through 9 to 11 years; the third group of 59 young adults were measured from childhood or early adolescence to the completion of growth. In the younger children the measurement was made between the epiphyseal plates, and in the older children the measurement includes the epiphyses. Included are the percentiles and the observed range of roentgenographic bone lengths.

TABLE 4. *Length of humerus, radius, and ulna in boys and girls*

BOYS

Age (yr–mo)	Humerus 10%	25%	50%	75%	90%	Range	Radius 10%	25%	50%	75%	90%	Range	Ulna 10%	25%	50%	75%	90%	Range
Measurements Between Epiphyseal Plates																		
0–2	6.68	7.02	7.28	7.47	7.65	6.3–7.9	5.54	5.68	5.85	6.16	6.30	5.4–6.4	6.29	6.48	6.66	6.89	7.04	6.1–7.2
0–4	7.43	7.78	8.05	8.29	8.52	7.3–9.0	6.14	6.29	6.52	6.70	6.95	6.1–7.0	6.82	7.04	7.22	7.42	7.61	6.8–7.8
0–6	8.13	8.50	8.80	9.06	9.33	7.8–9.4	6.60	6.76	7.02	7.24	7.51	6.4–7.9	7.31	7.55	7.71	7.95	8.22	7.0–8.7
1–0	9.91	10.25	10.48	10.77	11.20	9.4–11.6	7.68	7.86	8.17	8.42	8.73	7.6–9.3	8.63	8.85	9.08	9.35	9.69	8.5–10.3
1–6	11.25	11.58	11.84	12.12	12.58	11.0–12.8	8.53	8.73	9.06	9.34	9.67	8.4–10.2	9.55	9.80	10.06	10.37	10.69	9.4–11.4
2–0	12.29	12.72	12.97	13.26	13.71	12.1–14.1	9.23	9.45	9.80	10.10	10.44	9.0–11.0	10.35	10.62	10.90	11.22	11.55	10.1–12.3
2–6	13.12	13.56	13.84	14.13	14.58	12.9–15.0	9.90	10.13	10.47	10.76	11.12	9.6–11.8	11.05	11.33	11.63	11.96	12.29	10.6–13.0
3–0	13.92	14.42	14.65	14.96	15.41	13.6–16.1	10.55	10.78	11.09	11.38	11.75	10.1–12.4	11.70	11.99	12.30	12.64	12.98	11.2–13.6
3–6	14.68	15.21	15.44	15.75	16.21	14.3–16.9	11.13	11.38	11.69	11.97	12.35	10.7–13.0	12.30	12.60	12.93	13.27	13.65	11.8–14.2
4–0	15.41	15.97	16.21	16.52	17.00	15.0–18.0	11.68	11.96	12.26	12.54	12.94	11.1–13.8	12.88	13.19	13.54	13.88	14.30	12.2–15.1
4–6	16.12	16.70	16.95	17.28	17.79	15.8–18.5	12.21	12.51	12.80	13.09	13.51	11.6–14.2	13.44	13.76	14.13	14.48	14.92	12.8–15.5
5–0	16.80	17.39	17.66	18.03	18.57	16.1–19.4	12.73	13.04	13.32	13.61	14.06	11.9–15.0	13.98	14.32	14.70	15.06	15.52	13.1–16.4
5–6	17.47	18.07	18.35	18.76	19.32	17.3–20.3	13.23	13.55	13.82	14.12	14.59	12.8–15.5	14.50	14.86	15.25	15.62	16.08	14.1–17.0
6–0	18.14	18.73	19.03	19.47	20.05	17.4–21.2	13.72	14.01	14.32	14.63	15.12	13.3–16.1	15.00	15.38	15.77	16.15	16.63	14.9–17.6
6–6	18.81	19.38	19.69	20.17	20.76	18.6–22.0	14.19	14.47	14.79	15.13	15.65	13.8–16.8	15.48	15.87	16.27	16.66	17.17	15.2–18.7
7–0	19.46	20.00	20.34	20.86	21.44	19.0–22.9	14.64	14.93	15.26	15.63	16.18	14.1–17.4	15.95	16.35	16.76	17.16	17.71	15.6–18.9
7–6	20.06	20.61	20.97	21.53	22.10	19.6–23.6	15.08	15.38	15.72	16.12	16.69	14.5–18.0	16.41	16.81	17.24	17.66	18.24	16.0–19.5
8–0	20.64	21.19	21.59	22.19	22.75	19.9–24.6	15.50	15.82	16.18	16.60	17.19	14.9–18.6	16.86	17.26	17.70	18.15	18.76	16.3–20.1
8–6	21.19	21.74	22.21	22.83	23.40	20.6–24.4	15.91	16.25	16.63	17.08	17.70	15.5–18.0	17.29	17.71	18.15	18.64	19.28	17.0–19.5
9–0	21.74	22.28	22.81	23.45	24.05	21.2–25.7	16.32	16.68	17.08	17.56	18.21	15.8–19.5	17.72	18.15	18.60	19.13	19.80	17.5–21.2
9–6	22.28	22.82	23.40	24.06	24.69	21.8–26.5	16.72	17.10	17.53	18.04	18.72	16.1–20.0	18.14	18.59	19.05	19.62	20.32	17.8–21.7
10–0	22.79	23.37	23.98	24.67	25.33	22.0–26.9	17.11	17.50	17.97	18.52	19.20	16.9–20.4	18.56	19.03	19.50	20.10	20.84	18.3–22.1
10–6	23.30	23.91	24.56	25.27	25.96	22.6–27.4	17.50	17.90	18.39	18.97	19.68	17.1–20.9	18.97	19.47	19.95	20.58	21.35	18.6–22.5
11–0	23.79	24.44	25.13	25.87	26.59	23.4–28.1	17.88	18.30	18.79	19.40	20.18	17.5–21.4	19.38	19.90	20.39	21.06	21.85	19.0–23.2
11–6	24.27	24.97	25.70	26.48	27.22	22.4–28.5	18.25	18.69	19.19	19.83	20.67	17.8–21.8	19.79	20.31	20.83	21.54	22.35	19.3–23.0
12–0	24.74	25.49	26.28	27.09	27.84	22.8–29.5	18.60	19.07	19.60	20.26	21.15	18.2–22.2	20.20	20.72	21.26	22.01	22.85	19.8–24.0
Measurements Include Epiphyses																		
10–0	24.67	25.31	25.87	26.83	27.58	23.6–29.2	18.42	18.90	19.28	19.85	20.60	18.0–22.2	19.26	19.72	20.27	20.89	21.67	18.9–23.2
10–6	25.12	25.78	26.40	27.37	28.13	24.3–29.8	18.85	19.30	19.71	20.32	21.10	18.4–22.7	19.74	20.21	20.78	21.44	22.27	19.1–23.8
11–0	25.59	26.29	26.98	27.98	28.78	25.0–30.7	19.28	19.71	20.14	20.84	21.63	18.9–23.1	20.23	20.71	21.31	22.01	22.89	19.5–24.4
11–6	26.09	26.83	27.60	28.63	29.48	24.0–31.0	19.73	20.13	20.60	21.39	22.23	19.0–23.7	20.74	21.23	21.86	22.62	23.55	19.8–24.8
12–0	26.62	27.40	28.26	29.33	30.23	24.2–33.3	20.18	20.60	21.11	21.97	22.86	19.4–24.5	21.26	21.76	22.43	23.28	24.32	20.5–26.6
12–6	27.20	28.00	28.98	30.08	31.03	26.8–33.7	20.66	21.09	21.66	22.58	23.53	20.1–25.1	21.81	22.32	23.05	23.99	25.15	20.6–26.9
13–0	27.88	28.70	29.75	30.88	31.88	27.5–34.0	21.16	21.63	22.22	22.96	23.96	20.5–25.0	22.38	22.94	23.71	24.76	25.93	21.6–26.4
13–6	28.69	29.53	30.58	31.75	32.80	27.6–35.1	21.68	22.22	22.92	23.96	24.98	20.7–25.6	22.98	23.63	24.43	25.56	26.68	22.5–27.4
14–0	29.55	30.47	31.48	32.70	33.80	28.5–36.1	22.23	22.90	23.74	24.77	25.80	21.2–26.3	23.62	24.34	25.18	26.33	27.40	22.8–28.2
14–6	30.45	31.43	32.42	33.62	34.59	28.9–36.6	22.85	23.63	24.45	25.39	26.47	21.7–27.1	24.30	25.07	25.94	27.05	28.09	23.5–29.0
15–0	31.40	32.30	33.20	34.38	35.30	30.0–36.6	23.53	24.30	25.13	25.93	27.03	23.4–27.5	25.05	25.82	26.64	27.65	28.72	24.8–29.8
15–6	32.00	32.87	33.87	34.95	35.93	31.0–36.7	24.14	24.84	25.62	26.35	27.46	23.5–27.8	25.68	26.45	27.18	28.10	29.18	25.3–29.9
16–0	32.40	33.33	34.42	35.45	36.43	31.7–37.2	24.52	25.20	25.97	26.66	27.78	23.5–28.4	26.08	26.80	27.57	28.45	29.54	26.0–30.6
16–6	32.72	33.65	34.79	35.84	36.82	29.8–37.8	24.79	25.45	26.20	26.90	27.99	24.5–28.9	26.36	27.05	27.87	28.68	29.82	26.0–30.6
17–0	32.92	33.87	35.02	36.12	37.10	30.4–38.3	24.95	25.59	26.32	27.05	28.14	24.5–29.6	26.50	27.22	28.05	28.85	30.01	26.0–31.1
17–6	33.07	34.04	35.16	36.33	37.28	30.4–38.3	25.00	25.64	26.38	27.14	28.25	24.5–29.6	26.55	27.30	28.14	28.95	30.12	26.0–31.1
18–0	33.17	34.15	35.28	36.46	37.42	31.2–38.7	25.02	25.66	26.42	27.20	28.32	24.5–30.1	26.58	27.34	28.20	29.00	30.17	26.0–31.6

TABLE 4. *(cont'd).*

Age (yr–mo)	Humerus						Radius						Ulna					
	10%	25%	50%	75%	90%	Range	10%	25%	50%	75%	90%	Range	10%	25%	50%	75%	90%	Range
						Measurements Between Epiphyseal Plates												
0–2	6.72	6.91	7.12	7.30	7.50	6.0–7.7	5.43	5.58	5.72	5.88	6.05	5.2–6.5	6.08	6.30	6.50	6.65	6.82	5.8–7.2
0–4	7.52	7.73	8.00	8.17	8.38	7.4–8.8	5.93	6.11	6.28	6.46	6.64	5.7–7.0	6.59	6.84	7.05	7.21	7.38	6.4–7.9
0–6	8.22	8.44	8.74	8.89	9.12	7.7–9.5	6.37	6.56	6.74	6.95	7.14	6.0–7.5	7.09	7.35	7.58	7.75	7.92	6.7–8.2
1–0	9.77	10.04	10.38	10.60	10.86	8.8–11.4	7.42	7.64	7.85	8.10	8.31	7.1–8.6	8.27	8.56	8.82	9.06	9.32	7.9–9.7
1–6	11.02	11.32	11.70	11.98	12.27	10.6–12.7	8.22	8.48	8.74	9.00	9.24	7.9–9.7	9.24	9.55	9.84	10.11	10.41	8.8–10.9
2–0	12.07	12.40	12.80	13.10	13.42	11.5–14.0	8.92	9.20	9.50	9.77	10.04	8.5–10.4	10.00	10.34	10.66	10.95	11.27	9.3–11.6
2–6	12.94	13.32	13.75	14.09	14.44	12.6–14.9	9.55	9.85	10.18	10.47	10.75	8.7–11.1	10.69	11.05	11.39	11.70	12.04	9.8–12.4
3–0	13.73	14.13	14.58	14.99	15.39	13.2–15.7	10.12	10.45	10.80	11.12	11.41	9.9–11.8	11.32	11.70	12.07	12.39	12.75	11.0–13.2
3–6	14.49	14.91	15.38	15.84	16.28	13.8–16.7	10.66	11.01	11.39	11.73	12.05	10.3–12.5	11.90	12.31	12.71	13.04	13.42	11.6–13.9
4–0	15.21	15.66	16.15	16.66	17.14	14.3–17.4	11.18	11.55	11.95	12.33	12.68	10.8–12.9	12.45	12.88	13.32	13.67	14.06	12.1–14.4
4–6	15.90	16.37	16.89	17.44	17.97	15.0–18.5	11.68	12.06	12.48	12.91	13.30	11.3–13.8	12.98	13.43	13.90	14.29	14.69	12.6–15.2
5–0	16.56	17.05	17.60	18.21	18.77	15.8–19.5	12.16	12.55	12.99	13.47	13.90	11.8–14.9	13.49	13.96	14.45	14.89	15.30	13.1–16.5
5–6	17.19	17.71	18.29	18.94	19.54	16.1–20.1	12.62	13.02	13.48	14.01	14.48	12.3–15.0	13.99	14.47	14.98	15.46	15.90	13.5–16.5
6–0	17.80	18.35	18.95	19.64	20.29	16.8–20.7	13.06	13.49	13.97	14.53	15.03	12.7–15.4	14.47	14.96	15.50	16.02	16.48	14.0–17.0
6–6	18.40	18.98	19.60	20.32	21.01	17.4–22.2	13.49	13.95	14.45	15.05	15.55	13.1–16.5	14.94	15.45	16.01	16.56	17.05	14.6–18.4
7–0	18.99	19.60	20.25	20.99	21.71	18.2–23.3	13.91	14.41	14.92	15.56	16.06	13.6–17.2	15.41	15.94	16.51	17.09	17.60	15.0–19.1
7–6	19.56	20.21	20.89	21.65	22.40	18.6–23.1	14.33	14.86	15.39	16.05	16.56	13.9–16.9	15.87	16.42	17.01	17.62	18.13	15.5–18.6
8–0	20.12	20.82	21.51	22.30	23.07	19.4–24.4	14.74	15.29	15.86	16.58	17.04	14.5–18.1	16.32	16.90	17.50	18.14	18.65	15.9–20.1
8–6	20.66	21.42	22.13	22.94	23.73	19.8–24.4	15.15	15.71	16.33	17.00	17.51	14.9–18.1	16.77	17.38	17.99	18.66	19.16	16.4–19.6
9–0	21.19	22.01	22.75	23.58	24.40	20.3–25.1	15.55	16.13	16.80	17.47	18.00	15.1–18.5	17.20	17.85	18.47	19.18	19.68	16.8–20.4
9–6	21.71	22.59	23.38	24.24	25.08	20.8–26.5	15.96	16.54	17.26	17.96	18.50	15.6–19.7	17.62	18.30	18.94	19.70	20.22	17.2–21.7
10–0	22.23	23.17	24.03	24.91	25.78	21.4–26.4	16.38	16.97	17.72	18.45	19.02	16.0–19.7	18.04	18.73	19.44	20.23	20.79	17.7–21.5
10–6	22.77	23.76	24.70	25.60	26.51	21.7–28.2	16.81	17.42	18.20	18.95	19.55	16.4–21.4	18.50	19.20	19.99	20.78	21.40	18.0–23.6
11–0	23.32	24.36	25.38	26.31	27.25	22.0–28.0	17.25	17.89	18.70	19.48	20.13	16.7–21.1	18.97	19.69	20.57	21.37	22.03	18.5–23.6
11–6	23.88	24.98	26.07	27.08	28.01	22.4–29.5	17.72	18.39	19.23	20.03	20.77	17.0–21.9	19.46	20.24	21.17	21.98	22.68	19.1–24.5
12–0	24.45	25.62	26.78	27.76	28.78	22.8–30.0	18.22	18.93	19.80	20.63	21.44	17.5–22.3	19.98	20.82	21.80	22.60	23.33	19.6–25.1
						Measurements Include Epiphyses												
10–0	23.80	24.66	25.80	26.73	27.50	23.0–28.2	17.50	18.32	19.03	19.87	20.62	17.0–21.0	18.95	19.75	20.50	21.40	22.20	18.6–22.9
10–6	24.55	25.52	26.73	27.73	28.66	23.6–30.7	17.94	18.85	19.65	20.61	21.39	17.5–23.0	19.53	20.36	21.28	22.20	23.07	19.0–25.1
11–0	25.28	26.31	27.60	28.64	29.68	23.8–30.9	18.41	19.38	20.28	21.33	22.12	17.8–23.0	20.12	20.97	22.00	22.94	23.83	19.7–24.6
11–6	25.98	27.06	28.38	29.46	30.60	24.2–32.0	18.93	19.92	20.90	21.99	22.78	18.2–23.7	20.70	21.58	22.65	23.60	24.51	20.2–25.4
12–0	26.65	27.75	29.09	30.19	31.43	24.8–32.9	19.45	20.48	21.50	22.59	23.39	18.8–24.5	21.28	22.18	23.24	24.20	25.12	20.5–26.8
12–6	27.28	28.38	29.72	30.86	32.18	25.4–33.2	19.97	21.06	22.07	23.10	23.89	19.3–24.8	21.85	22.77	23.75	24.70	25.62	21.0–26.9
13–0	27.87	28.97	30.30	31.46	32.85	26.1–33.8	20.49	21.57	22.55	23.54	24.29	19.9–24.8	22.40	23.28	24.18	25.13	26.04	21.5–27.2
13–6	28.42	29.51	30.82	32.00	33.40	26.6–34.5	21.00	22.03	22.98	23.89	24.60	20.5–24.9	22.92	23.73	24.57	25.48	26.40	22.1–27.2
14–0	28.92	30.00	31.30	32.40	33.77	27.7–35.2	21.50	22.45	23.34	24.12	24.80	20.9–25.4	23.36	24.13	24.89	25.76	26.69	22.6–27.2
14–6	29.37	30.42	31.70	32.66	33.95	28.0–35.9	21.88	22.80	23.62	24.28	24.94	21.4–25.9	23.69	24.47	25.16	25.92	26.90	22.9–27.5
15–0	29.72	30.74	32.00	32.79	34.06	28.5–36.1	22.13	23.02	23.82	24.38	25.03	21.6–26.1	23.95	24.76	25.37	26.04	27.08	23.0–27.7
15–6	29.92	30.92	32.15	32.88	34.10	28.8–36.5	22.22	23.12	23.92	24.45	25.08	21.8–26.2	24.12	24.98	25.51	26.14	27.12	23.4–28.1
16–0	30.02	31.01	32.20	32.92	34.10	28.8–36.5	22.25	23.15	23.98	24.48	25.10	21.8–26.2	24.22	25.10	25.60	26.21	27.16	23.4–28.1

Source: Maresh, MM. Linear growth of long bones of the extremities from infancy through adolescence. *Am J Dis Child* 1955;89:725–42.

Mean Acromion-Olecranon Length of White and Black Children by Sex and Age

The data are from cycle two, a study conducted from July 1963 to December 1965. The study involved selection and examination of a probability sample of noninstitutionalized children in the United States, aged 6 to 11 years. This program succeeeded in examining 96% of the 7,417 children selected. The lengths here were measured as the distance from the acromial process of the right scapula (outer point of the shoulder) to the olecranon process of the ulna. The subjects were standing with the right arm at the side and the elbow flexed to 90 degrees. The fixed crossbar on the anthropometer was placed firmly at the right acromial process, and the movable crossbar was brought into firm contact with the olecranon process.

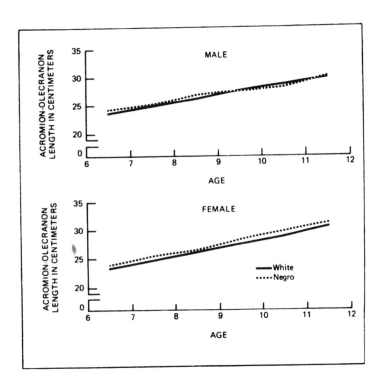

FIG. 8

Source: Malina RM, Hamill PVV, Lemeshow S. *Body dimensions and proportions of white and negro children 6 to 11 years.* Series 11, No. 143. DHEW Publication No. (HRA)75-1625, Washington, D.C.: U.S. Government Printing Office, 1974.

Shoulder-Elbow Length

The shoulder-elbow length was measured by the same method of Malina (see p. 146). The data comprise an eight-state random survey of 4,127 infants, children, and youths.

TABLE 5. *Shoulder–elbow length in males and females (in centimeters)*

Age (years)	No.	Mean	SD	Min.	5th	50th	95th	Max.
MALES								
2.0–3.5	114	18.8	1.4	15.0	16.6	18.7	21.1	22.3
3.5–4.5	118	20.2	1.2	17.8	18.4	20.0	22.2	23.6
4.5–5.5	143	22.0	1.3	18.8	20.0	21.7	24.3	27.1
5.5–6.5	108	23.5	1.4	20.3	21.0	23.4	25.8	27.1
6.5–7.5	105	25.0	1.4	22.3	22.7	24.9	27.4	28.6
7.5–8.5	98	26.3	1.4	22.1	24.1	26.2	28.5	31.0
8.5–9.5	114	27.8	1.5	24.0	25.3	27.6	30.1	31.5
9.5–10.5	124	28.7	1.6	25.1	26.2	28.5	31.6	33.7
10.5–11.5	140	29.7	1.4	26.0	27.1	29.6	31.8	33.8
11.5–12.5	154	31.0	1.7	26.0	28.6	30.7	33.8	36.5
12.5–13.5	153	32.4	2.0	28.3	29.0	32.1	35.8	38.8
13.5–14.5	155	33.9	2.1	29.2	30.4	33.8	36.9	38.5
14.5–15.5	130	35.1	2.0	30.3	31.6	35.1	37.8	39.4
15.5–16.5	99	36.6	1.8	30.3	33.1	36.9	38.9	41.9
16.5–17.5	104	36.9	1.8	32.8	33.9	36.8	39.6	40.9
17.5–19.0	88	37.4	2.2	33.7	34.3	37.1	40.1	48.4
FEMALES								
2.0–3.5	97	18.2	1.3	15.5	15.9	18.1	20.2	22.0
3.5–4.5	110	20.3	1.2	17.7	18.4	20.1	22.3	23.1
4.5–5.5	120	21.7	1.2	18.5	19.4	21.8	23.6	25.1
5.5–6.5	109	23.1	1.2	18.8	21.1	23.0	24.9	26.3
6.5–7.5	121	24.4	1.4	20.7	22.1	24.3	26.7	28.4
7.5–8.5	94	25.7	1.4	23.2	23.5	25.7	28.0	30.5
8.5–9.5	136	27.2	1.4	23.8	25.1	27.0	29.4	31.0
9.5–10.5	128	28.5	1.6	24.6	26.1	28.3	31.4	33.9
10.5–11.5	140	29.9	1.9	24.8	26.7	29.9	32.5	35.7
11.5–12.5	133	31.1	1.8	26.0	28.3	31.0	33.8	36.7
12.5–13.5	161	32.4	1.7	27.9	29.7	32.3	35.1	37.4
13.5–14.5	116	33.1	1.7	28.6	30.0	33.0	35.7	37.3
14.5–15.5	132	33.9	1.7	30.5	31.4	33.6	36.4	39.8
15.5–16.5	98	33.6	1.7	29.8	30.8	33.2	36.4	38.0
16.5–17.5	117	33.7	1.6	29.8	31.0	33.7	36.2	37.6
17.5–19.0	68	33.8	1.4	31.3	31.6	33.7	36.3	37.9

Source: Snyder RG, Schneider LW, Owings CL, Reynolds HJM, Golomb AH, Schork MA. *Anthropometry of Infants, Children and Youths to Age Eighteen*, SP450 Highway Safety Research Institute, University of Michigan. Warrendale, PA: Society of Automotive Engineers, Inc., 1977.

Mean Elbow-Wrist Length of White and Black Children by Sex and Age

The elbow-wrist length was measured as the distance from the olecranon process to the distal end of the styloid process of the ulna. With the subject seated, the elbow was flexed to 90 degrees, and the forearm and hand were pronated. The fixed arm of the anthropometer was firmly placed at the olecranon process, and the movable arm was firmly placed at the distal end of the styloid process of the ulna.

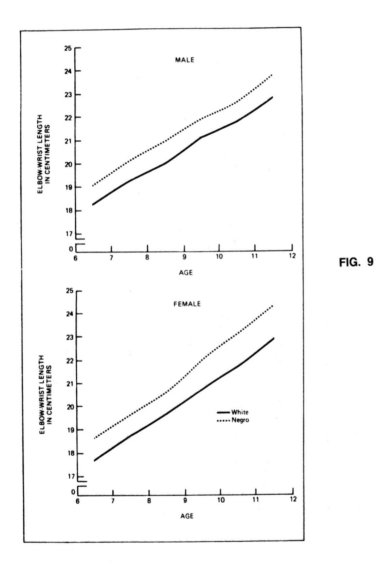

FIG. 9

Source: Malina et al., 1974 (see Fig. 8 of this chapter).

Elbow-Hand Length

The elbow-hand length is measured with the subject standing erect, the upper arm hanging at the side, the elbow flexed to 90 degrees, and the hands and fingers extended and to neutral rotation. The anthropometer measured the distance from the posterior surface of the right upper arm, just above the elbow, to the tip of the middle finger parallel to the long axis of the forearm.

TABLE 6. *Elbow–hand length in males and females (in centimeters)*

Age (years)	No.	Mean	SD	Min.	5th	50th	95th	Max.
			MALES					
2.0–3.5	114	24.8	1.7	20.5	21.7	24.8	27.7	28.9
3.5–4.5	118	26.6	1.5	23.4	24.4	26.4	29.6	31.1
4.5–5.5	143	28.7	1.4	25.1	26.4	28.7	31.0	32.7
5.5–6.5	108	30.6	1.8	26.9	27.7	30.4	33.6	36.5
6.5–7.5	105	32.2	1.9	28.1	28.9	32.1	35.3	36.9
7.5–8.5	98	33.8	1.7	28.4	31.4	33.5	36.3	38.9
8.5–9.5	114	35.6	2.0	30.6	32.9	35.2	39.2	40.7
9.5–10.5	124	36.8	2.1	32.2	33.1	36.7	40.5	42.0
10.5–11.5	140	38.2	2.0	33.1	34.9	38.1	41.5	43.8
11.5–12.5	154	40.0	2.3	34.6	36.6	39.6	44.0	47.0
12.5–13.5	152	41.7	2.7	35.9	37.5	41.3	46.4	49.8
13.5–14.5	154	44.2	2.8	37.9	39.6	43.9	48.5	51.7
14.5–15.5	130	45.5	2.7	37.5	40.5	45.5	49.1	50.7
15.5–16.5	100	47.3	2.3	41.0	43.4	47.2	50.7	52.7
16.5–17.5	104	47.7	2.1	42.6	44.4	47.6	50.8	54.1
17.5–19.0	88	48.3	2.3	43.1	44.4	47.8	52.7	53.2
			FEMALES					
2.0–3.5	96	24.0	1.5	21.0	21.8	23.6	26.4	28.3
3.5–4.5	110	26.8	1.6	23.1	24.3	26.6	29.4	31.8
4.5–5.5	120	28.3	1.5	24.7	26.1	28.2	31.0	32.3
5.5–6.5	109	29.9	1.6	25.4	27.2	29.8	32.5	34.5
6.5–7.5	120	31.5	1.8	28.2	28.9	31.2	35.2	37.0
7.5–8.5	94	32.9	1.7	29.2	30.2	32.9	35.6	38.3
8.5–9.5	137	34.9	2.0	30.6	32.0	34.6	38.2	41.6
9.5–10.5	128	36.6	2.2	31.9	33.4	36.3	40.3	44.4
10.5–11.5	140	38.2	2.6	32.2	34.2	37.9	42.6	45.9
11.5–12.5	133	39.9	2.5	34.6	35.5	39.9	43.9	48.6
12.5–13.5	161	41.4	2.3	34.9	37.6	41.4	44.8	48.4
13.5–14.5	116	42.0	2.0	37.4	38.7	41.9	45.5	47.1
14.5–15.5	132	43.0	2.3	37.3	39.6	42.9	46.9	49.6
15.5–16.5	98	42.7	2.2	38.1	39.3	42.5	46.0	49.3
16.5–17.5	117	42.7	1.9	38.4	39.3	42.7	45.6	48.2
17.5–19.0	68	42.9	1.8	37.2	40.0	42.8	45.6	49.1

Source: Snyder et al., 1977 (see Table 5 of this chapter).

HEIGHT AND WEIGHT

Serial Height Measurements of One Boy

Measurements of height were made at approximate semiannual intervals of a boy, de Montbeillard's son. de Montbeillard was an ornithologist in a small town northwest of Dijon. His son was of a high socioeconomic class and was reared in the country. He was also distinguished in that in 1776 his father inoculated him for smallpox. This was 50 years after the introduction of the practice of direct inoculation against smallpox into western Europe and 30 years before Jenner's discovery. The top curve indicates the height gain in centimeters by years, and the bottom chart is the centimeters of growth (the height velocity) in centimeters by years.

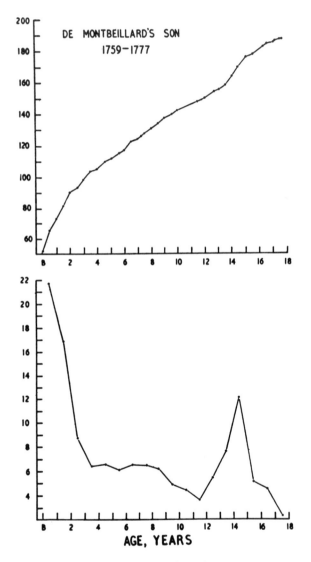

FIG. 1. Serial height measurements of one boy.

Source: Scammon RE. The first seriatim study of human growth. *Am J Phys Anthrop* 1927;10:329–36.

Intrauterine Growth

Head circumference was measured in 4,720 babies and length in 4,716 babies born at the Colorado General Hospital. Weight and length measurements were possible, and weight/length ratios for 4,706 infants were calculated based on measurements of infants born alive at various gestational ages (determined from the onset of the mother's last menstrual period).

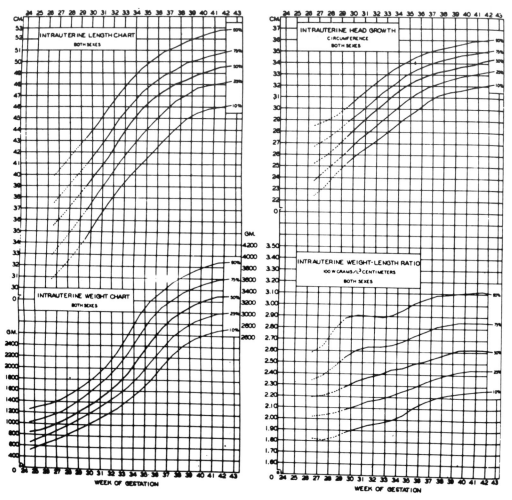

FIG. 2. Percentiles of intrauterine growth in weight, length, head circumference, and weight/length ratio as estimated from live births.

Source: Lubchenco L, Hansman C, Boyd E. Intrauterine growth in length and head circumference as estimated from live births at gestational ages from 26 to 42 weeks. *Pediatrics* 1966;37:403–8.

TABLE 1. *Intrauterine growth in length in 4,716 fetuses*

Gest. Age (wk)	No. Pts.	Mean	Smoothed Percentiles (cm) Both Sexes				
			10th	25th	50th	75th	90th
26	30	36.5	30.8	32.9	35.5	37.5	39.9
27	21	37.0	31.8	34.1	36.6	38.6	41.0
28	46	38.5	33.0	35.5	37.8	39.8	42.2
29	53	39.0	34.4	36.8	39.0	40.9	43.1
30	47	40.5	36.1	38.3	40.3	42.2	44.5
31	54	41.4	37.5	39.7	41.6	43.5	45.9
32	62	43.5	38.8	41.1	43.2	45.0	47.2
33	69	44.8	39.9	42.3	44.7	46.2	48.4
34	111	45.2	41.0	43.4	45.8	47.3	49.4
35	149	46.8	42.0	44.6	46.7	48.1	50.2
36	189	47.5	43.1	45.6	47.4	48.8	50.9
37	345	47.8	44.1	46.5	48.0	49.3	51.3
38	595	48.5	44.9	47.1	48.4	49.8	51.7
39	957	48.9	45.5	47.6	48.8	50.1	52.0
40	1,084	49.4	45.8	47.9	49.2	50.5	52.3
41	589	49.6	46.0	48.1	49.5	50.8	52.6
42	315	49.8	46.2	48.2	49.7	51.0	52.8
T	4,716						

Data used to construct the graphs in Fig. 2.

TABLE 2. *Intrauterine growth in head circumference in 4,720 fetuses*

Gest. Age (wk)	No. Pts	Mean	Smoothed Percentiles (cm) Both Sexes				
			10th	25th	50th	75th	90th
26	24	26.1	22.4	23.6	25.2	26.6	28.5
27	20	26.1	23.2	24.4	25.8	27.2	28.9
28	40	26.9	24.3	25.4	26.7	28.0	29.4
29	49	27.9	25.3	26.4	27.6	28.8	30.2
30	49	28.9	26.2	27.4	28.6	29.7	31.1
31	53	29.8	26.9	28.2	29.6	30.5	31.9
32	58	30.1	27.6	29.0	30.4	31.4	32.7
33	65	31.5	28.4	29.8	31.2	32.1	33.4
34	103	31.9	29.2	30.6	31.9	32.9	34.0
35	149	32.4	30.0	31.3	32.5	33.4	34.5
36	186	32.9	30.6	31.8	32.9	33.8	34.9
37	353	33.2	31.1	32.3	33.2	34.1	35.2
38	611	33.4	31.4	32.5	33.4	34.3	35.4
39	961	33.6	31.6	32.8	33.7	34.6	35.7
40	1,097	33.8	31.8	33.0	34.0	34.8	35.9
41	587	34.1	32.0	33.2	34.2	35.0	36.0
42	315	34.2	32.1	33.4	34.3	35.1	36.2
T	4,720						

Data used to construct the graphs in Fig. 2.

TABLE 3. *Intrauterine weight/length ratio in 4,706 fetuses*

Gest Age (wk)	No. Pts	Mean	Smoothed Percentiles Both Sexes				
			10th	25th	50th	75th	90th
26	29	2.22	1.82	2.02	2.19	2.34	2.58
27	20	2.22	1.81	2.03	2.21	2.38	2.66
28	46	2.22	1.83	2.05	2.24	2.46	2.79
29	54	2.37	1.88	2.09	2.29	2.55	2.88
30	51	2.41	1.93	2.13	2.33	2.61	2.91
31	62	2.45	1.95	2.16	2.37	2.63	2.90
32	72	2.31	1.96	2.17	2.39	2.63	2.89
33	70	2.45	1.99	2.21	2.42	2.65	2.91
34	111	2.47	2.04	2.25	2.45	2.68	2.95
35	152	2.54	2.11	2.30	2.49	2.73	3.01
36	188	2.56	2.16	2.33	2.51	2.77	3.05
37	344	2.61	2.20	2.37	2.55	2.81	3.08
38	589	2.61	2.22	2.40	2.59	2.83	3.09
39	950	2.66	2.24	2.43	2.62	2.85	3.10
40	1,076	2.66	2.25	2.44	2.62	2.85	3.11
41	579	2.67	2.26	2.44	2.62	2.85	3.11
42	313	2.65	2.26	2.44	2.61	2.84	3.10
T	4,706						

Data used to construct the graphs in Fig. 2.

Source: Lubchenco L., Hansman C, Boyd E. Intrauterine growth in length and head circumference as estimated from live births at gestational ages from 26 to 42 weeks. *Pediatrics* 1966;37:403–8.

Length and Weight of Children

These charts and tables were constructed using current body measurement data; they exploit the most recent advances in data analysis and computer technology. The data are derived either from studies done at the Fels Research Institute or from the health examination studies of the National Center for Health Statistics (NCHS). One set of charts for children from birth to 3 years is based on body measurements collected at the Fels Research Institute during 1929–1975. The set of charts for children 2 to 18 years of age is based on the NCHS data collected between 1963 and 1974.

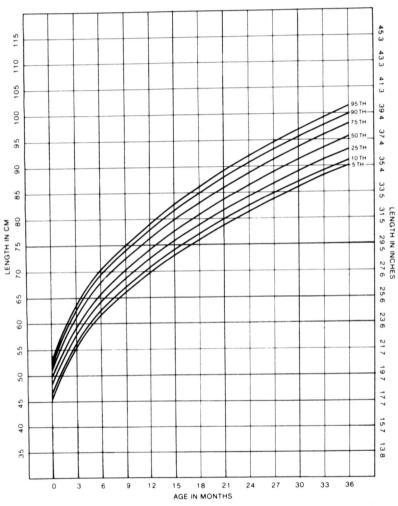

FIG. 3. Recumbent length by age percentiles for girls aged birth to 36 months.

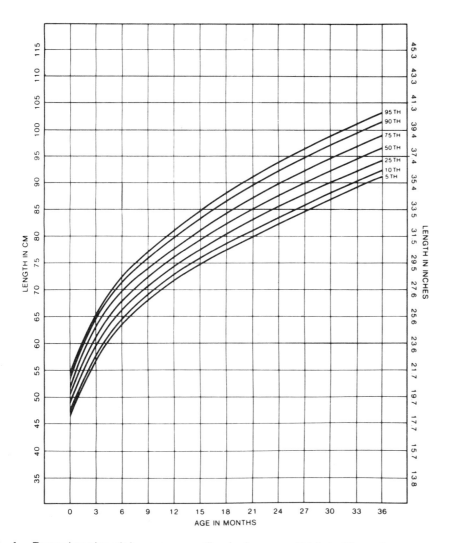

FIG. 4. Recumbent length by age percentiles for boys aged birth to 36 months.

Source: Hamill PVV, Drizd PA, Johnson CL, Reed RB, Roche AF. National Center for Health Statistics (NCHS) growth curves for children, birth to eighteen years. Washington, D.C.; U.S. Government Printing Office, 1977; DHEW publication no. (PHS)78-1650.

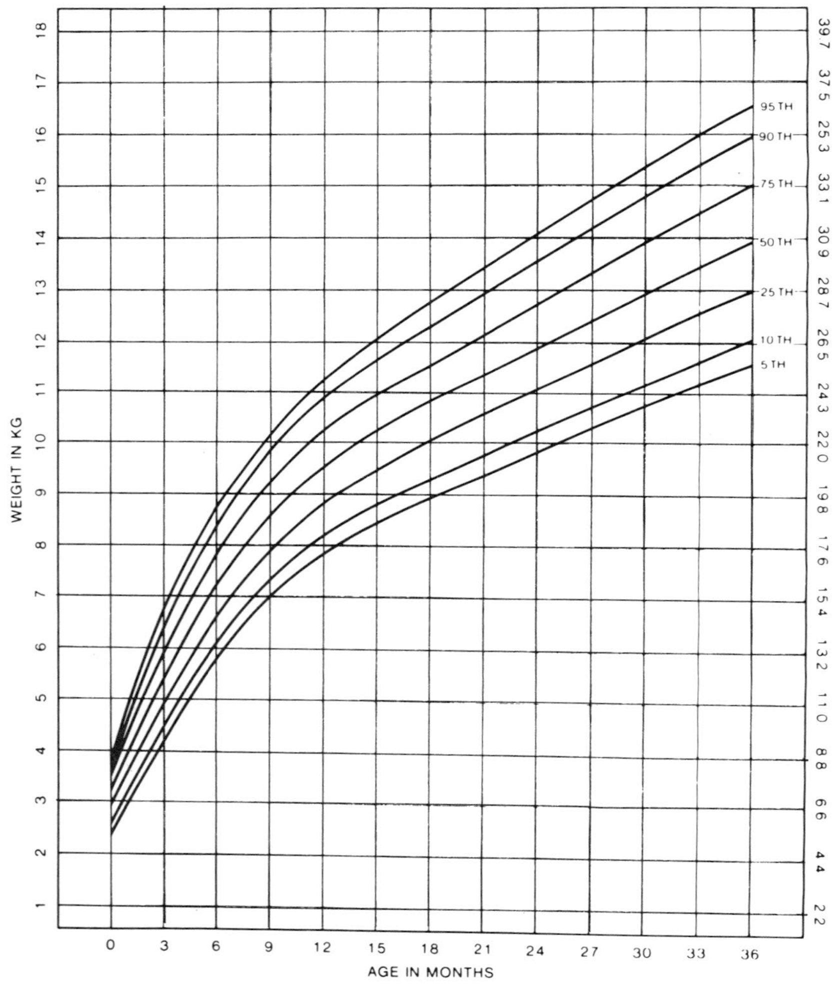

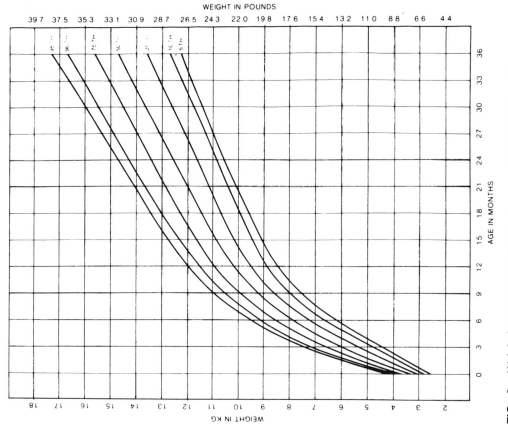

FIG. 6. Weight by age percentiles for boys aged birth to 36 months.

FIG. 5. Weight by age percentiles for girls aged birth to 36 months.

Source: Hamill PVV, Drizd PA, Johnson CL, Reed RB, Roche AF. National Center for Health Statistics (NCHS) growth curves for children, birth to eighteen years. Washington, D.C.; U.S. Government Printing Office, 1977; DHEW publication no. (PHS)78-1650.

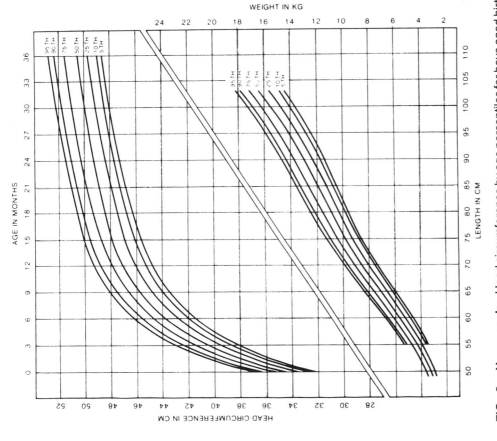

FIG. 7. Upper scale: Head circumference by age percentiles for girls aged birth to 36 months. **Lower scale:** Weight by length percentiles for girls aged birth to 36 months.

FIG. 8. Upper scale: Head circumference by age percentiles for boys aged birth to 36 months. **Lower scale:** Weight by length percentiles for boys aged birth to 36 months.

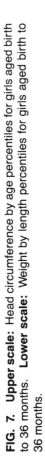

Source: Hamill PVV, Drizd PA, Johnson CL, Reed RB, Roche AF. National Center for Health Statistics (NCHS) growth curves for children, birth to eighteen years. Washington, D.C.; U.S. Government Printing Office, 1977; DHEW publication no. (PHS)78-1650.

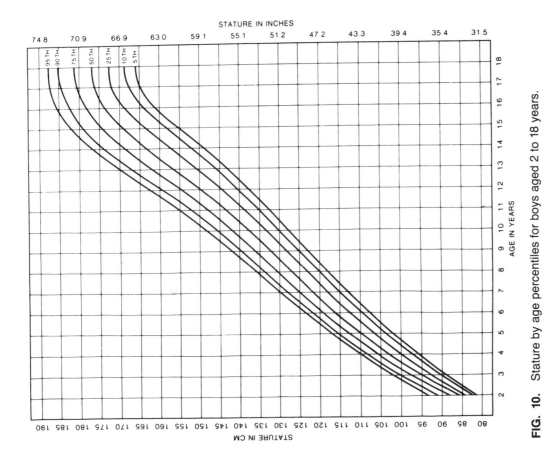

FIG. 10. Stature by age percentiles for boys aged 2 to 18 years.

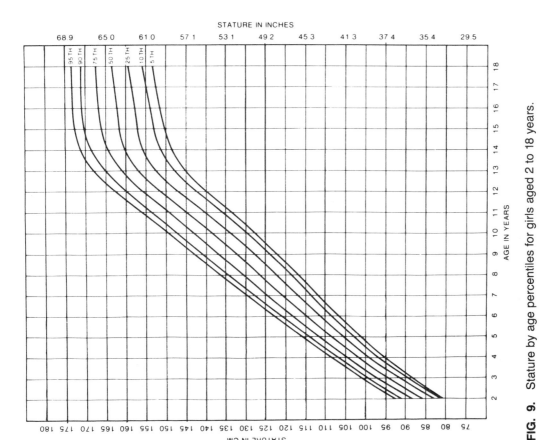

FIG. 9. Stature by age percentiles for girls aged 2 to 18 years.

Source: Hamill PVV, Drizd PA, Johnson CL, Reed RB, Roche AF. National Center for Health Statistics (NCHS) growth curves for children, birth to eighteen years. Washington, D.C.; U.S. Government Printing Office, 1977; DHEW publication no. (PHS)78-1650.

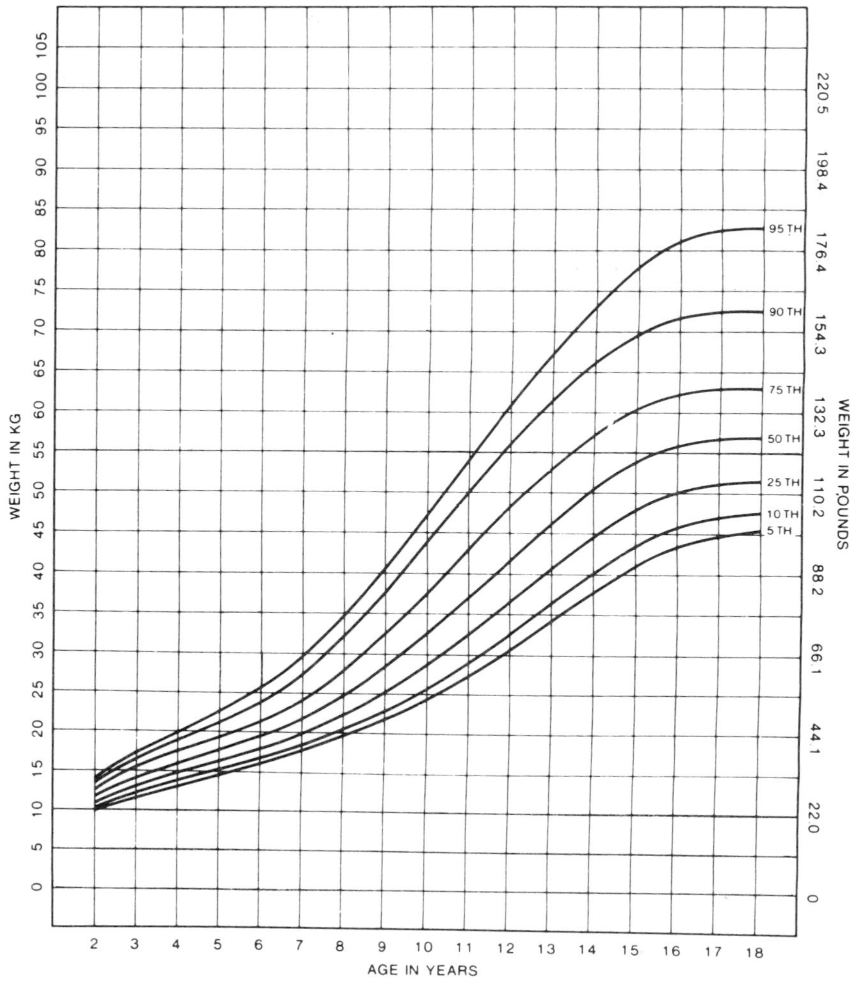

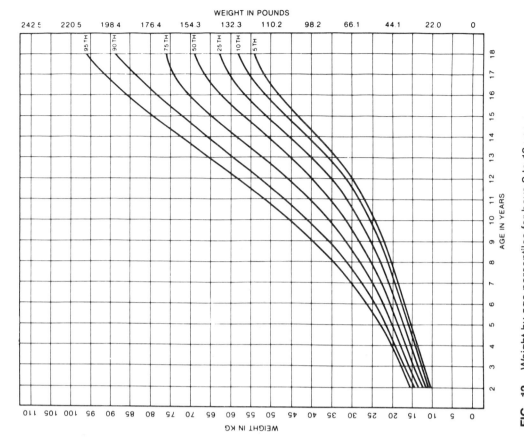

FIG. 12. Weight by age percentiles for boys 2 to 18 years.

FIG. 11. Weight by age percentiles for girls aged 2 to 18 years.

Source: Hamill PVV, Drizd PA, Johnson CL, Reed RB, Roche AF. National Center for Health Statistics (NCHS) growth curves for children, birth to eighteen years. Washington, D.C.; U.S. Government Printing Office, 1977; DHEW publication no. (PHS)78-1650.

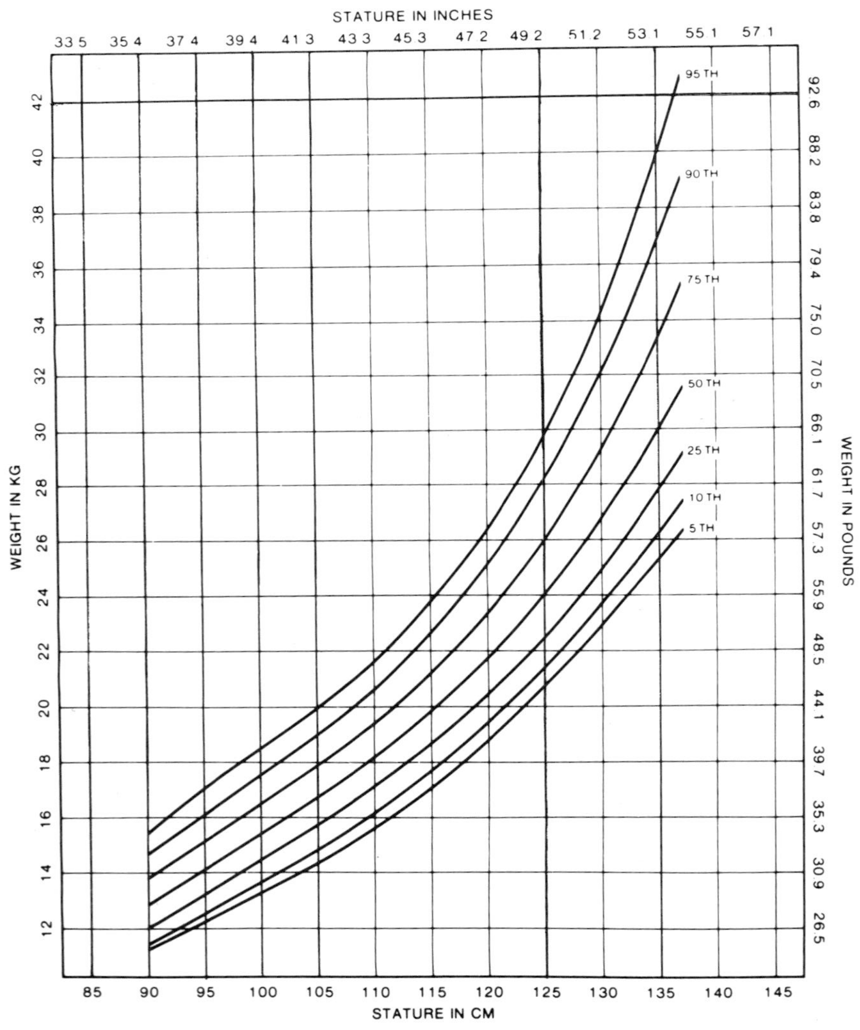

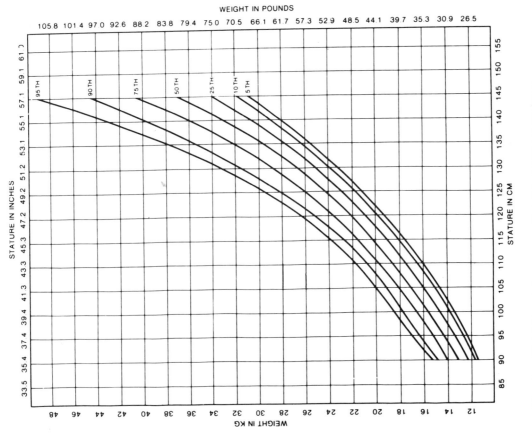

FIG. 14. Weight by stature percentiles for prepubescent boys.

FIG. 13. Weight by stature percentiles for prepubescent girls.

Source: Hamill PVV, Drizd PA, Johnson CL, Reed RB, Roche AF. National Center for Health Statistics (NCHS) growth curves for children, birth to eighteen years. Washington, D.C.; U.S. Government Printing Office, 1977; DHEW publication no. (PHS)78-1650.

Standard Growth Curves for Achondroplasia

Total height, upper and lower segments, and head circumference were measured in 403 patients with achondroplasia. The data were obtained through short stature clinics at UCLA-Harbor General Hospital; the University of Washington School of Medicine, Seattle, Washington; the University of Texas Medical School, Houston, Texas; and the 1976 national convention of Little People of America. The sample included 189 males and 214 females. Only those individuals satisfying strict diagnostic criteria for achondroplasia were included in the study.

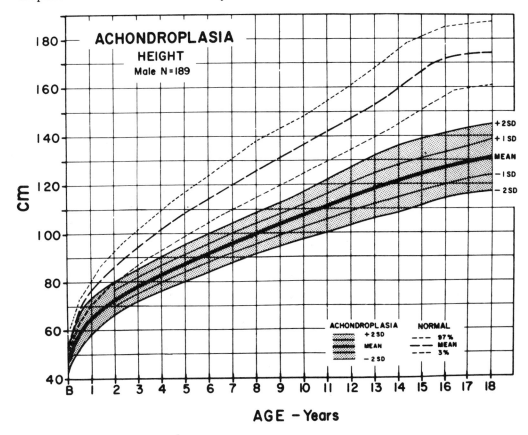

FIG. 15. Height of males with achondroplasia *(stippled area)* compared to normal male standard height curve (3rd, 50th, and 97th percentiles).

Source: Horton WA, Rotter JI, Rimoin DL, Scott CI. Standard growth curves for achondroplasia. *J Pediatr* 1978;93:435–8.

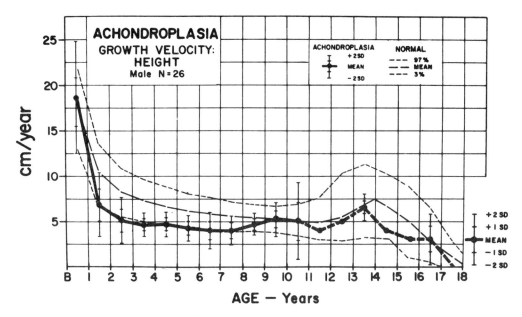

FIG. 16. Height growth velocity for males with achondroplasia compared to the normal male standard growth velocity curve.

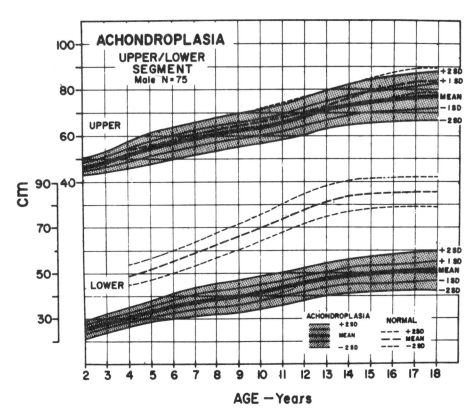

FIG. 17. Upper and lower segment length for males with achondroplasia *(stippled area)* compared to normal upper and lower segments.

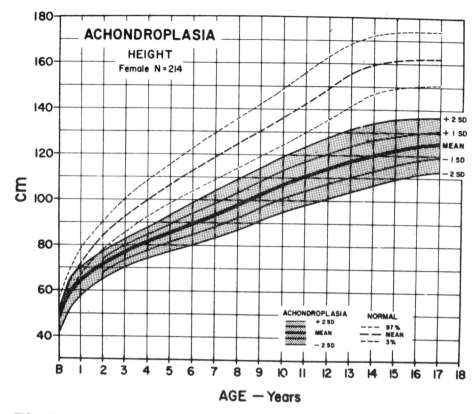

FIG. 18. Height for females with achondroplasia *(stippled area)* compared to the normal female standard height curve.

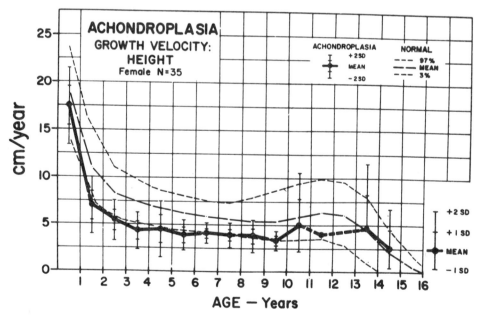

FIG. 19. Height velocity for females with achondroplasia compared to the normal female standard velocity curve.

Source: Horton WA, Rotter JI, Rimoin DL, Scott CI. Standard growth curves for achondroplasia. *J Pediatr* 1978;93:435–8.

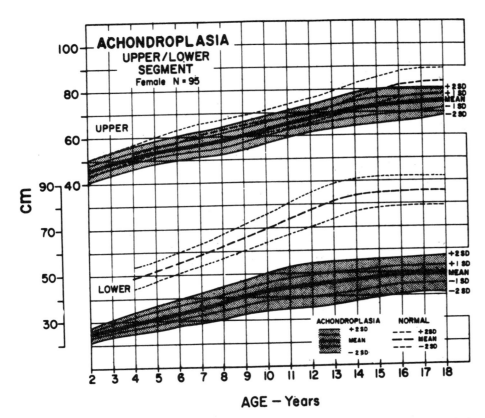

FIG. 20. Upper and lower segment lengths for females with achondroplasia *(stippled area)* compared to normal upper and lower segments.

Source: Horton WA, Rotter JI, Rimoin DL, Scott CI. Standard growth curves for achondroplasia. *J Pediatr* 1978;93:435–8.

Growth Curves for Height in Children with Bone Dysplasias; Diastrophic Dysplasia, Spondyloepiphyseal Dysplasia Congenita, and Pseudoachondroplasia

Data were obtained from 72 patients (38 boys and 34 girls) with diastrophic dysplasia, 62 patients (34 boys and 28 girls) with spondyloepiphyseal dysplasia, and 61 patients (28 boys and 33 girls) with pseudoachondroplasia. Longitudinal data were available for some patients. In most cases the data comprised either a single measurement or measurements separated by many years that were considered as isolated values. Measurements of total height were obtained from records at genetics clinics at five universities. Only patients meeting strict clinical and roentgenographic criteria for the diagnosis of each disorder were included.

TABLE 4. *Mean heights in diastrophic dysplasia, spondyloepiphyseal dysplasia, and pseudoachondroplasia*

	Diastrophic Dysplasia (n = 72)*			Spondyloepiphyseal Dysplasia (n = 62)*			Pseudoachondroplasia (n = 61)*		
	No. of OBS,	Height, cm		No. of OBS,	Height, cm		No. of OBS,	Height, cm	
Age, yr	M + F†	Mean	SD	M + F	Mean	SD	M + F	Mean	SD
Birth	12 + 12	41.67	4.69	9 + 5	42.14	2.66	8 + 10	49.39	1.97
6 mo	3 + 0	56.33	1.15	3 + 2	48.00	3.03	2 + 4	63.17	2.86
1	3 + 2	63.40	5.94	2 + 1	58.67	4.04	0 + 6	71.17	1.47
2	3 + 3	70.00	5.51	8 + 5	68.23	4.94	2 + 7	80.22	3.07
4	6 + 7	82.69	6.25	12 + 5	80.00	8.24	4 + 7	88.73	3.07
6	8 + 7	90.87	7.61	8 + 5	88.38	7.01	5 + 6	94.55	3.86
8	5 + 10	100.27	8.50	6 + 7	94.23	11.53	4 + 4	98.13	5.69
10	4 + 5	103.89	9.99	7 + 7	99.43	11.10	2 + 8	106.80	6.41
12	7 + 3	102.90	10.95	7 + 0	106.57	14.73	2 + 5	111.14	9.96
14	7 + 1	104.88	9.93	6 + 3	114.56	19.79	1 + 2	124.00	2.00
16	2 + 1	112.67	13.43	3 + 0	120.33	15.82	0 + 2	120.50	14.85
18	12 + 9	118.33	12.03	9 + 9	115.50	14.88	11 + 19	118.83	12.22

Figure in parentheses, the number of patients for whom measurements were made. + indicates number of observations (OBS) that contributed to means and SDs broken down by sex.

Source: Horton WA, Hall JG, Scott CI, Pyeritz RE, Rimoin DL. Growth curves for height for diastrophic dysplasia, spondyloepiphyseal dysplasia congenita, and pseudoachondroplasia. *Am J Dis Child* 1982;136:316–9.

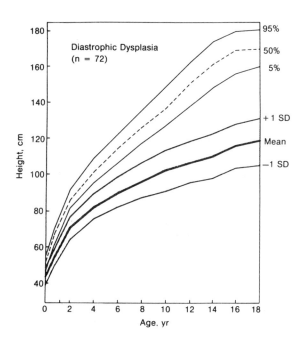

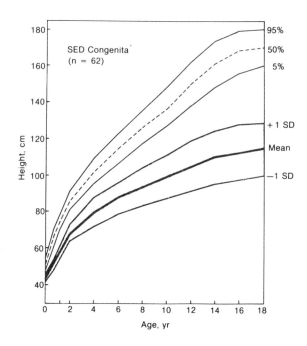

FIG. 21. Growth curve for height for patients (male and female combined) with diastrophic dysplasia. The means ± 1 SD are plotted. For comparison a standard normal curve depicting the 50th, 95th, and 5th percentiles was prepared by averaging normal male and female height derived from the National Center for Health Statistics (NCHS) growth curves.

FIG. 22. Growth curve for height of patients (male and female combined) with spondyloepiphyseal dysplasia (SED) congenita. For comparison a standard normal curve depicting the 50th, 95th, and 5th percentiles was prepared by averaging the normal male and female height derived from the National Center for Health Statistics (NCHS) growth curves. (From National Center for Health Statistics Growth Charts, National Center for Health Statistics, 1976, vol. 25, suppl. HRA 76-1120.)

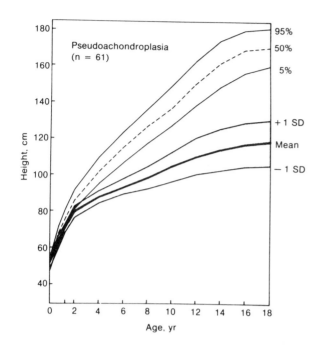

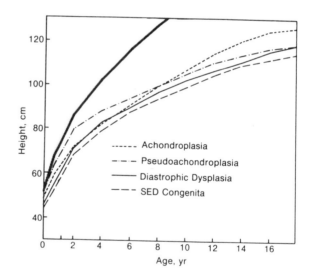

FIG 23. Growth curve for height for patients (male and female combined) with pseudoachondroplasia. The means ± 1 SD are plotted. For comparison a standard normal curve depicting the 50th, 95th, and 5th percentiles was prepared by averaging the normal male and female height derived from the National Center for Health Statistics (NCHS) growth curves.

FIG. 24. Curves depicting mean heights for patients with diastrophic dysplasia, spondyloepiphyseal dysplasia (SED) congenita, pseudoachondroplasia and achondroplasia. Shaded area indicates normal growth curve.

Source: Horton WA, Hall JG, Scott CI, Pyeritz RE, Rimoin DL. Growth curves for height for diastrophic dysplasia, spondyloepiphyseal dysplasia congenita, and pseudoachondroplasia. *Am J Dis Child* 1982;136:316–9.

Whole-Year Velocity Standards and Yearly Increments for Height in Boys and Girls

The standards were based on 80 children of each sex followed longitudinally at the Child Study Center in London from birth to 5.5 years. From 5.5 to 15 years the normal data were from the London Country Council Survey of 1959, which comprised approximately 1,000 boys and 1,000 girls at each year of age. The group of 16.5-year-olds and onward was compared with 30 children from the Harpenden Growth Study who were studied each year until age 20. Annual increments were available for children in the Child Study Center group up until age 11 to 12.

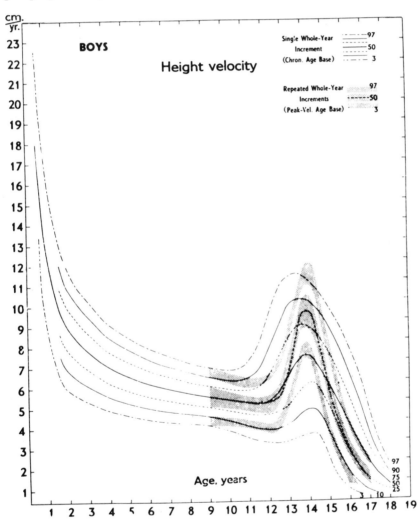

FIG. 25. Peak height velocity for boys. The graph is composed of single whole-year increments with a chronological age base displayed in a conventional manner by means of a continuous line indicating the 50th percentile, and broken lines indicating the 3rd and 97th percentiles. These are the standards used before and during adolescence if no data on developmental ages are available. Repeated whole-year increments (peak velocity age base) are plotted as shaded bands with a dashed line for the 50th percentile. This individual curve represents the velocity taken at each successive year by an individual who has his peak at the average age and an average velocity throughout adolescence. The shaded curves represent the shape of the individual child's growth spurt at adolescence better than the single-increment line.

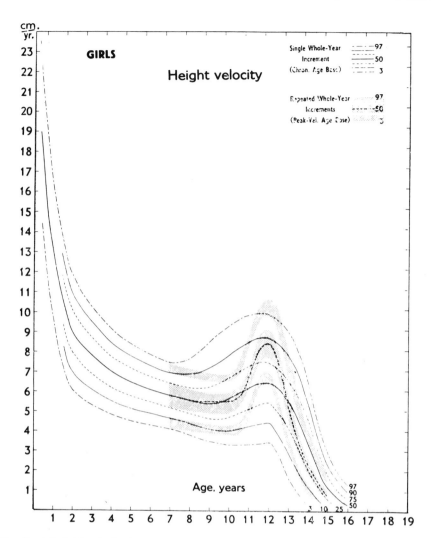

FIG. 26. Peak height velocity for girls. See Fig. 25 legend for further explanation.

Source: Tanner JM, Whitehouse RH, Takaishi M. Standards from birth to maturity for height, weight, height velocity and weight velocity; British children, 1956. Part II. *Arch Dis Child* 1966;41:613–35.

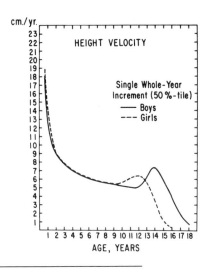

FIG. 27. Height velocity: single whole-year increment (50th percentile for boys and girls). This chart compares only the boy and girl means from the Tanner study (Table 4, Fig. 21). The standard deviations have been removed. The relative velocity for boys (7.3 cm) is greater than that for girls (6.5 cm) during the maximal year of growth. The data indicate a rapid deceleration following birth and a relatively short duration of acceleration during adolescence.

Source: Lowry GH. *Growth and development of children*, 7th ed. Chicago:Yearbook Medical Publishers Inc., 1978.

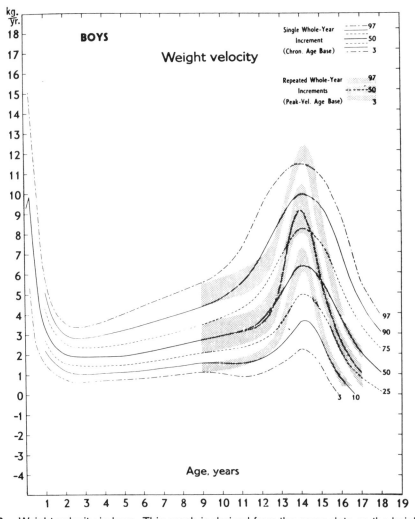

FIG. 28. Weight velocity in boys. This graph is derived from the same data as the height velocity standards, with the single whole-year increments noted at the 50th percentile as a smooth line and the 97th and 3rd percentiles as dotted lines; from birth to adolescence the peak velocity-centered curves whole-year peak increments are represented by the dotted 50th percentile and shaded areas.

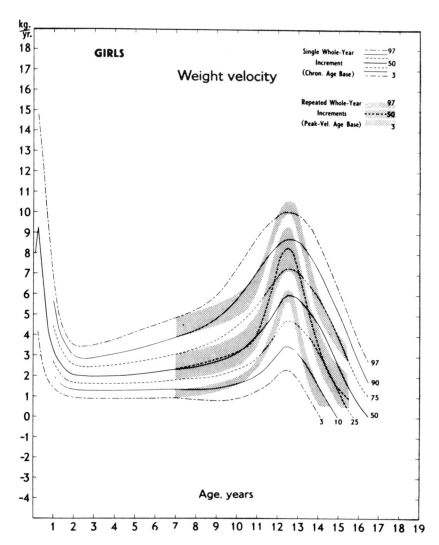

FIG. 29. Weight velocity for girls. See Fig. 28 legend for further explanation.

Source: Tanner JM, Whitehouse RH, Takaishi M. Standards from birth to maturity for height, weight, height velocity and weight velocity; British children, 1956. Part II. *Arch Dis Child* 1966;41:613–35.

Related Reference: Vickers VS, Stuart HC. Anthropometry in the pediatrician's office: Norms for selected body measurements: based on studies of children of North European stock. *J Pediatr* 1943;22:155–170.

Annual Increments in Standing Height Versus Menarcheal Age

This section is concerned with the interrelationships of certain maturational indicators, i.e., chronological age at menarche, assessments of skeletal maturation, and standing height and body weight together with their annual increments. The data are based on the analysis of records of 200 girls, the occurrence of menarche having been the only criterion of selection.

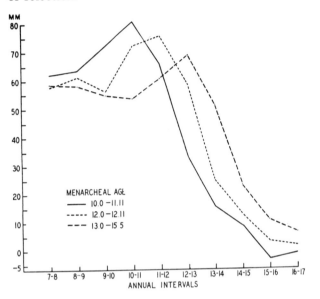

FIG. 30. Mean annual increment in standing height of girls in three menarcheal age groups.

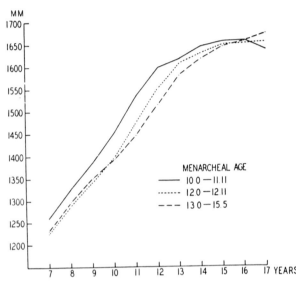

FIG. 31. Mean standing height of girls, 7 to 17 years of age, in three menarcheal age groups.

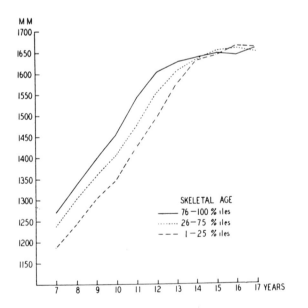

FIG. 32. Mean standing height of girls, 7 to 17 years of age, in three skeletal age groups.

Source: Simmons K, Gruelich WW. Menarcheal age and the height, weight and skeletal age of girls 7–17 years. *J Pediatr* 1943;22:518–48.

Correlation in Body Length: Siblings and Parent/Child

These correlations are drawn from the Fels Institute's longitudinal studies. The data show greater similarities between sisters of most ages considered. That is, sister-sister (SS) size correlations exceed age-matched brother-brother (BB) and sister-brother (SB) correlations, as might be expected for variables influenced at least in part by the X chromosome.

TABLE 5. *Sibling correlations in body length*

AGE (YEARS)	SISTER-SISTER		BROTHER-BROTHER		SISTER-BROTHER	
	N	r	N	r	N	r
Birth...........	45	0.52	59	0.52	113	0.34
0.5............	75	0.52	73	0.44	156	0.35
1.0............	74	0.54	74	0.49	154	0.39
2.0............	66	0.62	70	0.50	147	0.39
3.0............	63	0.62	70	0.68	137	0.47
4.0............	61	0.67	63	0.61	123	0.50
5.0............	53	0.73	68	0.57	116	0.54
6.0............	51	0.76	70	0.57	123	0.56
7.0............	52	0.70	67	0.51	114	0.46
8.0............	47	0.74	62	0.50	102	0.53
9.0............	43	0.72	62	0.50	102	0.49
10.0...........	40	0.71	60	0.45	90	0.47
11.0...........	37	0.66	52	0.48	84	0.41
12.0...........	37	0.70	50	0.48	82	0.34
13.0...........	36	0.67	50	0.34	77	0.28
14.0...........	34	0.59	46	0.26	69	0.28
15.0...........	30	0.43	40	0.10	63	0.29
16.0...........	29	0.41	40	0.07	59	0.36
17.0...........	25	0.58	31	0.10	48	0.40

Recumbent length to age 5.5, stature thereafter.

Source: Garn SM, Rohmann CG. Interaction of nutrition and genetics in the timing of growth and development. *Pediatr Clin North Am* 1966;13:353–78.

Parent-child correlations are positive and significant. These correlations, which tend to peak during late puberty and slowly thereafter, give full two-generation evidence for the genetic mediation of body size and serve to show that sibling correlations are not simply due to family line similarities and nutritional status.

TABLE 6. *Parent/child correlation in body length*

AGE (YEARS)	FATHER-SON	MOTHER-SON	FATHER-DAUGHTER	MOTHER-DAUGHTER	MIDPARENT-[*] SON	MIDPARENT-[*] DAUGHTER
Birth	0.14	0.15	0.14	−0.06	0.18	0.05
0.5	0.33	0.26	0.29	0.14	0.38	0.28
1.0	0.36	0.28	0.34	0.23	0.42	0.34
2.0	0.37	0.30	0.36	0.28	0.45	0.40
3.0	0.37	0.31	0.20	0.13	0.45	0.21
4.0	0.36	0.36	0.38	0.30	0.48	0.44
5.0	0.38	0.35	0.35	0.33	0.48	0.44
6.0	0.36	0.36	0.36	0.32	0.49	0.44
7.0	0.34	0.34	0.39	0.28	0.47	0.43
8.0	0.39	0.35	0.39	0.26	0.50	0.42
9.0	0.37	0.34	0.40	0.24	0.47	0.42
10.0	0.36	0.35	0.34	0.19	0.47	0.35
11.0	0.39	0.33	0.30	0.11	0.48	0.28
12.0	0.40	0.31	0.33	0.15	0.46	0.32
13.0	0.36	0.28	0.37	0.21	0.42	0.38
14.0	0.34	0.27	0.37	0.34	0.41	0.45
15.0	0.32	0.36	0.40	0.43	0.43	0.50
16.0	0.34	0.36	0.46	0.48	0.45	0.58
17.0	0.33	0.41	0.47	0.49	0.46	0.58

[*] Parental stature measured in fourth decade. Midparental stature is average of both parents.

Source: Garn SM, Rohmann CG. Interaction of nutrition and genetics in the timing of growth and development. *Pediatr Clin North Am* 1966;13:353–78.

TABLE 7. *Fels parent-specific standards for height in girls; children's stature by age and midparent stature*

GIRLS

Age	Parental Midpoint (cm.)									
	161	163	165	167	169	171	173	175	177	178
Birth..	47.3	48.9	49.0	49.2	49.2	48.8	49.7	49.1	49.0	47.5
0-1...	53.0	53.4	54.2	52.0	53.3	53.1	53.5	53.2	55.8	52.8
0-3...	57.4	58.4	59.6	57.4	59.4	59.6	59.4	58.0	61.3	57.6
0-6...	64.4	64.7	65.6	65.7	64.6	66.5	66.6	67.4	67.3	65.8
0-9...	68.2	69.0	70.2	70.1	69.8	71.5	71.5	71.0	72.2	69.8
1-0...	72.3	73.0	73.8	74.0	74.0	75.2	75.5	74.6	77.3	73.2
1-6...	78.8	79.5	80.6	81.4	80.2	81.7	82.6	81.6	84.0	81.0
2-0...	84.6	84.0	86.5	87.4	85.5	88.5	88.7	88.2	89.5	87.6
2-6...	89.1	87.2	91.0	91.6	89.9	93.2	92.9	92.6	93.9	92.0
3-0...	93.2	90.4	94.5	95.8	93.8	97.1	96.5	96.5	98.5	96.2
3-6...	96.7	93.5	98.3	99.6	97.8	101.4	100.3	102.0	102.4	103.0
4-0...	100.1	96.8	102.4	103.5	103.9	104.0	104.0	103.8	105.8	104.3
4-6...	103.5	100.2	106.0	106.7	105.8	108.6	107.5	107.4	109.4	108.0
5-0...	106.8	103.5	108.9	109.9	109.1	111.6	110.9	111.0	112.6	111.7
5-6...	110.0	107.0	112.2	113.2	112.0	114.8	114.4	114.2	115.8	115.4
6-0...	113.2	110.2	115.0	116.2	115.0	118.2	117.8	117.8	119.1	118.8
6-6...	116.1	113.4	117.8	119.4	117.6	121.2	121.2	120.8	122.6	122.3
7-0...	118.8	116.5	120.6	122.4	120.2	124.4	124.4	124.0	125.0	125.5
7-6...	121.7	119.4	123.5	125.7	122.9	127.6	127.6	127.3	127.8	128.7
8-0...	124.6	122.4	126.3	128.8	125.8	130.7	130.8	130.8	130.8	132.0
8-6...	127.3	125.5	129.4	131.8	128.5	133.8	133.8	133.3	133.9	135.0
9-0...	130.1	128.6	132.2	134.7	131.4	137.1	136.7	136.6	137.0	138.2
9-6...	132.7	131.6	135.6	137.5	134.2	140.2	139.8	139.9	139.9	140.9
10-0...	136.0	135.1	139.0	140.3	136.9	143.8	142.9	143.1	143.8	143.6
10-6...	139.1	138.5	142.3	143.2	140.0	147.4	146.0	143.1	147.4	146.4
11-0...	141.9	141.6	145.9	146.0	143.4	150.3	149.0	149.6	151.3	149.4
11-6...	145.0	144.8	149.4	148.9	146.6	153.2	152.1	152.8	155.3	152.2
12-0...	148.0	147.8	152.8	151.8	150.3	156.4	155.2	155.8	159.0	154.9
12-6...	150.8	151.1	155.8	154.4	154.0	159.0	158.2	158.8	161.1	158.0
13-0...	152.9	154.2	158.8	157.0	157.0	161.0	161.1	161.7	162.3	160.5
13-6...	154.5	157.2	161.0	159.1	159.0	163.0	163.3	164.0	163.0	162.5
14-0...	155.4	158.8	161.7	160.9	161.0	163.7	165.0	165.9	163.9	164.1
14-6...	155.7	159.4	162.6	162.5	161.5	164.0	166.2	167.4	164.5	165.5
15-0...	155.9	159.8	162.6	163.7	162.9	164.0	167.1	168.4	165.0	166.5
15-6...	156.1	160.1	162.7	164.7	162.9	164.0	167.5	169.2	165.3	167.8
16-0...	156.0	160.5	162.8	165.5	163.4	164.1	167.8	169.7	165.5	167.8
16-6...	156.1	160.7	162.9	166.1	163.8	164.2	167.8	170.3	165.6	168.7
17-0...	156.2	160.8	163.0	166.5	164.0	164.3	167.9	170.3	165.7	169.4
17-6...	156.2	160.9	163.0	166.9	164.2	164.4	167.9	171.4	165.7	170.4
18-0...	156.2	161.0	165.0	167.2	164.3	164.4	167.9	171.8	165.7	170.8

TABLE 8. *Fels parent-specific standards for height in boys; children's stature by age and midparent stature*

BOYS

Age	Parental Midpoint (cm.)									
	161	163	165	167	169	171	173	175	177	178
Birth.		47.1	49.7	50.3	50.0	48.3	50.7	50.0	51.5	51.4
0-1...		52.7	54.6	54.7	57.6	53.2	53.6	52.2	55.6	55.9
0-3...		58.9	60.8	60.0	62.2	57.4	60.8	61.2	61.4	62.6
0-6...		65.1	66.2	66.8	67.4	65.8	70.2	69.0	70.2	70.3
0-9...		70.7	72.9	73.8	73.2	71.0	74.8	75.2	77.1	75.7
1-0...		73.1	75.6	75.7	75.1	73.4	76.6	77.1	79.6	77.8
1-6...		79.9	82.4	81.7	82.0	81.2	82.6	83.4	86.8	85.2
2-0...		85.4	87.2	87.0	87.4	87.8	88.0	88.9	92.0	91.3
2-6...		88.8	91.3	92.0	92.1	93.2	93.5	94.0	96.7	96.0
3-0...		93.2	94.9	96.1	96.0	97.2	98.1	98.3	100.7	99.9
3-6...		96.3	98.4	100.0	99.5	101.0	102.3	102.6	104.5	103.5
4-0...		99.5	102.2	103.5	103.1	104.6	106.0	106.3	108.0	107.0
4-6...		102.7	105.4	107.1	106.6	108.0	109.6	109.6	111.4	110.4
5-0...		105.6	108.5	110.6	110.0	111.5	113.2	112.7	114.6	113.8
5-6...		108.3	111.3	113.4	112.7	114.5	116.3	115.8	117.4	116.8
6-0...		110.9	114.1	116.4	115.4	117.4	118.7	118.7	120.4	119.8
6-6...		113.6	116.9	119.3	118.4	120.3	122.4	121.7	123.4	122.8
7-0...		116.2	119.7	122.3	121.3	123.2	125.6	124.6	126.4	125.6
7-6...		118.9	122.5	125.1	124.3	126.1	128.8	127.6	129.5	128.4
8-0...		121.6	125.0	127.8	126.8	128.8	131.6	130.4	132.8	131.6
8-6...		124.2	127.6	130.7	129.3	131.5	134.0	133.2	135.9	134.6
9-0...		126.9	130.4	133.3	131.9	134.1	138.0	136.0	138.8	137.5
9-6...		129.9	132.9	136.1	134.6	136.9	141.0	138.8	142.0	140.5
10-0...		132.5	135.8	138.8	137.4	139.8	143.8	141.5	145.3	143.2
10-6...		135.6	138.8	141.5	140.3	142.6	144.8	144.3	148.6	146.0
11-0...		138.5	141.8	144.1	143.0	145.4	149.9	146.8	151.9	148.9
11-6...		141.6	144.9	146.9	145.6	148.3	152.8	149.6	155.4	151.6
12-0...		144.7	148.0	149.7	148.4	151.4	155.7	152.4	158.8	154.5
12-6...		147.7	151.1	152.6	151.6	154.6	158.3	155.8	162.3	157.5
13-0...		151.0	154.2	155.7	154.9	158.0	161.7	159.6	166.3	160.5
13-6...		154.5	157.7	158.9	158.1	161.6	164.6	163.6	170.1	163.8
14-0...		158.8	161.7	162.3	161.6	165.7	167.6	167.8	173.4	166.9
14-6...		162.6	164.9	165.5	164.8	169.6	170.3	172.0	173.4	171.3
15-0...		165.8	168.1	169.1	167.9	172.9	173.0	174.7	176.4	175.2
15-6...		168.0	171.3	172.0	170.6	174.5	175.6	175.8	177.0	179.6
16-0...		169.4	173.3	174.3	172.8	177.3	175.6	176.6	177.4	181.2
16-6...		170.3	174.2	175.8	174.4	178.4	178.7	177.3	177.4	182.8
17-0...		170.9	174.7	176.8	175.4	179.2	179.4	177.8	177.5	184.3
17-6...		171.2	174.9	174.4	176.0	180.0	179.9	178.2	177.6	185.4
18-0...		171.5	175.0	177.9	176.2	180.5	180.2	178.6	177.6	186.3

Note: no attempt to eliminate sampling fluctuations.

Tables 7 and 8 represent a parent-specific size standard, thus allowing one to incorporate parental size into height assessments rather than using a single value for children of all the tall and progeny of the short. Midparental stature is the average of the father's and mother's height in centimeters. Parental statures in each case are the size during the fourth decade. **Source:** Garn SM, Rohmann CG. Interaction of nutrition and genetics in the timing of growth and development. *Pediatr Clin North Am* 1966;13:353–78.

System of Predicting Adult Height

This system is based on the fact that there is a high correlation between the skeletal ages as read from standards of hand X-rays (Greulich, WW, Pyle SI. *Radiographic atlas of skeletal development of the hand and wrist.* Stanford, California; Stanford University Press, 1950) and the proportion of adult stature achieved by the children at the time their X-rays are taken. That is, skeletal age correlates with the percent of mature height (PMH) at about n = 0.86 at most ages after 9 years when chronological age is held constant. The tables have been constructed from data gathered at the University of California Institute of Child Welfare on 192 normal Berkeley children (103 girls and 89 boys) measured and X-rayed every 6 months from 8 through 18 years or until all epiphyses of the hand were closed. Tables were then validated by applying them to a different group of 46 children (23 boys and 23 girls). The child's height and maturity are taken at 100% and the fraction of his own mature height was computed for every earlier measuring. Tables 9–19 are used to estimate the mature height for both boys and girls using the skeletal age. The Tables have been divided into average (with the skeletal age within one year of the chronological age), accelerated (where the skeletal age is 1 year or more advanced over the chronological age), and retarded (where the skeletal age is one year or more retarded for the chronological age).

TABLE 9. *Average boys: percentage and estimated mature height for boys with skeletal age within one year of the chronological age (skeletal ages 7–12 years)*

Skeletal Age	7-0	7-3	7-6	7-9	8-0	8-3	8-6	8-9	9-0	9-3	9-6	9-9	10-0	10-3	10-6	10-9	11-0	11-3	11-6	11-9	12-0	12-3	12-6	12-9
% of Mature Height	69.5	70.2	70.9	71.6	72.3	73.1	73.9	74.6	75.2	76.1	76.9	77.7	78.4	79.1	79.5	80.0	80.4	81.2	81.8	82.7	83.4	84.3	85.3	86.3
Ht. (inches)																								
42	60.4																							
43	61.9	61.3	60.6	60.1																				
44	63.3	62.7	62.1	61.5	60.9	60.2																		
45	64.7	64.1	63.5	62.8	62.2	61.6	60.9	60.3																
46	66.2	65.5	64.9	64.2	63.6	62.9	62.2	61.7	61.2	60.4														
47	67.6	67.0	66.3	65.6	65.0	64.3	63.6	63.0	62.5	61.8	61.1	60.5												
48	69.1	68.4	67.7	67.0	66.4	65.7	65.0	64.3	63.8	63.1	62.4	61.8	61.2	60.7	60.4	60.0								
49	70.5	69.8	69.1	68.4	67.8	67.0	66.3	65.7	65.2	64.4	63.7	63.1	62.5	61.9	61.6	61.3	60.9	60.3						
50	71.9	71.2	70.5	69.8	69.2	68.4	67.7	67.0	66.5	65.7	65.0	64.4	63.8	63.2	62.9	62.5	62.2	61.6	61.1	60.5				
51	73.4	72.6	71.9	71.2	70.5	69.8	69.0	68.4	67.8	67.0	66.3	65.6	65.1	64.5	64.2	63.8	63.4	62.8	62.3	61.7	61.1	60.5	59.8	
52	74.8	74.1	73.3	72.6	71.9	71.1	70.4	69.7	69.1	68.3	67.6	66.9	66.3	65.7	65.4	65.0	64.7	64.0	63.6	62.9	62.3	61.7	61.0	60.3
53	76.3	75.5	74.8	74.0	73.3	72.5	71.7	71.0	70.5	69.6	68.9	68.2	67.6	67.0	66.7	66.3	65.9	65.3	64.8	64.1	63.5	62.9	62.1	61.4
54	77.7	76.9	76.2	75.4	74.7	73.9	73.1	72.4	71.8	71.0	70.2	69.5	68.9	68.3	67.9	67.5	67.2	66.5	66.0	65.3	64.7	64.1	63.3	62.6
55	79.1	78.3	77.6	76.8	76.1	75.2	74.4	73.7	73.1	72.3	71.5	70.8	70.2	69.5	69.2	68.8	68.4	67.7	67.2	66.5	65.9	65.2	64.5	63.7
56	80.6	79.8	79.0	78.2	77.5	76.6	75.8	75.1	74.5	73.6	72.8	72.1	71.4	70.8	70.4	70.0	69.5	69.0	68.5	67.7	67.1	66.4	65.6	64.9
57			80.4	79.6	78.8	78.0	77.1	76.4	75.8	74.9	74.1	73.4	72.7	72.1	71.7	71.3	70.9	70.2	69.7	68.9	68.3	67.6	66.8	66.0
58					80.2	79.3	78.5	77.7	77.1	76.2	75.4	74.6	74.0	73.3	73.0	72.5	72.1	71.4	70.9	70.1	69.5	68.8	68.0	67.2
59						80.7	79.8	79.1	78.5	77.5	76.7	75.9	75.3	74.6	74.2	73.8	73.4	72.7	72.1	71.3	70.7	70.0	69.2	68.4
60								80.4	79.8	78.8	78.0	77.2	76.5	75.9	75.5	75.0	74.6	73.9	73.3	72.6	71.9	71.2	70.3	69.5
61										80.2	79.3	78.5	77.8	77.1	76.7	76.3	75.9	75.1	74.6	73.8	73.1	72.4	71.5	70.7
62											80.6	79.8	79.1	78.4	78.0	77.5	77.1	76.4	75.8	75.0	74.3	73.5	72.7	71.8
63													80.4	79.6	79.2	78.8	78.4	77.6	77.0	76.2	75.5	74.7	73.9	73.0
64														80.9	80.5	80.0	79.6	78.8	78.2	77.4	76.7	75.9	75.0	74.2
65																	80.8	80.0	79.5	78.6	77.9	77.1	76.2	75.3
66																			80.7	79.8	79.1	78.3	77.4	76.5
67																					80.3	79.5	78.5	77.6
68																						80.7	79.7	78.8
69																							80.9	80.0

TABLE 10. *Average boys: percentage and estimated mature height for boys with skeletal age within one year of the chronological age (skeletal ages 13 years to maturity)*

Skeletal Age	13-0	13-3	13-6	13-9	14-0	14-3	14-6	14-9	15-0	15-3	15-6	15-9	16-0	16-3	16-6	16-9	17-0	17-3	17-6	17-9	18-0	18-3	18-6
% of Mature Height	87.6	89.0	90.2	91.4	92.7	93.8	94.8	95.8	96.8	97.3	97.6	98.0	98.2	98.5	98.7	98.9	99.1	99.3	99.4	99.5	99.6	99.8	100.0
Ht. (inches)																							
53	60.5																						
54	61.6	60.7																					
55	62.8	61.8	61.0	60.2																			
56	63.9	62.9	62.1	61.3	60.4																		
57	65.1	64.0	63.2	62.4	61.5	60.8	60.1																
58	66.2	65.2	64.3	63.5	62.6	61.8	61.2	60.5															
59	67.4	66.3	65.4	64.6	63.6	62.9	62.2	61.6	61.0	60.6	60.5	60.2	60.1										
60	68.5	67.4	66.5	65.6	64.7	64.0	63.3	62.6	62.0	61.7	61.5	61.2	61.1	60.9	60.8	60.7	60.5	60.4	60.4	60.3	60.2	60.1	60.0
61	69.6	68.5	67.6	66.7	65.8	65.0	64.3	63.7	63.0	62.7	62.5	62.2	62.1	61.9	61.8	61.7	61.6	61.4	61.4	61.3	61.2	61.1	61.0
62	70.8	69.7	68.7	67.8	66.9	66.1	65.4	64.7	64.1	63.7	63.5	63.3	63.1	62.9	62.8	62.7	62.6	62.4	62.4	62.3	62.2	62.1	62.0
63	71.9	70.8	69.8	68.9	68.0	67.2	66.5	65.8	65.1	64.7	64.5	64.3	64.2	64.0	63.8	63.7	63.6	63.4	63.4	63.3	63.3	63.1	63.0
64	73.1	71.9	71.0	70.0	69.0	68.2	67.5	66.8	66.1	65.8	65.6	65.3	65.2	65.0	64.8	64.7	64.6	64.4	64.4	64.3	64.3	64.1	64.0
65	74.2	73.0	72.1	71.1	70.1	69.3	68.6	67.8	67.2	66.8	66.6	66.3	66.2	66.0	65.9	65.7	65.6	65.5	65.4	65.3	65.3	65.1	65.0
66	75.3	74.2	73.2	72.2	71.2	70.4	69.6	68.9	68.2	67.8	67.6	67.3	67.2	67.0	66.9	66.7	66.6	66.5	66.4	66.3	66.3	66.1	66.0
67	76.5	75.3	74.3	73.3	72.3	71.4	70.7	69.9	69.2	68.9	68.6	68.4	68.2	68.0	67.9	67.7	67.6	67.5	67.4	67.3	67.3	67.1	67.0
68	77.6	76.4	75.4	74.4	73.4	72.5	71.7	71.0	70.3	69.9	69.7	69.4	69.2	69.0	68.9	68.8	68.6	68.5	68.4	68.3	68.3	68.1	68.0
69	78.8	77.5	76.5	75.5	74.4	73.6	72.8	72.0	71.3	70.9	70.7	70.4	70.3	70.0	69.9	69.8	69.6	69.5	69.4	69.3	69.3	69.1	69.0
70	79.9	78.7	77.6	76.6	75.5	74.6	73.8	73.1	72.3	71.9	71.7	71.4	71.3	71.1	70.9	70.8	70.6	70.5	70.4	70.4	70.3	70.1	70.0
71		79.8	78.7	77.7	76.6	75.7	74.9	74.1	73.4	73.0	72.7	72.4	72.3	72.1	71.9	71.8	71.6	71.5	71.4	71.4	71.3	71.1	71.0
72		80.9	79.8	78.8	77.7	76.8	75.9	75.2	74.4	74.0	73.8	73.5	73.3	73.1	73.0	72.8	72.7	72.5	72.4	72.4	72.3	72.1	72.0
73			80.9	79.9	78.8	77.8	77.0	76.2	75.4	75.0	74.8	74.5	74.3	74.1	74.0	73.8	73.7	73.5	73.4	73.4	73.3	73.1	73.0
74					79.8	78.9	78.1	77.2	76.4	76.0	75.8	75.5	75.4	75.1	75.0	74.8	74.7	74.5	74.4	74.4	74.3	74.1	74.0
75					80.9	80.0	79.1	78.3	77.5	77.1	76.8	76.5	76.4	76.1	76.0	75.8	75.7	75.5	75.5	75.4	75.3	75.2	75.0
76							80.2	79.3	78.5	78.1	77.9	77.6	77.4	77.2	77.0	76.8	76.7	76.5	76.5	76.4	76.3	76.2	76.0
77								80.4	79.5	79.1	78.9	78.6	78.4	78.2	78.0	77.9	77.7	77.5	77.5	77.4	77.3	77.2	77.0
78									80.6	80.2	79.9	79.6	79.4	79.2	79.0	78.9	78.7	78.5	78.5	78.4	78.3	78.2	78.0

TABLE 11. *Accelerated boys: percentage of estimated mature height for boys with skeletal age one year or more advanced over the chronological age (skeletal ages 7–11 years)*

Skeletal Age	7-0	7-3	7-6	7-9	8-0	8-3	8-6	8-9	9-0	9-3	9-6	9-9	10-0	10-3	10-6	10-9	11-0	11-3	11-6	11-9
% of Mature Height	67.0	67.6	68.3	68.9	69.6	70.3	70.9	71.5	72.0	72.8	73.4	74.1	74.7	75.3	75.8	76.3	76.7	77.6	78.6	80.0
Ht. (inches)																				
41	61.2	60.7	60.0																	
42	62.7	62.1	61.5	61.0	60.3															
43	64.2	63.6	63.0	62.4	61.8	61.2	60.6	60.1												
44	65.7	65.1	64.4	63.9	63.2	62.6	62.1	61.5	61.1	60.4										
45	67.2	66.6	65.9	65.3	64.7	64.0	63.5	62.9	62.5	61.8	61.3	60.7	60.2							
46	68.7	68.0	67.3	66.8	66.1	65.4	64.9	64.3	63.9	63.2	62.7	62.1	61.6	61.1	60.7	60.3	60.0			
47	70.1	69.5	68.8	68.2	67.5	66.9	66.3	65.7	65.3	64.6	64.0	63.4	62.9	62.4	62.0	61.6	61.3	60.6		
48	71.6	71.0	70.3	69.7	69.0	68.3	67.7	67.1	66.7	65.9	65.4	64.8	64.3	63.7	63.3	62.9	62.6	61.9	61.1	60.0
49	73.1	72.5	71.7	71.1	70.4	69.7	69.1	68.5	68.1	67.3	66.8	66.1	65.6	65.1	64.6	64.2	63.9	63.1	62.3	61.3
50	74.6	74.0	73.2	72.6	71.8	71.1	70.5	69.9	69.4	68.7	68.1	67.5	66.9	66.4	66.0	65.5	65.2	64.4	63.6	62.5
51	76.1	75.4	74.7	74.0	73.3	72.5	71.9	71.3	70.8	70.1	69.5	68.8	68.3	67.7	67.3	66.8	66.5	65.7	64.9	63.8
52	77.6	76.9	76.1	75.5	74.7	74.0	73.3	72.7	72.2	71.4	70.8	70.2	69.6	69.1	68.6	68.2	67.8	67.0	66.2	65.0
53	79.1	78.4	77.6	76.9	76.2	75.4	74.8	74.1	73.6	72.8	72.2	71.5	71.0	70.4	69.9	69.5	69.1	68.3	67.4	66.3
54	80.6	79.9	79.1	78.4	77.6	76.8	76.2	75.5	75.0	74.2	73.6	72.9	72.3	71.7	71.2	70.8	70.4	69.6	68.7	67.5
55			80.5	79.8	79.0	78.2	77.6	76.9	76.4	75.5	74.9	74.2	73.6	73.0	72.6	72.1	71.7	70.9	70.0	68.8
56					80.5	79.7	79.0	78.3	77.8	76.9	76.3	75.6	75.0	74.4	73.9	73.4	73.0	72.2	71.2	70.0
57							80.4	79.7	79.2	78.3	77.7	76.9	76.3	75.7	75.2	74.7	74.3	73.5	72.5	71.3
58									80.6	79.7	79.0	78.3	77.6	77.0	76.5	76.0	75.6	74.7	73.8	72.5
59											80.4	79.6	79.0	78.4	77.8	77.3	76.9	76.0	75.1	73.8
60													80.3	79.7	79.2	78.6	78.2	77.3	76.3	75.0
61															80.5	79.9	79.5	78.6	77.6	76.3
62																81.3	80.8	79.9	78.9	77.5
63																			80.2	78.8
64																				80.0

Source: Bayley N, Pinneau SR. Tables for predicting adult height from skeletal age: revised for use with the Greulich-Pyle hand standards. *J Pediatr* 1952;40:423–41.

TABLE 12. *Accelerated boys: percentage and estimated mature height for boys with skeletal age one year or more advanced over the chronological age (skeletal ages 12–17 years)*

Skeletal Age Ht. (inches)	12-0	12-3	**12-6**	12-9	13.0	**13-3**	13-6	13-9	**14-0**	14-3	**14-6**	14-9	**15-0**	15-3	**15-6**	15-9	**16-0**	16-3	**16-6**	16-9	**17-0**
% of Mature Height	80.9	81.8	82.8	83.9	85.0	86.3	87.5	89.0	90.5	91.8	93.0	94.3	95.8	96.7	97.1	97.6	98.0	98.3	98.5	98.8	99.0
49	60.6																				
50	61.8	61.1	60.4																		
51	63.0	62.3	61.6	60.8	60.0																
52	64.3	63.6	62.8	62.0	61.2	60.3															
53	65.5	64.8	64.0	63.2	62.4	61.4	60.6														
54	66.7	66.0	65.2	64.4	63.5	62.6	61.7	60.7													
55	68.0	67.2	66.4	65.6	64.7	63.7	62.9	61.8	60.8												
56	69.2	68.5	67.6	66.7	65.9	64.9	64.0	62.9	61.9	61.0	60.2										
57	70.5	69.7	68.8	67.9	67.1	66.0	65.1	64.0	63.0	62.1	61.3	60.4									
58	71.7	70.9	70.0	69.1	68.2	67.2	66.3	65.2	64.1	63.2	62.4	61.5	60.5	60.0							
59	72.9	72.1	71.3	70.3	69.4	68.4	67.4	66.3	65.2	64.3	63.4	62.6	61.6	61.0	60.8	60.5	60.2	60.0			
60	74.2	73.4	72.5	71.5	70.6	69.5	68.6	67.4	66.3	65.4	64.5	63.6	62.6	62.0	61.8	61.5	61.2	61.0	60.9	60.7	60.6
61	75.4	74.6	73.7	72.7	71.8	70.7	69.7	68.5	67.4	66.4	65.6	64.7	63.7	63.1	62.8	62.5	62.2	62.1	61.9	61.7	61.6
62	76.6	75.8	74.9	73.9	72.9	71.8	70.9	69.7	68.5	67.5	66.7	65.7	64.7	64.1	63.9	63.5	63.3	63.1	62.9	62.8	62.6
63	77.9	77.0	76.1	75.1	74.1	73.0	72.0	70.8	69.6	68.6	67.7	66.8	65.8	65.1	64.9	64.5	64.3	64.1	64.0	63.8	63.6
64	79.1	78.2	77.3	76.3	75.3	74.2	73.1	71.9	70.7	69.7	68.8	67.9	66.8	66.2	65.9	65.6	65.3	65.1	65.0	64.8	64.6
65	80.3	79.5	78.5	77.5	76.5	75.3	74.3	73.0	71.8	70.8	69.9	68.9	67.8	67.2	66.9	66.6	66.3	66.1	66.0	65.8	65.7
66		80.7	79.7	78.7	77.6	76.5	75.4	74.2	72.9	71.9	71.0	70.0	68.9	68.3	68.0	67.6	67.3	67.1	67.0	66.8	66.7
67			80.9	79.9	78.8	77.6	76.6	75.3	74.0	73.0	72.0	71.1	69.9	69.3	69.0	68.6	68.4	68.2	68.0	67.8	67.7
68					80.0	78.8	77.7	76.4	75.1	74.1	73.1	72.1	71.0	70.3	70.0	69.7	69.4	69.2	69.0	68.8	68.7
69						80.0	78.9	77.5	76.2	75.2	74.2	73.2	72.0	71.4	71.1	70.7	70.4	70.2	70.1	69.8	69.7
70							80.0	78.7	77.3	76.3	75.3	74.2	73.1	72.4	72.1	71.7	71.4	71.2	71.1	70.9	70.7
71								79.8	78.5	77.3	76.3	75.3	74.1	73.4	73.1	72.7	72.4	72.2	72.1	71.9	71.7
72								80.9	79.6	78.4	77.4	76.4	75.2	74.5	74.2	73.8	73.5	73.2	73.1	72.9	72.7
73									80.7	79.5	78.5	77.4	76.2	75.5	75.2	74.8	74.5	74.3	74.1	73.9	73.7
74										80.6	79.6	78.5	77.2	76.5	76.2	75.8	75.5	75.3	75.1	74.9	74.7
75											80.6	79.5	78.3	77.6	77.2	76.8	76.5	76.3	76.1	75.9	75.8
76												80.6	79.3	78.6	78.3	77.9	77.6	77.3	77.2	76.9	76.8
77													80.4	79.6	79.3	78.9	78.6	78.3	78.2	77.9	77.8
78														80.7	80.3	79.9	79.6	79.3	79.2	78.9	78.8

TABLE 13. *Retarded boys: percentage and estimated mature height for boys with skeletal age one year or more retarded for the chronological age (skeletal ages 6–13 years).*

Skeletal Age Ht. (inches)	6-0	6-3	6-6	6-9	**7-0**	7-3	7-6	7-9	**8-0**	8-3	8-6	8-9	**9-0**	9-3	9-6	9-9	**10-0**	10-3	10-6	10-9	**11-0**	11-3	11-6	11-9	**12-0**	12-3	**12-6**	12-9	13-0
% of Mature Height	68.0	69.0	70.0	70.9	71.8	72.8	73.8	74.7	75.6	76.5	77.3	77.9	78.6	79.4	80.0	80.7	81.2	81.6	81.9	82.1	82.3	82.7	83.2	83.9	84.5	85.2	86.0	86.9	88.0
41	60.3																												
42	61.8	60.9	60.0																										
43	63.2	62.3	61.4	60.6																									
44	64.7	63.8	62.9	62.1	61.3	60.4																							
45	66.2	65.2	64.3	63.5	62.7	61.8	61.0	60.2																					
46	67.6	66.7	65.7	64.9	64.1	63.2	62.3	61.6	60.8	60.1																			
47	69.1	68.1	67.1	66.3	65.5	64.6	63.7	62.9	62.2	61.4	60.8	60.3																	
48	70.6	69.6	68.6	67.7	66.9	65.9	65.0	64.3	63.5	62.7	62.1	61.6	61.1	60.5	60.0														
49	72.1	71.0	70.0	69.1	68.3	67.3	66.4	65.6	64.8	64.1	63.4	62.9	62.3	61.7	61.3	60.7	60.3	60.0											
50	73.5	72.5	71.4	70.5	69.6	68.7	67.8	66.9	66.1	65.4	64.7	64.2	63.6	63.0	62.5	62.0	61.6	61.3	61.1	60.9	60.8	60.5	60.1						
51	75.0	73.9	72.9	71.9	71.0	70.1	69.1	68.3	67.5	66.7	66.0	65.5	64.9	64.2	63.8	63.2	62.8	62.5	62.3	62.1	62.0	61.7	61.3	60.8	60.4				
52	76.5	75.4	74.3	73.3	72.4	71.4	70.5	69.6	68.8	68.0	67.3	66.8	66.2	65.5	65.0	64.4	64.0	63.7	63.5	63.3	63.2	62.9	62.5	62.0	61.5	61.0	60.5		
53	77.9	76.8	75.7	74.8	73.8	72.8	71.8	71.0	70.1	69.3	68.6	68.0	67.4	66.8	66.3	65.7	65.3	65.0	64.7	64.6	64.4	64.1	63.7	63.2	62.7	62.2	61.6	61.0	60.2
54	79.4	78.3	77.1	76.2	75.2	74.2	73.2	72.3	71.4	70.6	69.9	69.3	68.7	68.0	67.5	66.9	66.5	66.2	65.9	65.8	65.6	65.3	64.9	64.4	63.9	63.4	62.8	62.1	61.4
55	80.9	79.7	78.6	77.6	76.6	75.5	74.5	73.6	72.8	71.9	71.2	70.6	70.0	69.3	68.8	68.2	67.7	67.4	67.2	67.0	66.8	66.5	66.1	65.6	65.1	64.6	64.0	63.3	62.5
56			80.0	79.0	78.0	76.9	75.9	75.0	74.1	73.2	72.4	71.9	71.2	70.5	70.0	69.4	69.0	68.6	68.4	68.2	68.0	67.7	67.3	66.7	66.3	65.7	65.1	64.4	63.6
57				80.4	79.4	78.3	77.2	76.3	75.4	74.5	73.7	73.2	72.5	71.8	71.3	70.6	70.2	69.9	69.6	69.4	69.3	68.9	68.5	67.9	67.5	66.9	66.3	65.6	64.8
58					80.8	79.7	78.6	77.6	76.7	75.8	75.0	74.5	73.8	73.0	72.5	71.9	71.4	71.1	70.8	70.6	70.5	70.1	69.7	69.1	68.6	68.1	67.4	66.7	65.9
59							79.9	79.0	78.0	77.1	76.3	75.7	75.1	74.3	73.8	73.1	72.7	72.3	72.0	71.9	71.7	71.3	70.9	70.3	69.8	69.2	68.6	67.9	67.0
60								80.3	79.4	78.4	77.6	77.0	76.3	75.6	75.0	74.3	73.9	73.5	73.3	73.1	72.9	72.6	72.1	71.5	71.0	70.4	69.8	69.0	68.2
61									80.7	79.7	78.9	78.3	77.6	76.8	76.3	75.6	75.1	74.8	74.5	74.3	74.1	73.8	73.3	72.7	72.2	71.6	70.9	70.2	69.3
62											80.2	79.6	78.9	78.1	77.5	76.8	76.4	76.0	75.7	75.5	75.3	75.0	74.5	73.9	73.4	72.8	72.1	71.3	70.5
63												80.9	80.2	79.3	78.8	78.1	77.6	77.2	76.9	76.7	76.5	76.2	75.7	75.1	74.6	73.9	73.3	72.5	71.6
64														80.6	80.0	79.3	78.8	78.4	78.1	78.0	77.8	77.4	76.9	76.3	75.7	75.1	74.4	73.6	72.7
65																80.5	80.0	79.7	79.4	79.2	79.0	78.6	78.1	77.5	76.9	76.3	75.6	74.8	73.9
66																		80.9	80.6	80.4	80.2	79.8	79.3	78.7	78.1	77.5	76.7	75.9	75.0
67																							80.5	79.9	79.3	78.6	77.9	77.1	76.1

TABLE 14. *Average girls: percentage and estimated mature height for girls with skeletal age within one year of the chronological age (skeletal ages 6–11 years)*

Skeletal Age / Ht. (inches)	6-0	6-3	6-6	6-10	7-0	7-3	7-6	7-10	8-0	8-3	8-6	8-10	9-0	9-3	9-6	9-9	10-0	10-3	10-6	10-9	11-0	11-3	11-6	11-9
% of Mature Height	72.0	72.9	73.8	75.1	75.7	76.5	77.2	78.2	79.0	80.1	81.0	82.1	82.7	83.6	84.4	85.3	86.2	87.4	88.4	89.6	90.6	91.0	91.4	91.8
37	51.4																							
38	52.8	52.1	51.5																					
39	54.2	53.5	52.8	51.9	51.5	51.0																		
40	55.6	54.9	54.2	53.3	52.8	52.3	51.8	51.2																
41	56.9	56.2	55.6	54.6	54.2	53.6	53.1	52.4	51.9	51.2														
42	58.3	57.6	56.9	55.9	55.5	54.9	54.4	53.7	53.2	52.4	51.9	51.2												
43	59.7	59.0	58.3	57.3	56.8	56.2	55.7	55.0	54.4	53.7	53.1	52.4	52.0	51.4										
44	61.1	60.4	59.6	58.6	58.1	57.5	57.0	56.3	55.7	54.9	54.3	53.6	53.2	52.6	52.1	51.6	51.0							
45	62.5	61.7	61.0	59.9	59.4	58.8	58.3	57.5	57.0	56.2	55.6	54.8	54.4	53.8	53.3	52.8	52.2	51.5						
46	63.9	63.1	62.3	61.3	60.8	60.1	59.6	58.8	58.2	57.4	56.8	56.0	55.6	55.0	54.5	53.9	53.4	52.6	52.0	51.3				
47	65.3	64.5	63.7	62.6	62.1	61.4	60.9	60.1	59.5	58.7	58.0	57.2	56.8	56.2	55.7	55.1	54.5	53.8	53.2	52.5	51.9	51.6	51.4	51.2
48	66.7	65.8	65.0	63.9	63.4	62.7	62.2	61.4	60.8	59.9	59.3	58.5	58.0	57.4	56.9	56.3	55.7	54.9	54.3	53.6	53.0	52.7	52.5	52.3
49	68.1	67.2	66.4	65.2	64.7	64.1	63.5	62.7	62.0	61.2	60.5	59.7	59.3	58.6	58.1	57.4	56.8	56.1	55.4	54.7	54.1	53.8	53.6	53.4
50	69.4	68.6	67.8	66.6	66.1	65.4	64.8	63.9	63.3	62.4	61.7	60.9	60.5	59.8	59.2	58.6	58.0	57.2	56.6	55.8	55.2	54.9	54.7	54.5
51	70.8	70.0	69.1	67.9	67.4	66.7	66.1	65.2	64.6	63.7	63.0	62.1	61.7	61.0	60.4	59.8	59.2	58.4	57.7	56.9	56.3	56.0	55.8	55.6
52	72.2	71.3	70.5	69.2	68.7	68.0	67.4	66.5	65.8	64.9	64.2	63.3	62.9	62.2	61.6	61.0	60.3	59.5	58.8	58.0	57.4	57.1	56.9	56.6
53	73.6	72.7	71.8	70.6	70.0	69.3	68.7	67.8	67.1	66.2	65.4	64.6	64.1	63.4	62.8	62.1	61.5	60.6	60.0	59.2	58.5	58.2	58.0	57.7
54		74.1	73.2	71.9	71.3	70.6	69.9	69.1	68.4	67.4	66.7	65.8	65.3	64.6	64.0	63.3	62.6	61.8	61.1	60.3	59.6	59.3	59.1	58.8
55			74.5	73.2	72.7	71.9	71.2	70.3	69.6	68.7	67.9	67.0	66.5	65.8	65.2	64.5	63.8	62.9	62.2	61.4	60.7	60.4	60.2	59.9
56				74.6	74.0	73.2	72.5	71.6	70.9	69.9	69.1	68.2	67.7	67.0	66.4	65.7	65.0	64.1	63.3	62.5	61.8	61.5	61.3	61.0
57						74.5	73.8	72.9	72.2	71.2	70.4	69.4	68.9	68.2	67.5	66.8	66.1	65.2	64.5	63.6	62.9	62.6	62.4	62.1
58								74.2	73.4	72.4	71.6	70.6	70.1	69.4	68.7	68.0	67.3	66.4	65.6	64.7	64.0	63.7	63.5	63.2
59									74.7	73.7	72.8	71.9	71.3	70.6	69.9	69.2	68.4	67.5	66.7	65.8	65.1	64.8	64.6	64.3
60										74.9	74.1	73.1	72.6	71.8	71.1	70.3	69.6	68.7	67.9	67.0	66.2	65.9	65.6	65.4
61												74.3	73.8	73.0	72.3	71.5	70.8	69.8	69.0	68.1	67.3	67.0	66.7	66.4
62														74.2	73.5	72.7	71.9	70.9	70.1	69.2	68.4	68.1	67.8	67.5
63															74.6	73.9	73.1	72.1	71.3	70.3	69.5	69.2	68.9	68.6
64																	74.2	73.2	72.4	71.4	70.6	70.3	70.0	69.7
65																		74.4	73.5	72.5	71.7	71.4	71.1	70.8
66																			74.7	73.7	72.9	72.5	72.2	71.9
67																				74.8	74.0	73.6	73.3	73.0
68																						74.7	74.4	74.1

TABLE 15. *Average girls: percentage and estimated mature height for girls with skeletal age within one year of chronological age (skeletal ages 12–18 years)*

Skeletal Age / Ht. (inches)	12-0	12-3	12-6	12-9	13-0	13-3	13-6	13-9	14-0	14-3	14-6	14-9	15-0	15-3	15-6	15-9	16-0	16-3	16-6	16-9	17-0	17-6	18-0
% of Mature Height	92.2	93.2	94.1	95.0	95.8	96.7	97.4	97.8	98.0	98.3	98.6	98.8	99.0	99.1	99.3	99.4	99.6	99.6	99.7	99.8	99.9	99.95	100.0
47	51.0																						
48	52.1	51.5	51.0																				
49	53.1	52.6	52.1	51.6	51.1																		
50	54.2	53.6	53.1	52.6	52.2	51.7	51.3	51.1	51.0														
51	55.3	54.7	54.2	53.7	53.2	52.7	52.4	52.1	52.0	51.9	51.7	51.6	51.5	51.5	51.4	51.3	51.2	51.2	51.2	51.1	51.1	51.0	51.0
52	56.4	55.8	55.3	54.7	54.3	53.8	53.4	53.2	53.1	52.9	52.7	52.6	52.5	52.5	52.4	52.3	52.2	52.2	52.2	52.1	52.1	52.0	52.0
53	57.5	56.9	56.3	55.8	55.3	54.8	54.4	54.2	54.1	53.9	53.8	53.6	53.5	53.5	53.4	53.3	53.2	53.2	53.2	53.1	53.1	53.0	53.0
54	58.6	57.9	57.4	56.8	56.4	55.8	55.4	55.2	55.1	54.9	54.8	54.7	54.5	54.5	54.4	54.3	54.2	54.2	54.2	54.1	54.1	54.0	54.0
55	59.7	59.0	58.4	57.9	57.4	56.9	56.5	56.2	56.1	56.0	55.8	55.7	55.6	55.5	55.4	55.3	55.2	55.2	55.2	55.1	55.1	55.0	55.0
56	60.7	60.1	59.5	58.9	58.5	57.9	57.5	57.3	57.1	57.0	56.8	56.7	56.6	56.5	56.4	56.3	56.2	56.2	56.2	56.1	56.1	56.0	56.0
57	61.8	61.2	60.6	60.0	59.5	58.9	58.5	58.3	58.2	58.0	57.8	57.7	57.6	57.5	57.4	57.3	57.2	57.2	57.2	57.1	57.1	57.0	57.0
58	62.9	62.2	61.6	61.1	60.5	60.0	59.5	59.3	59.2	59.0	58.8	58.7	58.6	58.5	58.4	58.3	58.2	58.2	58.2	58.1	58.1	58.0	58.0
59	64.0	63.3	62.7	62.1	61.6	61.0	60.6	60.3	60.2	60.0	59.8	59.7	59.6	59.5	59.4	59.4	59.2	59.2	59.2	59.1	59.1	59.0	59.0
60	65.1	64.4	63.8	63.2	62.6	62.0	61.6	61.3	61.2	61.0	60.9	60.7	60.6	60.5	60.4	60.4	60.2	60.2	60.2	60.1	60.1	60.0	60.0
61	66.2	65.5	64.8	64.2	63.7	63.1	62.6	62.4	62.2	62.1	61.9	61.7	61.6	61.6	61.4	61.4	61.2	61.2	61.2	61.1	61.1	61.0	61.0
62	67.2	66.5	65.9	65.3	64.7	64.1	63.7	63.4	63.3	63.1	62.9	62.8	62.6	62.6	62.4	62.4	62.2	62.2	62.2	62.1	62.1	62.0	62.0
63	68.3	67.6	67.0	66.3	65.8	65.1	64.7	64.4	64.3	64.1	63.9	63.8	63.6	63.6	63.4	63.4	63.3	63.3	63.2	63.1	63.1	63.0	63.0
64	69.4	68.7	68.0	67.4	66.8	66.2	65.7	65.4	65.3	65.1	64.9	64.8	64.6	64.6	64.4	64.4	64.3	64.3	64.2	64.1	64.1	64.0	64.0
65	70.5	69.7	69.1	68.4	67.8	67.2	66.7	66.5	66.3	66.1	65.9	65.8	65.7	65.6	65.5	65.4	65.3	65.3	65.2	65.1	65.1	65.0	65.0
66	71.6	70.8	70.1	69.5	68.9	68.3	67.8	67.5	67.3	67.1	66.9	66.8	66.7	66.6	66.5	66.4	66.3	66.3	66.2	66.1	66.1	66.0	66.0
67	72.7	71.9	71.2	70.5	69.9	69.3	68.8	68.5	68.4	68.2	68.0	67.8	67.7	67.6	67.5	67.4	67.3	67.3	67.2	67.1	67.1	67.0	67.0
68	73.8	73.0	72.3	71.6	71.0	70.3	69.8	69.5	69.4	69.2	69.0	68.8	68.7	68.6	68.5	68.4	68.3	68.3	68.2	68.1	68.1	68.0	68.0
69	74.8	74.0	73.3	72.6	72.0	71.4	70.8	70.6	70.4	70.2	70.0	69.8	69.7	69.6	69.5	69.4	69.3	69.3	69.2	69.1	69.1	69.0	69.0
70			74.4	73.7	73.1	72.4	71.9	71.6	71.4	71.2	71.0	70.8	70.7	70.6	70.5	70.4	70.3	70.3	70.2	70.1	70.1	70.0	70.0
71				74.7	74.1	73.4	72.9	72.6	72.4	72.2	72.0	71.9	71.7	71.6	71.5	71.4	71.3	71.3	71.2	71.1	71.1	71.0	71.0
72						74.5	73.9	73.6	73.5	73.2	73.0	72.9	72.7	72.7	72.5	72.4	72.3	72.3	72.2	72.1	72.1	72.0	72.0
73							74.9	74.6	74.5	74.3	74.0	73.9	73.7	73.7	73.5	73.4	73.3	73.3	73.2	73.1	73.1	73.0	73.0
74												74.9	74.7	74.7	74.5	74.4	74.3	74.3	74.2	74.1	74.1	74.0	74.0

Source: Bayley N, Pinneau SR. Tables for predicting adult height from skeletal age: revised for use with the Greulich-Pyle hand standards. *J Pediatr* 1952;40:423–41.

TABLE 16. *Accelerated girls: percentage and estimated mature height for girls with skeletal age one year or more advanced over the chronological age (skeletal ages 7–11 years)*

Skeletal Age → % of Mature Height / Ht. (inches) ↓	7-0	7-3	7-6	7-10	8-0	8-3	8-6	8-10	9-0	9-3	9-6	9-9	10-0	10-3	10-6	10-9	11-0	11-3	11-6	11-9
(%)	71.2	72.2	73.2	74.2	75.0	76.0	77.1	78.4	79.0	80.0	80.9	81.9	82.8	84.1	85.6	87.0	88.3	88.7	89.1	89.7
37	52.0	51.2																		
38	53.4	52.6	51.9	51.2																
39	54.8	54.0	53.3	52.6	52.0	51.3														
40	56.2	55.4	54.6	53.9	53.3	52.6	51.9	51.0												
41	57.6	56.8	56.0	55.3	54.7	53.9	53.2	52.3	51.9	51.3										
42	59.0	58.2	57.4	56.6	56.0	55.3	54.5	53.6	53.2	52.5	51.9	51.3								
43	60.4	59.6	58.7	58.0	57.3	56.6	55.8	54.8	54.4	53.8	53.2	52.5	51.9	51.1						
44	61.8	60.9	60.1	59.3	58.7	57.9	57.1	56.1	55.7	55.0	54.4	53.7	53.1	52.3	51.4					
45	63.2	62.3	61.5	60.6	60.0	59.2	58.4	57.4	57.0	56.3	55.6	54.9	54.3	53.5	52.6	51.7	51.0			
46	64.6	63.7	62.8	62.0	61.3	60.5	59.7	58.7	58.2	57.5	56.9	56.2	55.6	54.7	53.7	52.9	52.1	51.9	51.6	51.3
47	66.0	65.1	64.2	63.3	62.7	61.8	61.0	59.9	59.5	58.8	58.1	57.4	56.8	55.9	54.9	54.0	53.2	53.0	52.7	52.4
48	67.4	66.5	65.6	64.7	64.0	63.2	62.3	61.2	60.8	60.0	59.3	58.6	58.0	57.1	56.1	55.2	54.4	54.1	53.9	53.5
49	68.8	67.9	66.9	66.0	65.3	64.5	63.6	62.5	62.0	61.3	60.6	59.8	59.2	58.3	57.2	56.3	55.5	55.2	55.0	54.6
50	70.2	69.3	68.3	67.4	66.7	65.8	64.9	63.8	63.3	62.5	61.8	61.1	60.4	59.5	58.4	57.5	56.6	56.4	56.1	55.7
51	71.6	70.6	69.7	68.7	68.0	67.1	66.1	65.1	64.6	63.8	63.0	62.3	61.6	60.6	59.6	58.6	57.8	57.5	57.2	56.9
52	73.0	72.0	71.0	70.1	69.3	68.4	67.4	66.3	65.8	65.0	64.3	63.5	62.8	61.8	60.7	59.8	58.9	58.6	58.4	58.0
53	74.4	73.4	72.4	71.4	70.7	69.7	68.7	67.6	67.1	66.3	65.5	64.7	64.0	63.0	61.9	60.9	60.0	59.8	59.5	59.1
54		74.8	73.8	72.8	72.0	71.1	70.0	68.9	68.4	67.5	66.7	65.9	65.2	64.2	63.1	62.1	61.2	60.9	60.6	60.2
55				74.1	73.3	72.4	71.3	70.2	69.6	68.8	68.0	67.2	66.4	65.4	64.3	63.2	62.3	62.0	61.7	61.3
56					74.7	73.7	72.6	71.4	70.9	70.0	69.2	68.4	67.6	66.6	65.4	64.4	63.4	63.1	62.8	62.4
57							73.9	72.7	72.2	71.3	70.5	69.6	68.8	67.8	66.6	65.5	64.6	64.3	64.0	63.5
58								74.0	73.4	72.5	71.7	70.8	70.0	69.0	67.8	66.7	65.7	65.4	65.1	64.7
59									74.7	73.8	72.9	72.0	71.3	70.2	68.9	67.8	66.8	66.5	66.2	65.8
60											74.2	73.3	72.5	71.3	70.1	69.0	68.0	67.6	67.3	66.9
61												74.5	73.7	72.5	71.3	70.1	69.1	68.8	68.5	68.0
62													74.9	73.7	72.4	71.3	70.2	69.9	69.6	69.1
63														74.9	73.6	72.4	71.3	71.0	70.7	70.2
64															74.8	73.6	72.5	72.2	71.8	71.3
65																74.7	73.6	73.3	72.9	72.5
66																	74.7	74.4	74.1	73.6
67																				74.7

TABLE 17. *Accelerated girls: percentage and estimated mature height for girls with skeletal age one year or more advanced over the chronological age (skeletal ages 12–17 years)*

Skeletal Age → % of Mature Height / Ht. (inches) ↓	12-0	12-3	12-6	12-9	13-0	13-3	13-6	13-9	14-0	14-3	14-6	14-9	15-0	15-3	15-6	15-9	16-0	16-3	16-6	16-9	17-0	17-6
(%)	90.1	91.3	92.4	93.5	94.5	95.5	96.3	96.8	97.2	97.7	98.0	98.3	98.6	98.8	99.0	99.2	99.3	99.4	99.5	99.7	99.8	99.95
46	51.1																					
47	52.2	51.5																				
48	53.3	52.6	51.9	51.3																		
49	54.4	53.7	53.0	52.4	51.9	51.3	50.9															
50	55.5	54.8	54.1	53.5	52.9	52.4	51.9	51.7	51.4	51.2	51.0											
51	56.6	55.9	55.2	54.5	54.0	53.4	53.0	52.7	52.5	52.2	52.0	51.9	51.7	51.6	51.5	51.4	51.4	51.3	51.3	51.2	51.1	51.0
52	57.7	57.0	56.3	55.6	55.0	54.5	54.0	53.7	53.5	53.2	53.1	52.9	52.7	52.6	52.5	52.4	52.4	52.3	52.3	52.2	52.1	52.0
53	58.8	58.1	57.4	56.7	56.1	55.5	55.0	54.8	54.5	54.2	54.1	53.9	53.8	53.6	53.5	53.4	53.4	53.3	53.3	53.2	53.1	53.0
54	59.9	59.1	58.4	57.8	57.1	56.5	56.1	55.8	55.6	55.3	55.1	54.9	54.8	54.7	54.5	54.4	54.4	54.3	54.3	54.2	54.1	54.0
55	61.0	60.2	59.5	58.8	58.2	57.6	57.1	56.8	56.6	56.3	56.1	56.0	55.8	55.7	55.6	55.4	55.4	55.3	55.3	55.2	55.1	55.0
56	62.2	61.3	60.6	59.9	59.3	58.6	58.2	57.9	57.6	57.3	57.1	57.0	56.8	56.7	56.6	56.5	56.4	56.3	56.3	56.2	56.1	56.0
57	63.3	62.4	61.7	61.0	60.3	59.7	59.2	58.9	58.6	58.3	58.2	58.0	57.8	57.7	57.6	57.5	57.4	57.3	57.3	57.2	57.1	57.0
58	64.4	63.5	62.8	62.0	61.4	60.7	60.2	59.9	59.7	59.4	59.2	59.0	58.8	58.7	58.6	58.5	58.4	58.4	58.3	58.2	58.1	58.0
59	65.5	64.6	63.9	63.1	62.4	61.8	61.3	61.0	60.7	60.4	60.2	60.0	59.8	59.7	59.6	59.5	59.4	59.4	59.3	59.2	59.1	59.0
60	66.6	65.7	64.9	64.2	63.5	62.8	62.3	62.0	61.7	61.4	61.2	61.0	60.9	60.7	60.6	60.5	60.4	60.4	60.3	60.2	60.1	60.0
61	67.7	66.8	66.0	65.2	64.6	63.9	63.3	63.0	62.8	62.4	62.2	62.1	61.9	61.7	61.6	61.5	61.4	61.4	61.3	61.2	61.1	61.0
62	68.8	67.9	67.1	66.3	65.6	64.9	64.4	64.0	63.8	63.5	63.3	63.1	62.9	62.8	62.6	62.5	62.4	62.4	62.3	62.2	62.1	62.0
63	69.9	69.0	68.2	67.4	66.7	66.0	65.4	65.1	64.8	64.5	64.3	64.1	63.9	63.8	63.6	63.5	63.4	63.4	63.3	63.2	63.1	63.0
64	71.0	70.1	69.3	68.4	67.7	67.0	66.5	66.1	65.8	65.5	65.3	65.1	64.9	64.8	64.6	64.5	64.5	64.4	64.3	64.2	64.1	64.0
65	72.1	71.2	70.3	69.5	68.8	68.1	67.5	67.1	66.9	66.5	66.3	66.1	65.9	65.8	65.7	65.5	65.5	65.4	65.3	65.2	65.1	65.0
66	73.3	72.3	71.4	70.6	69.8	69.1	68.5	68.2	67.9	67.6	67.3	67.1	66.9	66.8	66.7	66.5	66.5	66.4	66.3	66.2	66.1	66.0
67	74.4	73.4	72.5	71.7	70.9	70.2	69.6	69.2	68.9	68.6	68.4	68.2	68.0	67.8	67.7	67.5	67.5	67.4	67.3	67.2	67.1	67.0
68		74.5	73.6	72.7	72.0	71.2	70.6	70.2	70.0	69.6	69.4	69.2	69.0	68.8	68.7	68.5	68.5	68.4	68.3	68.2	68.1	68.0
69			74.7	73.8	73.0	72.3	71.7	71.3	71.0	70.6	70.4	70.2	70.0	69.8	69.7	69.6	69.5	69.4	69.3	69.2	69.1	69.0
70				74.9	74.1	73.3	72.7	72.3	72.0	71.6	71.4	71.2	71.0	70.9	70.7	70.6	70.5	70.4	70.4	70.2	70.1	70.0
71						74.3	73.7	73.3	73.0	72.7	72.4	72.2	72.0	71.9	71.7	71.6	71.5	71.4	71.4	71.2	71.1	71.0
72							74.8	74.4	74.1	73.7	73.5	73.2	73.0	72.9	72.7	72.6	72.5	72.4	72.4	72.2	72.1	72.0
73										74.7	74.5	74.3	74.0	73.9	73.7	73.6	73.5	73.4	73.4	73.2	73.1	73.0
74														74.9	74.7	74.6	74.5	74.4	74.4	74.2	74.1	74.0

TABLE 18. *Retarded girls: percentage and estimated mature height for girls with skeletal age one year or more retarded for the chronological age (skeletal ages 6–11 years)*

Skeletal Age	6-0	6-3	6-6	6-10	7-0	7-3	7-6	7-10	8-0	8-3	8-6	8-10	9-0	9-3	9-6	9-9	10-0	10-3	10-6	10-9	11-0	11-3	11-6	11-9
% of Mature Height	73.3	74.2	75.1	76.3	77.0	77.9	78.8	79.7	80.4	81.3	82.3	83.6	84.1	85.1	85.8	86.6	87.4	88.4	89.6	90.7	91.8	92.2	92.6	92.9
Ht. (inches) 38	51.8	51.2																						
39	53.2	52.6	51.9	51.1																				
40	54.6	53.9	53.3	52.4	51.9	51.3																		
41	55.9	55.3	54.6	53.7	53.2	52.6	52.0	51.4																
42	57.3	56.6	55.9	55.0	54.5	53.9	53.3	52.7	52.2	51.7	51.0													
43	58.7	58.0	57.3	56.4	55.8	55.2	54.6	54.0	53.5	52.9	52.2	51.4	51.1											
44	60.0	59.3	58.6	57.7	57.1	56.5	55.8	55.2	54.7	54.1	53.5	52.6	52.3	51.7	51.3									
45	61.4	60.6	59.9	59.0	58.4	57.8	57.1	56.5	56.0	55.4	54.7	53.8	53.5	52.9	52.4	52.0	51.5							
46	62.8	62.0	61.3	60.3	59.7	59.1	58.4	57.7	57.2	56.6	55.9	55.0	54.7	54.1	53.6	53.1	52.6	52.0	51.3					
47	64.1	63.3	62.6	61.6	61.0	60.3	59.6	59.0	58.5	57.8	57.1	56.2	55.9	55.2	54.8	54.3	53.8	53.2	52.5	51.8	51.2	51.0		
48	65.5	64.7	63.9	62.9	62.3	61.6	60.9	60.2	59.7	59.0	58.3	57.4	57.1	56.4	55.9	55.4	54.9	54.3	53.6	52.9	52.3	52.1	51.8	51.7
49	66.9	66.0	65.2	64.2	63.6	62.9	62.2	61.5	60.9	60.3	59.5	58.6	58.3	57.6	57.1	56.6	56.1	55.4	54.7	54.0	53.4	53.1	52.9	52.7
50	68.2	67.4	66.6	65.5	64.9	64.2	63.5	62.7	62.2	61.5	60.8	59.8	59.5	58.8	58.3	57.7	57.2	56.6	55.8	55.1	54.5	54.2	54.0	53.8
51	69.6	68.7	67.9	66.8	66.2	65.5	64.7	64.0	63.4	62.7	62.0	61.0	60.6	59.9	59.4	58.9	58.4	57.7	56.9	56.2	55.6	55.3	55.1	54.9
52	70.9	70.1	69.2	68.2	67.5	66.8	66.0	65.2	64.7	64.0	63.2	62.2	61.8	61.1	60.6	60.0	59.5	58.8	58.0	57.3	56.6	56.4	56.2	56.0
53	72.3	71.4	70.6	69.5	68.8	68.0	67.3	66.5	65.9	65.2	64.4	63.4	63.0	62.3	61.8	61.2	60.6	60.0	59.2	58.4	57.7	57.5	57.2	57.1
54	73.7	72.8	71.9	70.8	70.1	69.3	68.5	67.8	67.2	66.4	65.6	64.6	64.2	63.5	62.9	62.4	61.8	61.1	60.3	59.5	58.8	58.6	58.3	58.1
55		74.1	73.2	72.1	71.4	70.6	69.8	69.0	68.4	67.7	66.8	65.8	65.4	64.6	64.1	63.5	62.9	62.2	61.4	60.6	59.9	59.7	59.4	59.2
56			74.6	73.4	72.7	71.9	71.1	70.3	69.7	68.9	68.0	67.0	66.6	65.8	65.3	64.7	64.1	63.3	62.5	61.7	61.0	60.7	60.5	60.3
57				74.7	74.0	73.2	72.3	71.5	70.9	70.1	69.3	68.2	67.8	67.0	66.4	65.8	65.2	64.5	63.6	62.8	62.1	61.8	61.6	61.4
58						74.5	73.6	72.8	72.1	71.3	70.5	69.4	69.0	68.2	67.6	67.0	66.4	65.6	64.7	63.9	63.2	62.9	62.6	62.4
59							74.9	74.0	73.4	72.6	71.7	70.6	70.2	69.3	68.8	68.1	67.5	66.7	65.8	65.0	64.3	64.0	63.7	63.5
60									74.6	73.8	72.9	71.8	71.3	70.5	69.9	69.3	68.7	67.9	67.0	66.2	65.4	65.1	64.8	64.6
61											74.1	73.0	72.5	71.7	71.1	70.4	69.8	69.0	68.1	67.3	66.4	66.2	65.9	65.7
62												74.2	73.7	72.9	72.3	71.6	70.9	70.1	69.2	68.4	67.5	67.2	67.0	66.7
63													74.7	74.0	73.4	72.7	72.1	71.3	70.3	69.5	68.6	68.3	68.0	67.8
64															74.6	73.9	73.2	72.4	71.4	70.6	69.7	69.4	69.1	68.9
65																	74.4	73.5	72.5	71.7	70.8	70.5	70.2	70.0
66																		74.7	73.7	72.8	71.9	71.6	71.3	71.0
67																			74.8	73.9	73.0	72.7	72.4	72.1
68																					74.1	73.8	73.4	73.2
69																						74.8	74.5	74.3

TABLE 19. *Retarded girls: percentage and estimated mature height for girls with skeletal age one year or more retarded for the chronological age (skeletal ages 12–17 years)*

Skeletal Age	12-0	12-3	12-6	12-9	13-0	13-3	13-6	13-9	14-0	14-3	14-6	14-9	15-0	15-3	15-6	15-9	16-0	16-3	16-6	16-9	17-0
% of Mature Height	93.2	94.2	94.9	95.7	96.4	97.1	97.7	98.1	98.3	98.6	98.9	99.2	99.4	99.5	99.6	99.7	99.8	99.9	99.9	99.95	100.0
Ht. (inches) 48	51.5	51.0																			
49	52.6	52.0	51.6	51.2																	
50	53.6	53.1	52.7	52.2	51.9	51.5	51.2	51.0													
51	54.7	54.1	53.7	53.3	52.9	52.5	52.2	52.0	51.9	51.7	51.6	51.4	51.3	51.3	51.2	51.2	51.1	51.1	51.1	51.0	51.0
52	55.8	55.2	54.8	54.3	53.9	53.6	53.2	53.0	52.9	52.7	52.6	52.4	52.3	52.3	52.2	52.2	52.1	52.1	52.1	52.0	52.0
53	56.9	56.3	55.8	55.4	55.0	54.6	54.2	54.0	53.9	53.8	53.6	53.4	53.3	53.3	53.2	53.2	53.1	53.1	53.1	53.0	53.0
54	57.9	57.3	56.9	56.4	56.0	55.6	55.3	55.0	54.9	54.8	54.6	54.4	54.3	54.3	54.2	54.2	54.1	54.1	54.1	54.0	54.0
55	59.0	58.4	58.0	57.5	57.1	56.6	56.3	56.1	56.0	55.8	55.6	55.4	55.3	55.3	55.2	55.2	55.1	55.1	55.1	55.0	55.0
56	60.1	59.4	59.0	58.5	58.1	57.7	57.3	57.1	57.0	56.8	56.6	56.5	56.3	56.2	56.2	56.1	56.1	56.1	56.1	56.0	56.0
57	61.2	60.5	60.1	59.6	59.1	58.7	58.3	58.1	58.0	57.8	57.6	57.5	57.3	57.3	57.2	57.2	57.1	57.1	57.1	57.0	57.0
58	62.2	61.6	61.1	60.6	60.2	59.7	59.4	59.1	59.0	58.8	58.6	58.5	58.3	58.3	58.2	58.2	58.1	58.1	58.1	58.0	58.0
59	63.3	62.6	62.2	61.7	61.2	60.8	60.4	60.1	60.0	59.8	59.7	59.5	59.4	59.3	59.2	59.2	59.1	59.1	59.1	59.0	59.0
60	64.4	63.7	63.2	62.7	62.2	61.8	61.4	61.2	61.0	60.9	60.7	60.5	60.4	60.3	60.2	60.2	60.1	60.1	60.1	60.0	60.0
61	65.5	64.8	64.3	63.7	63.3	62.8	62.4	62.2	62.1	61.9	61.7	61.5	61.4	61.3	61.2	61.2	61.1	61.1	61.1	61.0	61.0
62	66.5	65.8	65.3	64.8	64.3	63.9	63.5	63.2	63.1	62.9	62.7	62.5	62.4	62.3	62.2	62.2	62.1	62.1	62.1	62.0	62.0
63	67.6	66.9	66.4	65.8	65.3	64.9	64.5	64.2	64.1	63.9	63.7	63.5	63.4	63.3	63.3	63.2	63.1	63.1	63.1	63.0	63.0
64	68.7	67.9	67.4	66.9	66.4	65.9	65.5	65.2	65.1	64.9	64.7	64.5	64.4	64.3	64.3	64.2	64.1	64.1	64.1	64.0	64.0
65	69.7	69.0	68.5	67.9	67.4	66.9	66.5	66.3	66.1	65.9	65.7	65.5	65.4	65.3	65.3	65.2	65.1	65.1	65.1	65.0	65.0
66	70.8	70.1	69.5	69.0	68.5	68.0	67.6	67.3	67.1	66.9	66.7	66.5	66.4	66.3	66.3	66.2	66.1	66.1	66.1	66.0	66.0
67	71.9	71.1	70.6	70.0	69.5	69.0	68.6	68.3	68.2	68.0	67.7	67.5	67.4	67.3	67.3	67.2	67.1	67.1	67.1	67.0	67.0
68	73.0	72.2	71.7	71.1	70.5	70.0	69.6	69.3	69.2	69.0	68.8	68.6	68.4	68.3	68.2	68.1	68.1	68.1	68.1	68.0	68.0
69	74.0	73.2	72.7	72.1	71.6	71.1	70.6	70.3	70.2	70.0	69.8	69.6	69.4	69.3	69.3	69.2	69.1	69.1	69.1	69.0	69.0
70		74.3	73.8	73.1	72.6	72.1	71.6	71.4	71.2	71.0	70.8	70.6	70.4	70.4	70.3	70.2	70.1	70.1	70.1	70.0	70.0
71			74.8	74.2	73.6	73.1	72.7	72.4	72.2	72.0	71.8	71.6	71.4	71.4	71.3	71.2	71.1	71.1	71.1	71.0	71.0
72					74.7	74.2	73.7	73.4	73.3	73.0	72.8	72.6	72.4	72.4	72.3	72.2	72.2	72.1	72.1	72.1	72.0
73							74.7	74.4	74.3	74.0	73.8	73.6	73.4	73.4	73.3	73.2	73.2	73.1	73.1	73.1	73.0
74											74.8	74.6	74.4	74.4	74.3	74.2	74.1	74.1	74.1	74.0	74.0

Source: Bayley N, Pinneau SR. Tables for predicting adult height from skeletal age: revised for use with the Greulich-Pyle hand standards. *J Pediatr* 1952;40:423–41.

Center of Gravity

This section represents a series of measurements of 1,172 living subjects (596 males and 576 females) whose ages ranged from birth to 20 years, and of 18 fetal cadavers having body lengths of 25 to 55 cm. The material was collected in Minneapolis and St. Paul, Minnesota, and Moose Heart, Illinois.

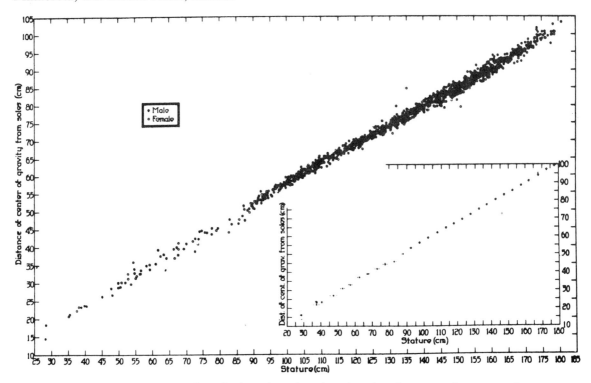

FIG. 33. Distance of the center of gravity from the soles plotted against the stature from approximately the sixth fetal month to maturity. The inset represents the relationship between the distance of the center of gravity from the soles versus stature. Dots in this graph mark the intersection of the mean height of the center of gravity and the mean stature for each 5 cm interval of stature.

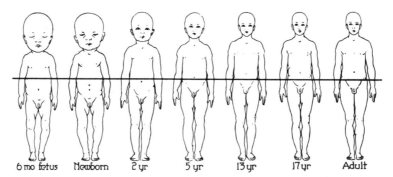

FIG. 34. Ventral aspect of the body at intervals from the sixth fetal month to maturity. Body lengths are reduced to the same scale, and the transverse plane of gravity is represented by a transverse line. The distance of the center of gravity above the soles is expressed as an index or percent of stature and maintains a fairly constant ratio, ranging from 55.0 to 59.0 during the whole of the developmental period. The coefficient of correlation (r) between the distance of the center of gravity above the soles and the stature was 0.99. The most precise statement of this relationship between the distance and the stature was expressed by the analytical equation $y = 0.557x + 1.4$ cm, where y equals the distance from the center of the soles and x equals stature.

Source: Palmer CE. Studies of the center of gravity in the human body. *Child Dev* 1944;15:99–180.

TABLE 20. Intervals of stature: means and variability of height of transverse plane of gravity from soles (females)

Interval of stature (cm.)	Number of cases	Mean and probable error (cm.)	Standard deviation (cm.)	Coefficient of variability (percent)
25– 30	0	-	-	-
30– 35	0	-	-	-
35– 40	4	22.03 ± 0.40	1.20	5.44
40– 45	0	-	-	-
45– 50	1	28.70 +	-	-
50– 55	8	30.95 + 0.53	2.23	7.21
55– 60	3	32.83 + 0.88	2.26	6.88
60– 65	2	38.60 + 0.40	0.85	2.20
65– 70	5	37.00 + 0.69	2.28	6.16
70– 75	2	41.25 + 0.23	0.49	1.88
75– 30	1	44.80 +	-	-
80– 85	1	44.10 +	-	-
85– 90	9	50.78 + 0.37	1.63	3.21
90– 95	16	53.93 + 0.21	1.25	2.32
95–100	15	56.33 + 0.18	1.03	1.83
100–105	21	58.97 + 0.18	1.22	2.06
105–110	31	62.20 + 0.13	1.08	1.73
110–115	16	65.13 + 0.11	0.66	1.01
115–120	18	67.02 + 0.20	1.25	1.86
120–125	30	69.67 + 0.12	0.94	1.35
125–130	25	72.46 + 0.13	0.99	1.37
130–135	38	74.94 + 0.15	1.35	1.80
135–140	30	77.67 + 0.22	1.75	2.25
140–145	40	80.37 + 0.14	1.31	1.63
145–150	54	82.78 + 0.15	1.58	1.91
150–155	60	85.28 + 0.15	1.76	2.06
155–160	70	83.37 + 0.10	1.22	1.38
160–165	57	90.47 + 0.12	1.30	1.43
165–170	18	93.83 + 0.22	1.36	1.45
170–175	6	97.12 + 0.81	2.95	3.04
175–180	3	99.20 + 0.51	1.31	1.32
180–185	-	-	-	-

TABLE 21. Intervals of stature: means and variability of height of transverse plane of gravity from soles (males)

Interval of stature (cm.)	Number of cases	Mean and probable error (cm.)	Standard deviation (cm.)	Coefficient of variability (percent)
25– 30	2	16.5 ± 0.86	0.18	10.91
30– 35	0	-	-	-
35– 40	1	23.3 +	-	-
40– 45	2	23.75 + 0.06	0.06	2.53
45– 50	2	26.60 + 0.43	0.90	3.38
50– 55	3	32.23 + 0.55	1.42	4.41
55– 60	5	33.42 + 0.30	0.91	2.72
60– 65	3	36.57 + 0.47	1.21	3.31
65– 70	2	39.70 + 0.09	0.20	1.40
70– 75	6	42.27 + 0.60	2.17	5.13
75– 80	5	44.52 + 0.24	0.80	1.80
80– 85	2	47.05 + 0.57	1.20	2.55
85– 90	5	49.50 + 0.74	2.20	4.44
90– 95	15	53.47 + 0.21	1.20	2.34
95–100	18	56.82 + 0.15	0.92	1.62
100–105	35	59.62 + 0.12	1.09	1.83
105–110	27	62.31 + 0.15	1.16	1.86
110–115	27	64.87 + 0.15	1.18	1.82
115–120	25	67.45 + 0.14	0.99	1.47
120–125	26	69.93 + 0.13	0.95	1.36
125–130	29	72.30 + 0.17	1.39	1.92
130–135	44	75.37 + 0.11	1.10	1.46
135–140	47	77.84 + 0.10	1.04	1.34
140–145	55	80.68 + 0.11	1.26	1.56
145–150	48	83.54 + 0.12	1.27	1.52
150–155	39	85.97 + 0.13	1.18	1.37
155–160	18	89.24 + 0.22	1.41	1.58
160–165	25	92.16 + 0.14	1.05	1.13
165–170	45	94.14 + 0.13	1.30	1.38
170–175	31	97.25 + 0.18	1.51	1.55
175–180	16	99.67 + 0.22	1.29	1.29
180–185	1	103.1 +	-	-

Source: Palmer CE. Studies of the center of gravity in the human body. *Child Dev* 1944;15:99–180.

Standing Center of Gravity

Data in this section are from a national sample representative of the United States population consisting of 74 primary sampling units: 4,027 infants and children in schools from eight states. Children 2 to 18 years of age were selected and measured by sophisticated electronic and computer systems. The group is thought to represent a true random survey of children in these age ranges.

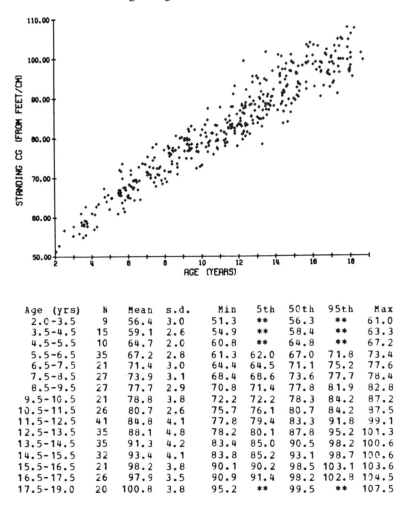

Age (yrs)	N	Mean	s.d.	Min	5th	50th	95th	Max
2.0-3.5	9	56.4	3.0	51.3	**	56.3	**	61.0
3.5-4.5	15	59.1	2.6	54.9	**	58.4	**	63.3
4.5-5.5	10	64.7	2.0	60.8	**	64.8	**	67.2
5.5-6.5	35	67.2	2.8	61.3	62.0	67.0	71.8	73.4
6.5-7.5	21	71.4	3.0	64.4	64.5	71.1	75.2	77.6
7.5-8.5	27	73.9	3.1	68.4	68.6	73.6	77.7	78.4
8.5-9.5	27	77.7	2.9	70.8	71.4	77.8	81.9	82.8
9.5-10.5	21	78.8	3.8	72.2	72.2	78.3	84.2	87.2
10.5-11.5	26	80.7	2.6	75.7	76.1	80.7	84.2	87.5
11.5-12.5	41	84.8	4.1	77.8	79.4	83.3	91.8	99.1
12.5-13.5	35	88.1	4.8	78.2	80.1	87.8	95.2	101.3
13.5-14.5	35	91.3	4.2	83.4	85.0	90.5	98.2	100.6
14.5-15.5	32	93.4	4.1	83.8	85.2	93.1	98.7	100.6
15.5-16.5	21	98.2	3.8	90.1	90.2	98.5	103.1	103.6
16.5-17.5	26	97.9	3.5	90.9	91.4	98.2	102.8	104.5
17.5-19.0	20	100.8	3.8	95.2	**	99.5	**	107.5

FIG. 35.   Standing center of gravity in males versus age.

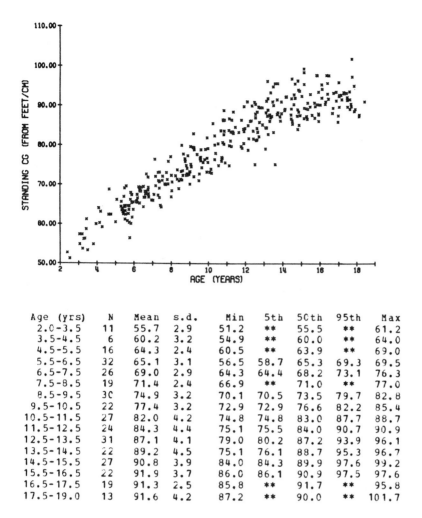

Age (yrs)	N	Mean	s.d.	Min	5th	50th	95th	Max
2.0-3.5	11	55.7	2.9	51.2	**	55.5	**	61.2
3.5-4.5	6	60.2	3.2	54.9	**	60.0	**	64.0
4.5-5.5	16	64.3	2.4	60.5	**	63.9	**	69.0
5.5-6.5	32	65.1	3.1	56.5	58.7	65.3	69.3	69.5
6.5-7.5	26	69.0	2.9	64.3	64.4	68.2	73.1	76.3
7.5-8.5	19	71.4	2.4	66.9	**	71.0	**	77.0
8.5-9.5	30	74.9	3.2	70.1	70.5	73.5	79.7	82.8
9.5-10.5	22	77.4	3.2	72.9	72.9	76.6	82.2	85.4
10.5-11.5	27	82.0	4.2	74.8	74.8	83.0	87.7	88.7
11.5-12.5	24	84.3	4.4	75.1	75.5	84.0	90.7	90.9
12.5-13.5	31	87.1	4.1	79.0	80.2	87.2	93.9	96.1
13.5-14.5	22	89.2	4.5	75.1	76.1	88.7	95.3	96.7
14.5-15.5	27	90.8	3.9	84.0	84.3	89.9	97.6	99.2
15.5-16.5	22	91.9	3.7	86.0	86.1	90.9	97.5	97.6
16.5-17.5	19	91.3	2.5	85.8	**	91.7	**	95.8
17.5-19.0	13	91.6	4.2	87.2	**	90.0	**	101.7

FIG. 36. Standing center of gravity from the feet in females versus age.

Source: Snyder RS, Schneider LW, Owings CL, Reynolds HM, Golomb DH, Schork MA. Anthropometry of infants, children and youths, to age eighteen, for product safety design. SP-450, sponsored by the Highway Safety Research Institute, University of Michigan. Published by the Society of Automotive Engineers, Warrendale, PA.

Mean Sitting Height

The data in this section were obtained from the cycle 2 study of the health examination survey conducted from 1963 to 1965. This involved selection and examination of a probability sample of noninstitutionalized children in the United States aged 6–11 years. This program succeeded in examining 96% of the 7,417 children selected for this sample.

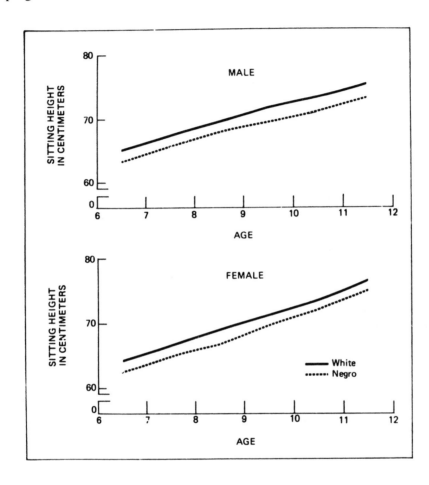

FIG. 37.   Mean sitting height of white and black children by sex and age.

TABLE 22. *Sitting height of children by race, sex, and age at last birthday*

Race, sex, and age	n	N	$\bar{X}$	s	$s_{\bar{x}}$	Percentile						
						5th	10th	25th	50th	75th	90th	95th
WHITE						In centimeters						
Boys												
6 years-----------------	489	1,787	65.0	2.68	0.13	60.4	61.4	63.2	65.1	66.7	68.5	69.7
7 years-----------------	551	1,781	67.2	2.74	0.15	63.0	64.0	65.4	67.2	68.9	70.8	71.8
8 years-----------------	537	1,739	69.5	2.94	0.12	65.1	65.7	67.6	69.6	71.5	73.3	74.3
9 years-----------------	525	1,730	71.6	3.15	0.19	66.4	67.4	69.6	71.6	73.7	75.6	76.7
10 years---------------	509	1,692	73.3	3.07	0.20	68.3	69.5	71.4	73.3	75.4	77.3	78.7
11 years---------------	542	1,662	75.6	3.10	0.13	70.6	71.5	73.5	75.5	77.7	79.6	80.7
Girls												
6 years-----------------	461	1,722	64.2	3.00	0.18	59.2	60.4	62.3	64.3	66.1	68.2	69.1
7 years-----------------	512	1,716	66.4	2.99	0.12	61.5	62.6	64.3	66.5	68.4	70.4	71.4
8 years-----------------	498	1,674	68.8	2.89	0.13	63.7	64.8	67.1	68.9	70.8	72.4	73.3
9 years-----------------	494	1,663	71.1	3.19	0.17	65.8	67.1	68.9	71.1	73.4	75.3	76.3
10 years---------------	505	1,632	73.5	3.39	0.14	68.2	69.2	71.1	73.5	75.7	77.6	79.1
11 years---------------	477	1,605	76.5	3.96	0.15	70.4	72.0	74.2	76.2	78.8	81.6	83.7
NEGRO												
Boys												
6 years-----------------	84	289	63.2	2.48	0.35	59.2	59.7	61.4	63.2	64.8	66.5	68.1
7 years-----------------	79	286	65.6	2.58	0.29	61.6	62.3	63.5	65.6	67.5	69.1	70.1
8 years-----------------	79	279	67.8	2.81	0.29	63.5	64.3	66.2	67.5	71.8	72.7	72.7
9 years-----------------	74	269	69.3	3.69	0.40	63.7	64.5	66.7	68.6	71.7	74.5	75.8
10 years---------------	65	264	70.9	3.54	0.33	64.8	66.1	68.3	70.6	73.2	75.4	77.5
11 years---------------	83	255	73.4	3.36	0.37	67.8	68.7	71.4	73.6	74.8	77.5	79.3
Girls												
6 years-----------------	72	281	62.3	2.78	0.35	57.4	58.8	60.4	62.3	64.5	66.2	66.6
7 years-----------------	93	284	64.9	3.05	0.40	60.0	61.2	62.7	64.7	67.0	69.3	70.5
8 years-----------------	113	281	66.6	3.50	0.26	61.5	62.4	64.5	66.3	68.6	71.5	73.4
9 years-----------------	84	265	69.6	3.43	0.44	64.2	65.4	67.4	69.5	71.6	74.4	75.5
10 years---------------	77	266	71.9	3.77	0.48	66.3	67.6	69.3	71.5	74.4	76.8	78.9
11 years---------------	84	253	75.1	4.08	0.38	68.3	69.3	72.5	75.3	78.4	80.3	81.4

These are the data from which the graph in Fig. 37 was constructed. n = sample size; N = estimated number of children in population in thousands; $\bar{X}$ = mean; s = standard deviation; $s_{\bar{x}}$ = standard error of the mean.

Source: Hamill PV, Johnston FE, Gram W. Height and weight of children, United States: height and weight measurements by age, sex, race, geographic region of children 6 to 11 years of age, United States 1963–65. National Center for Health Statistics, Series II, No. 104; Public Health Service Publication No. 1011, No. 104, U.S. Government Printing Office, Washington, D.C., 1970.

Related Reference: Hamill PVV, Johnson FE, Lemeshow S. Body weight, stature and sitting height: White and Negro youths 12 to 17 years, United States. DHEW Publication No. (HRA) 74-1608, U.S. Government Printing Office, Washington, D.C., 1973.

Erect Sitting Height of Males and Females

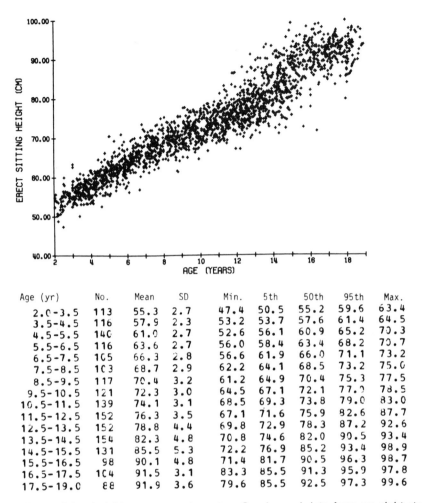

Age (yr)	No.	Mean	SD	Min.	5th	50th	95th	Max.
2.0-3.5	113	55.3	2.7	47.4	50.5	55.2	59.6	63.4
3.5-4.5	116	57.9	2.3	53.2	53.7	57.6	61.4	64.5
4.5-5.5	140	61.0	2.7	52.6	56.1	60.9	65.2	70.3
5.5-6.5	116	63.6	2.7	56.0	58.4	63.4	68.2	70.7
6.5-7.5	105	66.3	2.8	56.6	61.9	66.0	71.1	73.2
7.5-8.5	103	68.7	2.9	62.2	64.1	68.5	73.2	75.0
8.5-9.5	117	70.4	3.2	61.2	64.9	70.4	75.3	77.5
9.5-10.5	121	72.3	3.0	64.5	67.1	72.1	77.0	78.5
10.5-11.5	139	74.1	3.1	68.5	69.3	73.8	79.0	83.0
11.5-12.5	152	76.3	3.5	67.1	71.6	75.9	82.6	87.7
12.5-13.5	152	78.8	4.4	69.8	72.9	78.3	87.2	92.6
13.5-14.5	154	82.3	4.8	70.8	74.6	82.0	90.5	93.4
14.5-15.5	131	85.5	5.3	72.2	76.9	85.2	93.4	98.9
15.5-16.5	98	90.1	4.8	71.4	81.7	90.5	96.3	98.7
16.5-17.5	104	91.5	3.1	83.3	85.5	91.3	95.9	97.8
17.5-19.0	88	91.9	3.6	79.6	85.5	92.5	97.3	99.6

FIG. 38. Erect sitting height versus age in males. Graphs and data from an eight-state random survey of children thought to be representative of the United States population (see *Standing Center of Gravity* section).

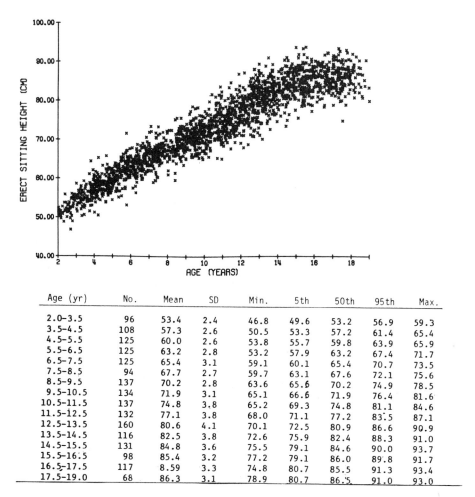

Age (yr)	No.	Mean	SD	Min.	5th	50th	95th	Max.
2.0–3.5	96	53.4	2.4	46.8	49.6	53.2	56.9	59.3
3.5–4.5	108	57.3	2.6	50.5	53.3	57.2	61.4	65.4
4.5–5.5	125	60.0	2.6	53.8	55.7	59.8	63.9	65.9
5.5–6.5	125	63.2	2.8	53.2	57.9	63.2	67.4	71.7
6.5–7.5	125	65.4	3.1	59.1	60.1	65.4	70.7	73.5
7.5–8.5	94	67.7	2.7	59.7	63.1	67.6	72.1	75.6
8.5–9.5	137	70.2	2.8	63.6	65.6	70.2	74.9	78.5
9.5–10.5	134	71.9	3.1	65.1	66.6	71.9	76.4	81.6
10.5–11.5	137	74.8	3.8	65.2	69.3	74.8	81.1	84.6
11.5–12.5	132	77.1	3.8	68.0	71.1	77.2	83.5	87.1
12.5–13.5	160	80.6	4.1	70.1	72.5	80.9	86.6	90.9
13.5–14.5	116	82.5	3.8	72.6	75.9	82.4	88.3	91.0
14.5–15.5	131	84.8	3.6	75.5	79.1	84.6	90.0	93.7
15.5–16.5	98	85.4	3.2	77.2	79.1	86.0	89.8	91.7
16.5–17.5	117	8.59	3.3	74.8	80.7	85.5	91.3	93.4
17.5–19.0	68	86.3	3.1	78.9	80.7	86.5	91.0	93.0

FIG. 39. Erect sitting height versus age in females.

Source: Snyder RS, Schneider LW, Owings CL, Reynolds HM, Golomb DH, Schork MA. Anthropometry of infants, children and youths, to age eighteen, for product safety design. SP-450, sponsored by the Highway Safety Research Institute, University of Michigan. Published by the Society of Automotive Engineers, Warrendale, PA.

Growth Remaining in Sitting Height

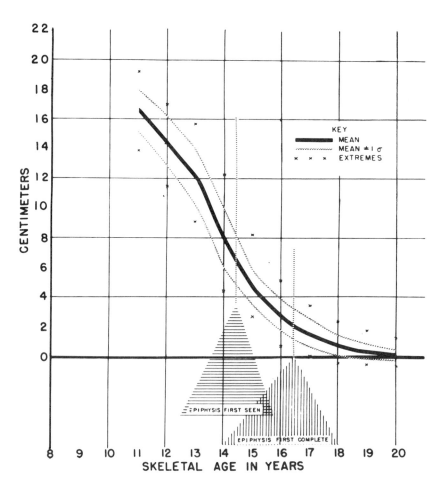

FIG. 40. Growth remaining in the trunk (sitting height) at consecutive skeletal age levels for 24 boys. The curves indicate averages and ranges for the residual growth observed after the attainment of given skeletal ages. Superimposed on these curves for comparison purposes are the ranges of skeletal age in the same children at which the two stages of ossification of the iliac epiphyses appeared (indicated by the location and length of the bases of the shaded areas). The length of the associated vertical bars, positioned at the average skeletal age when these events were observed, indicate the range of growth after this time in the individual children. Skeletal age seems to be the better index of the two for estimating the amount of future growth of the individual child

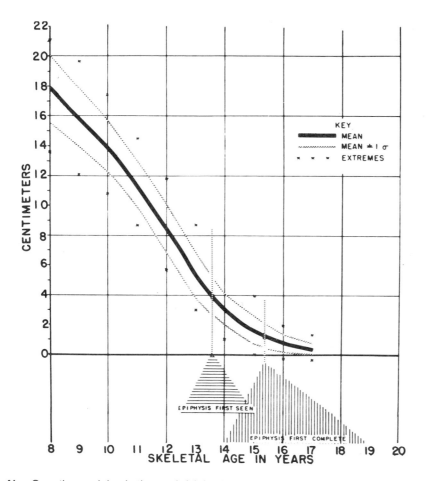

FIG. 41. Growth remaining in the trunk (sitting height) at consecutive skeletal age levels for 31 girls. (See legend to Fig. 40 for further explanation.)

Source: Anderson M, Hwang S-C, Green WT. Growth of the normal trunk in boys and girls during the second decade of life, related to age, maturity and ossification of the iliac epiphyses. *J Bone Joint Surg (Am)* 1965;47:1554–63.

TABLE 23. *Age at first appearance of four commonly used indicators of maturity and observed amounts of growth in sitting height following each variant*

		Chronological Age (Years)	Skeletal Age (Years)	Growth of Trunk Remaining (Centimeters)
First ossification iliac epiphysis				
31 girls:	earliest	10.00	12.50	8.40 max.
	average	13.29	13.57	4.05 aver.
	latest	16.50	15.00	0.10 min.
24 boys:	earliest	11.50	12.50	16.20 max.
	average	14.27	14.43	6.54 aver.
	latest	15.50	15.75	3.50 min.
Ossification completed in iliac epiphysis				
31 girls:	earliest	11.50	14.00	3.70 max.
	average	15.15	15.63	1.20 aver.
	latest	>19.00	>18.00	−0.50 min.
24 boys:	earliest	14.00	14.00	7.30 máx.
	average	16.00	16.45	2.51 aver.
	latest	18.50	18.00	0.00 min.
Year maximum growth				
31 girls:	earliest	9–10	9–10	10.4 max.
	average	12–13	12–13	5.6 aver.
	latest	15–16	13–14	1.7 min.
24 boys:	earliest	12–13	12–13	10.1 max.
	average	13–14	13–14	7.0 aver.
	latest	15–16	15–16	1.9 min.
Menarche				
31 girls:	earliest	10.08	11.50	9.5 max.
	average	13.04	13.17	4.6 aver.
	latest	15.83	14.50	2.1 min.

Values are derived from a longitudinal series of 55 children with normal trunks.

Source: Anderson M, Hwang S-C, Green WT. Growth of the normal trunk in boys and girls during the second decade of life, related to age, maturity and ossification of the iliac epiphyses. *J Bone Joint Surg (Am)* 1965;47:1554–63.

Diurnal Height Differences

All measurements were made immediately upon the child rising from bed in the morning and again at 4:00 or 5:00 in the afternoon. The differences in a.m. and p.m. heights were recorded in centimeters. Height differences were obtained on ambulatory children (ages 3 to 14 years) admitted to the pediatric ward of Walter Reed General Hospital over a 3-month period.

TABLE 24. *Diurnal a.m. and p.m. height differences of 100 children*

Variable	Value
Range of variation (cm)	0.80–2.8
Mean difference (cm)	1.54
Standard deviation (cm)	0.46
Standard error (cm)	0.04
No. of observations	100

Source: Strickland AL, Shearn RB. Diurnal height variation in children. *J Pediatr* 1972;80:1023–5.

HAND

Early Development

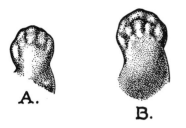

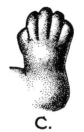

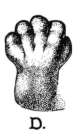

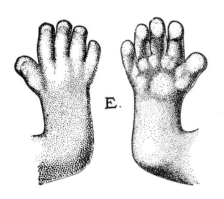

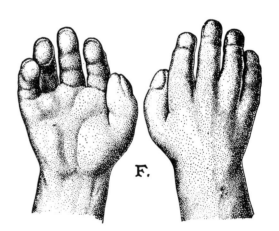

FIG. 1. Series showing various stages of early development of the upper extremity, after Retzius (Retzius G. Zur kenntnis der entwichlung der Korperforman des menschen wahrend der fotalen lebensstuben *Biol Untersuch NF* 1904;11:33–76). **A:** Anterior limb bud of an embryo 12 mm long. **B:** Anterior limb bud of an embryo 15 mm long. **C:** Anterior limb bud of an embryo 17 mm long. **D:** Hand and forearm of an embryo 20 mm long. **E:** Two views of a hand and forearm of an embryo 25 mm long. **F:** Two views of the hand of a fetus 52 mm long.

Source: Morris H. *Human anatomy, a complete systematic treatise.* 11th Ed. New York: McGraw-Hill Book Company, 1953.

Appearance of Ossification Centers

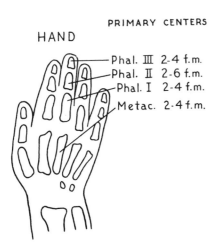

PRIMARY CENTERS

HAND

Phal. III 2-4 f.m.
Phal. II 2-6 f.m.
Phal. I 2-4 f.m.
Metac. 2-4 f.m.

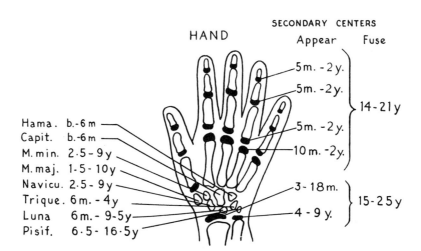

SECONDARY CENTERS

HAND   Appear   Fuse

5m. -2y.
5m. -2y.
}14-21y
5m. -2y.
10m. -2y.

Hama. b.-6m
Capit. b.-6m
M. min. 2.5-9y
M. maj. 1.5-10y
Navicu. 2.5-9y
Trique. 6m. -4y
Luna 6m.- 9.5y
Pisif. 6.5- 16.5y

3-18m.
}15-25y
4-9 y.

FIG. 2. Time schedule for appearance of the primary and secondary ossification centers and fusion of secondary centers with shafts of the hands. f.m. = Fetal months; m = months; y = year.

Source: Caffey J. *Pediatric x-ray diagnosis.* 7th Ed, 1978.

Appearance of the Ossification Centers of the Hand

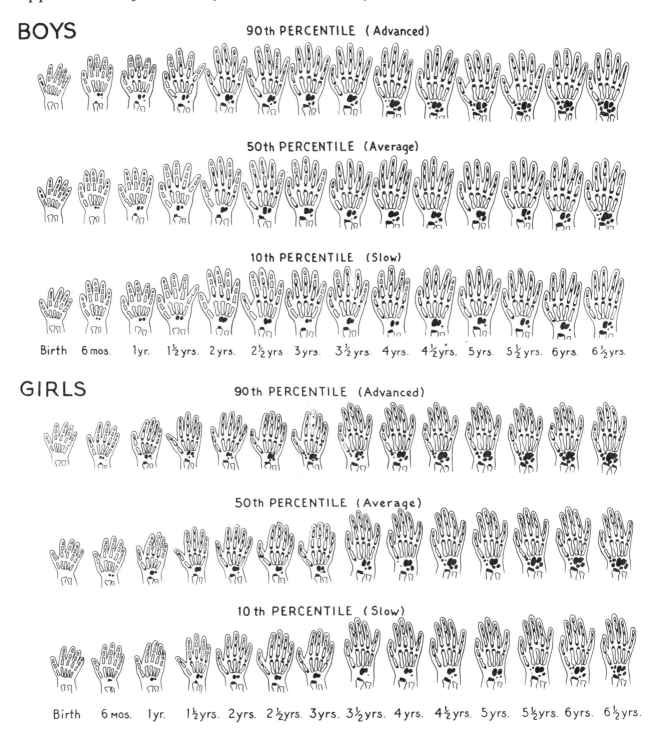

FIG. 3. Appearance of hand roentgenograms for boys and girls. A total of 228 infants were roentgenographed at birth (112 girls, 116 boys) and then at 3-month intervals during the first year, and thereafter at 6-month intervals. In the top row are advanced (90th percentile), middle row, average (50th percentile), and the bottom row, slowest (10th percentile).

Source: Vogt EC, Vickers VS. Osseous growth and development. *Radiology* 1938;31:441– 4.

Appearance of Metacarpal and Metatarsal Centers

Figures 4 and 5, and Tables 1 and 2 are based on the data of Francis and Werle, who studied a selected group of 307 boys and 315 girls in Cleveland, Ohio. The data represent a total of 1,728 observations at varying intervals over a period of 5 years.

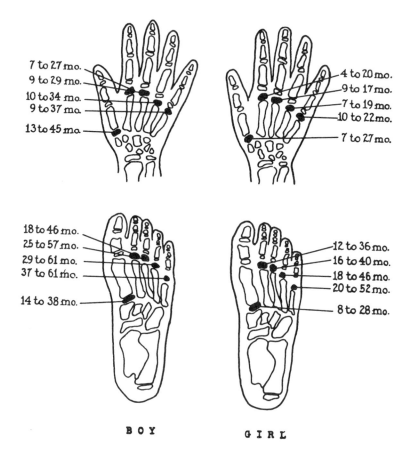

FIG. 4. Age ranges for the appearance of the metacarpal and metatarsal centers. Age ranges include the two standard deviations above and below the means.

Source: Francis CC, and Werle PP. The appearance of centers of ossification from birth to five years. *Am J Phys Anthropol* 1939;24:273.

TABLE 1. *Percentage of children with ossified centers by age*

Bone	Age (mo) 6	9	Age (yr) 1	1 1/2	2	2 1/2	3	3 1/2	4	4 1/2	5
Girls											
Metacarpal II	2	12	48	96	100						
Metacarpal III	2	9	43	95	99	100					
Metacarpal IV	1	5	32	88	99	100					
Metacarpal V	1	3	14	78	96	99	100				
Metacarpal I	1	1	8	65	94	99	100				
Metatarsal I		1	4	49	89	97	100				
Metatarsal II				14	60	90	97	98	100		
Metatarsal III				3	31	69	94	97	99	100	
Metatarsal IV					11	38	76	93	97	100	
Metatarsal V					4	24	44	72	89	92	95
Boys											
Metacarpal II		1	13	62	94	99	100				
Metacarpal III			6	38	86	97	98	100			
Metacarpal IV			4	26	72	93	96	100			
Metacarpal V			1	18	57	88	91	100			
Metacarpal I				6	29	74	80	98	95	98	100
Metatarsal I				2	31	75	87	98	100		
Metatarsal II				3	10	45	70	94	95	98	100
Metatarsal III					4	10	20	57	87	96	100
Metatarsal IV						3	7	32	56	86	98
Metatarsal V						3	4	13	41	78	94

The most useful bones are in boldface.

TABLE 2. *Age of appearance of centers of ossification*

Bone	Age (mo) males Mean	SD	Age (mo) females Mean	SD
Metacarpal II	17	5	12	4
Metacarpal III	19	5	13	2
Metacarpal IV	22	6	13	3
Metacarpal V	23	7	16	3
Metacarpal I	29	8	17	5
Metatarsal I	26	6	18	5
Metatarsal II	32	7	24	6
Metatarsal III	41	8	28	6
Metatarsal IV	45	8	32	7
Metatarsal V	49	6	36	8

The most useful bones are in boldface.

Source: Milman DH, Bakwin H. Ossification of the metacarpal and metatarsal centers as a measure of maturation. *J Pediatr* 1950;36:617–20.

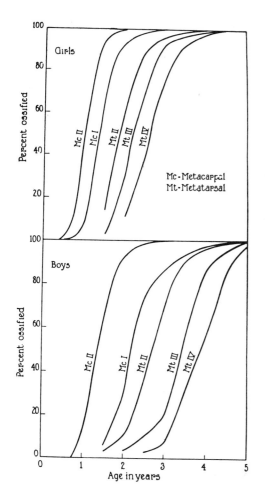

FIG. 5. Percentage of children with ossified centers by ages, from 6 months to 5 years. This is a graphic representation of the data in Table 1.

Source: Milman DH, Bakwin H. Ossification of the metacarpal and metatarsal centers as a measure of maturation. *J Pediatr* 1950;36:617–20.

Comparison of the Incidence and Degree of Inequality of Maturational Status in Right and Left Hand in 450 Children

TABLE 3. *Bilateral symmetry of skeletal maturation*

Osseous center	Right>Left (mo)											
	1–3			4–6			7–9			10–12		
	Boys	Girls	Total	Boys	Girls	Total	Boys	Girls	Total	Boys	Girls	Total
Capitate	41	41	82	20	28	48	5	4	9	4	2	6
Hamate	44	37	81	18	29	47	6	4	10	3	1	4
Triquetrum	24	33	57	25	28	53	6	2	8	5	2	7
Lunate	16	23	39	22	14	36	6	6	12	5	2	7
Navicular	13	28	41	21	25	46	9	4	13	3	6	9
Gtr. Multangular	17	19	36	9	14	23	8	3	11	5	3	8
Lsr. Multangular	16	13	29	14	21	35	7	2	9	5	2	7
Metacarpal I	45	60	105	31	22	53	11	3	14	3	2	5
II	51	63	114	19	23	42	9	7	16	3	4	7
III	54	61	115	19	21	40	9	6	15	0	5	5
IV	60	52	112	12	22	34	7	6	13	6	3	9
V	44	56	110	19	25	44	7	7	14	5	2	7
Prox. Phalanx I	45	51	96	21	19	40	6	6	12	8	4	12
II	42	50	92	15	22	37	12	7	19	6	5	11
III	48	46	94	28	22	50	8	6	14	5	6	11
IV	51	48	99	25	33	58	13	7	20	6	5	11
V	57	57	114	22	29	51	9	6	15	6	6	12
Mid. Phalanx II	58	71	129	29	27	56	14	14	28	5	2	7
III	56	64	120	30	31	61	14	12	26	5	3	8
IV	50	63	113	29	31	50	17	11	28	5	2	7
V	41	65	106	39	25	64	13	13	26	11	3	14
Dist. Phalanx I	49	40	89	22	20	42	9	6	15	6	4	10
II	40	47	87	38	21	59	11	6	17	4	3	7
III	47	45	92	20	21	41	14	6	20	5	1	6
IV	43	45	88	16	24	40	11	7	18	6	2	8
V	48	45	93	22	25	47	6	6	12	7	2	9
Radius	42	53	95	38	35	73	12	20	32	19	14	33
Ulna	18	24	42	15	11	26	12	4	16	7	9	16
Range	45	48	93	22	26	48	9	10	19	8	3	11
Skeletal Age	106	97	203	17	10	27	1	2	3	0	1	1

A total of 450 children were seen consecutively in Birmingham, Alabama. Roentgenograms of the right and left hands and wrists of each child were taken at the same visit, using identical procedures for each. Subjects ranged in age from 1 month to 16 years, 11 months, and included 227 boys and 223 girls.

The table demonstrates that in 291 (87%) of the 333 cases of inequality in skeletal age between the two sides, the difference was between 1 and 3 months. In 37 (11.5%) instances the difference was between 4 and 6 months, and in only five (1.5%) of the children did the discrepancy exceed 6 months. Deviations greater than 6 months were encountered more frequently in the lunate, metacarpal II, proximal phalanx I, middle phalanx, distal phalanx I, and the radius. Differences greater than 12 months were noted most commonly in the carpal area.

								Right<Left (mo)									
>12			1–3			4–6			7–9			10–12			>12		
Boys	Girls	Total	Boys	Girls	Total	Boys	Girls	Total	Boys	Girls	Total	Boys	Girls	Total	Boys	Girls	Total
0	2	2	33	17	50	12	24	36	8	5	13	7	6	13	3	2	5
0	2	2	28	41	69	21	18	39	6	5	11	4	5	9	0	1	1
1	4	5	20	33	53	16	12	28	5	4	9	1	5	6	2	1	3
2	4	6	22	31	53	15	24	39	10	12	22	12	5	17	4	5	9
1	0	1	12	26	38	9	7	16	2	0	2	5	3	8	1	5	6
2	2	4	14	22	36	16	20	36	13	6	19	5	8	13	2	6	8
0	3	3	11	20	31	17	13	30	9	6	15	6	6	12	2	4	6
2	2	4	32	35	67	9	10	19	7	3	10	3	1	4	0	2	2
2	1	3	37	35	72	17	11	28	11	4	15	1	1	2	1	1	2
1	4	5	42	26	68	24	12	36	5	3	8	5	2	7	3	1	4
0	4	4	40	37	77	21	17	38	7	6	13	5	1	6	0	1	1
1	1	2	39	37	76	22	17	39	6	2	8	2	1	3	0	1	1
1	1	2	30	38	68	22	21	43	10	9	19	9	6	15	4	1	5
0	2	2	47	35	82	10	13	23	9	3	12	3	4	7	1	0	1
1	1	2	43	29	72	16	17	33	4	2	6	4	2	6	0	1	1
0	1	1	37	25	62	13	10	23	8	3	11	3	0	3	1	0	1
1	1	2	39	25	64	18	15	33	2	1	3	5	1	6	0	0	0
2	1	3	28	22	50	9	8	17	6	2	8	2	3	5	0	0	0
2	1	3	23	21	44	15	15	30	5	0	5	1	3	4	1	0	1
0	1	1	20	27	47	15	14	29	8	3	11	1	2	3	1	0	1
4	1	5	30	17	47	12	17	29	6	5	11	3	3	6	2	1	3
6	3	9	27	26	53	17	12	29	9	10	19	7	9	16	1	0	1
4	1	5	23	28	51	11	17	28	6	2	8	2	1	3	0	1	1
1	1	2	30	34	64	12	15	27	7	3	10	4	1	5	0	0	0
1	2	3	25	38	63	20	12	32	5	2	7	6	3	9	0	0	0
1	2	3	23	24	47	18	19	37	4	4	8	6	0	6	0	0	0
5	7	12	27	22	49	18	11	29	2	6	8	2	1	3	1	0	1
8	5	13	9	8	17	10	5	15	4	4	8	3	0	3	1	0	1
4	7	11	45	42	87	26	30	56	11	8	19	8	4	12	7	5	12
0	1	1	46	42	88	6	4	10	0	0	0	0	0	0	0	0	0

Source: Dreizen S. Bilateral symmetry of skeletal maturation of the human hand and wrist. *Am J Dis Child* 1957;93:112–27.

Ossification of 29 Bone Growth Centers

TABLE 4. *Onset, completion, and span of ossification of 29 bone growth centers in the hand and wrist*

Bone growth center	Boys								Girls							
	Mean onset, order		Onset		Completion		Span		Mean onset, order		Onset		Completion		Span	
		No.	Mean	S.D.	Mean	S.D.	Mean	S.D.		No.	Mean	S.D.	Mean	S.D.	Mean	S.D
Capitate	1	56	2.9	1.7	183	12	180	12	1	53	2.5	1.8	159	10	157	10
Hamate	2	56	4.2	2.7	183	12	179	11	2	53	3.1	2.2	159	10	156	10
Radius, distal epiphysis	3	25	12.3	5.3	208	8	196	11	3	44	10.0	4.1	200	12	190	12
Finger 3, prox. phal. epiph.	4	57	16.4	4.6	191	12	175	12	4	56	10.6	3.2	166	12	155	11
Finger 2, prox. phal. epiph.	5	56	17.2	4.8	191	13	174	13	5	56	10.9	2.9	166	12	155	11
Finger 4, prox. phal. epiph.	6	56	18.1	5.0	191	13	173	13	6	56	11.0	3.2	166	12	155	11
Metacarpal 2, epiphysis	7	56	19.3	5.5	194	13	175	13	7	53	13.1	3.3	170	13	156	13
Finger 1, distal phal. epiph.	8	58	20.6	6.8	184	13	163	14	8	56	13.2	5.5	157	11	144	10
Metacarpal 3, epiphysis	9	56	21.8	6.9	195	13	173	14	9	53	14.4	3.9	170	13	156	13
Finger 5, prox. phal. epiph.	10	56	23.8	6.7	191	13	167	14	10	56	14.7	3.8	164	12	150	11
Metacarpal 4, epiphysis	11	56	24.8	7.3	194	13	170	14	11	53	15.5	3.8	169	14	153	14
Finger 3, middle phal. epiph.	12	56	25.1	6.2	192	13	167	14	12	56	15.7	5.4	167	12	152	11
Finger 4, middle phal. epiph.	13	56	26.0	6.7	192	13	166	14	13	55	16.0	5.2	168	12	152	11
Finger 2, middle phal. epiph.	14	56	27.1	7.1	191	12	164	14	14	56	17.0	5.4	166	12	149	11
Metacarpal 5, epiphysis	15	56	27.1	8.6	196	14	168	15	15	53	17.0	5.0	170	13	153	12
Triquetral	16	57	29.5	16.2	183	12	153	20	23	55	26.6	14.0	160	9	133	15
Finger 3, distal phal. epiph.	17	57	30.7	7.1	186	13	156	13	16	57	19.1	6.0	159	11	140	11
Finger 4, distal phal. epiph.	18	57	31.2	7.4	186	13	155	14	17	57	19.6	5.9	159	12	139	11
Metacarpal 1, epiphysis	19	56	34.8	11.1	187	14	152	16	18	55	19.9	5.4	164	13	144	12
Finger 1, prox. phal. epiph.	20	56	36.3	9.1	191	13	155	15	19	57	21.6	6.4	165	11	144	11
Finger 2, distal phal. epiph.	21	57	41.2	9.0	185	13	144	14	20	57	25.0	6.8	158	11	133	11
Finger 5, distal phal. epiph.	22	57	41.9	10.1	186	13	144	15	21	57	25.0	6.7	160	15	135	15
Lunate	23	58	43.5	14.7	183	11	140	16	24	55	36.1	17.3	160	9	124	16
Finger 5, middle phal. epiph.	24	56	44.4	11.9	190	13	146	15	22	55	25.9	8.3	165	12	139	12
Scaphoid	25	58	69.6	15.4	183	11	113	17	27	54	53.7	13.8	160	9	106	15
Trapezoid	26	58	72.0	16.1	183	11	111	15	26	55	51.8	12.3	160	9	108	13
Trapezium	27	58	72.7	18.4	183	11	110	19	25	54	51.6	16.4	160	9	108	18
Ulna, distal epiphysis	28	26	80.3	13.4	205	10	124	16	28	51	72.4	12.1	191	12	119	12
Adductor sesamoid (thumb)	29	50	150.8	13.7	192	14	41	14	29	47	127.8	10.3	167	14	39	13

Means and standard deviations are expressed in months.

The data are derived from longitudinal studies of child health and development at the Harvard School of Public Health between 1930 and 1956. Roentgenograms of the hand and wrist were obtained periodically between the ages of 3 months and 18 years in 66 boys and 67 girls.

Source: Stuart HC, Pyle, SI, Cornol J, Reed RB. Onsets, completions and spans of ossification in the 29 bone-growth centers of the hand and wrist. *Pediatrics*, 1962;29:237–49.

Mean Differences Between Skeletal Age and Chronological Age in Right and Left Hands of 450 Children

TABLE 5. *Skeletal age versus chronological age*

| Chronological age | Mean difference (mo) | | | | | |
| | Right hand | | | Left hand | | |
	Boys	Girls	Total	Boys	Girls	Total
1 mo–11 mo	1.55	1.17	1.39	1.73	1.33	1.52
1 yr–1 yr 11 mo	3.22	4.78	3.90	3.43	4.22	3.78
2 yr–2 yr 11 mo	6.68	6.09	6.36	6.76	6.91	6.86
3 yr–3 yr 11 mo	11.07	11.56	11.25	11.80	10.89	11.46
4 yr–4 yr 11 mo	11.20	9.87	10.40	10.80	9.93	10.28
5 yr–5 yr 11 mo	13.69	13.31	13.50	15.15	13.08	14.12
6 yr–6 yr 11 mo	16.25	16.85	16.18	15.92	17.23	16.19
7 yr–7 yr 11 mo	12.73	13.15	12.93	13.45	13.38	13.43
8 yr–8 yr 11 mo	9.06	8.69	8.88	10.75	9.13	9.94
9 yr–9 yr 11 mo	11.80	14.27	13.28	12.60	15.00	14.04
10 yr–10 yr 11 mo	10.05	12.95	11.54	10.84	13.85	12.38
11 yr–11 yr 11 mo	6.15	9.06	7.76	8.08	9.75	9.00
12 yr–12 yr 11 mo	9.94	10.27	10.09	10.82	10.60	10.72
13 yr–13 yr 11 mo	8.20	11.40	9.93	8.20	13.20	9.87
14 yr–14 yr 11 mo	8.18	6.67	7.50	7.55	6.22	6.95
15 yr–15 yr 11 mo	12.71	13.71	13.13	13.00	16.11	14.75
16 yr–16 yr 11 mo	10.83	7.50	10.00	10.67	9.50	10.37

The values represent the summation of both positive and negative differences, regardless of size. Only in age group 1 through 11 months did the mean difference fall below 3 months. Beginning with age group 2 years through 2 years 11 months did the mean deviation exceed 6 months in every instance. The peak mean difference of slightly more than 16 months was obtained for age group 6 years through 6 years, 11 months.

Source: Dreizen S, Bilateral symmetry of skeletal maturation of the human hand and wrist. *Am J Dis Child* 1957;93:112–27.

Epiphyseal Fusion

TABLE 6. *Modal ages for epiphyseal fusion in the hand-wrist of United States white youths*

| Hand-wrist bone | Modal age | | United States (1966–1970) | |
	Boys (refs.)	Girls (refs.)	Boys	Girls
Radius	18.0 (2)	15.8 (2)	—	—
Ulna	17.8 (2)	15.9 (2)	—	16.2
Metacarpal I	16.3 (1,2)	14.1 (1,2)	15.8	13.8
Metacarpal II	16.4 (1), 16.5 (2)	14.5 (2), 14.6 (1)	16.5	14.8
Metacarpal III	16.4 (1), 16.5 (2)	14.5 (2), 14.6 (1)	16.6	14.8
Metacarpal IV	16.4 (1,2)	14.4 (2), 14.6 (1)	16.6	14.9
Metacarpal V	16.5 (1,2)	14.4 (2), 15.0 (1)	16.6	15.0
Proximal phalanx I	16.2 (2,3), 16.3 (1)	14.2 (2), 14.3 (3), 14.4 (1)	16.3	14.0
Proximal phalanx II	16.3 (1), 16.4 (2)	14.2 (1,2)	15.9	14.0
Proximal phalanx III	16.2 (3), 16.3 (1,2)	14.2 (2), 14.5 (1)	16.1	14.1
Proximal phalanx IV	16.2 (1), 16.5 (2)	14.2 (1,2)	16.1	14.1
Poroximal phalanx V	16.2 (1,2)	14.2 (1,2)	15.8	14.0
Middle phalanx II	16.4 (1,2)	14.2 (1,2)	16.1	13.9
Middle phalanx III	16.4 (1), 16.5 (2)	14.4 (2), 14.5 (1)	16.3	14.1
Middle phalanx IV	16.4 (1,2)	14.3 (2), 14.5 (1)	16.3	14.1
Middle phalanx V	16.3 (2), 16.4 (1)	14.2 (2), 14.3 (1)	16.3	14.0
Distal phalanx I	15.7 (1), 15.9 (2)	13.5 (1), 13.6 (2)	15.7	13.5
Distal phalanx II	15.7 (3), 15.8 (2), 16.0 (1)	12.5 (2), 13.6 (1,2), 13.7 (3)	15.8	13.5
Distal phalanx III	16.0 (1,2)	13.6 (1,2)	15.8	13.5
Distal phalanx IV	15.8 (2), 16.0 (1)	13.6 (1,2)	15.6	13.4
Distal phalanx V	15.9 (2), 16.0 (1)	13.6 (1,2)	15.7	13.4

These figures represent the national estimates of the levels of hand-wrist skeletal maturity among noninstitutionalized youths aged 12 to 17 years in the United States. They are based on the findings from the health examination survey of 1966–1970. Table 6 includes data from this survey, as well as previous data.

Source: Roche AS, Roberts J, Hamill, PVV. Skeletal maturity of youths 12 to 17 years; racial, geographic area, and socioeconomic differentials. United States, 1966–1970. Washington, D.C.: U.S. Government Printing Office, 1978; DHEW Publication no. (PHS)79-1654.

Related References:

1. Garn SM, Rohmann CG, Apfelbaum B. Complete epiphyseal union of the hand. *Am J Phys Anthropol* 1961;19:365.
2. Hansman, CF. Appearance and fusion of ossification centers in the human skeleton. *AJR* 1962;88:476–482.
3. Pyle SI, Stuart HC, Corononi J, Reed RB. Onsets, completions and spans of the osseous stage of development in representative bone growth centers of the extremities. *Soc Res Child Develop Monogr* 1961;26:Serial No. 79.

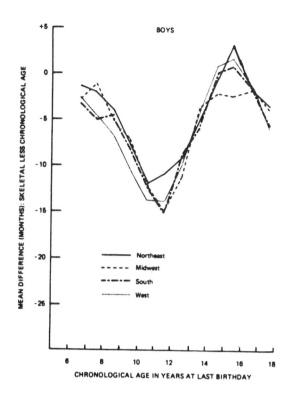

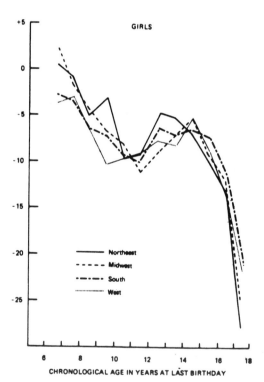

FIG. 6. Mean difference between skeletal age (hand-wrist) and chronological age for boys and girls aged 6 to 17 years by region and chronological age.

Source: Roche AS, Roberts J, Hamill, PVV. Skeletal maturity of youths 12 to 17 years; racial, geographic area, and socioeconomic differentials. United States, 1966–1970. Washington, D.C.: U.S. Government Printing Office, 1978; DHEW Publication no. (PHS)79-1654.

Metacarpal and Phalangeal Lengths

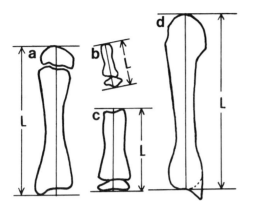

FIG. 7. Length measurements of **(a)** metacarpals, **(b)** distal phalanges, and **(c)** proximal phalanges made at right angles to the long axis and including the epiphysis, when separate. The exception is the third metacarpal excluding the styloid process as in **(d)**.

TABLE 7. *Standards for metacarpal and phalangeal lengths and variability (age 2–10)*

BONES		2 MEAN	S.D.	3 MEAN	S.D.	4 MEAN	S.D.	5 MEAN	S.D.	6 MEAN	S.D.	7 MEAN	S.D.	8 MEAN	S.D.	9 MEAN	S.D.	10 MEAN	S.D.
								Males											
Distal	5	8.8	...	8.4	0.6	9.0	0.7	9.9	0.6	10.7	0.6	11.4	0.8	12.2	0.9	12.6	1.0	13.5	0.9
	4	9.2	0.7	9.9	0.8	10.5	0.8	11.5	0.9	12.3	0.9	13.1	1.0	13.9	1.0	14.4	1.0	15.3	1.2
	3	8.7	0.9	9.5	0.8	10.2	0.8	11.1	0.8	11.8	0.9	12.7	1.0	13.4	1.0	14.0	1.0	14.8	1.2
	2	8.2	0.5	8.8	1.1	9.1	0.8	10.1	0.9	10.8	0.9	11.6	1.0	12.4	1.0	13.0	1.0	13.7	1.1
	1	11.1	0.6	12.3	0.8	13.2	1.0	14.4	0.9	15.4	0.9	16.5	1.0	17.4	1.0	17.9	1.2	19.0	1.2
Middle	5	8.8	0.9	9.8	0.8	10.6	1.0	11.2	1.0	12.0	1.0	12.7	1.1	13.5	1.1	14.3	1.2	15.0	1.2
	4	13.5	0.9	14.5	1.0	15.8	0.9	16.7	0.9	17.7	1.0	18.7	1.1	19.8	1.1	20.9	1.3	21.6	1.4
	3	14.1	0.8	15.1	1.1	16.5	1.0	17.6	1.0	18.7	1.1	19.8	1.2	20.9	1.2	22.0	1.4	22.9	1.4
	2	11.2	0.8	12.3	1.1	13.5	1.0	14.4	0.9	15.3	1.0	16.1	1.1	17.1	1.1	18.1	1.2	18.8	1.2
Proximal	5	16.1	0.7	17.8	0.9	19.2	1.0	20.6	1.0	21.8	1.0	23.0	1.1	24.2	1.3	25.2	1.5	26.4	1.5
	4	20.5	0.9	22.8	1.0	24.7	1.2	26.4	1.2	27.9	1.3	29.5	1.4	31.0	1.6	32.3	1.9	33.9	1.8
	3	21.8	1.0	24.2	1.1	26.3	1.4	28.1	1.4	29.8	1.4	31.5	1.6	33.2	1.8	34.7	2.2	36.1	1.9
	2	19.5	1.0	21.9	1.2	23.7	1.3	25.4	1.4	26.8	1.5	28.3	1.6	29.7	1.8	31.4	1.9	32.5	1.9
	1	15.2	...	15.9	1.1	17.2	1.1	18.3	1.2	19.6	1.2	20.8	1.3	21.8	1.3	23.1	1.5	24.2	1.4
Metacarpal	5	23.9	1.0	26.3	1.5	28.9	1.9	32.1	2.2	34.6	2.2	36.7	2.1	38.8	2.5	40.6	2.5	42.7	2.9
	4	25.5	1.4	28.9	1.5	31.7	2.1	35.0	2.5	37.9	2.7	40.1	2.5	42.2	3.1	44.1	2.8	46.5	3.5
	3	28.6	1.8	32.3	1.8	35.6	2.3	39.3	2.8	42.6	2.9	45.3	2.8	47.6	3.5	49.8	3.0	52.3	3.7
	2	30.6	1.5	34.5	1.7	37.9	2.3	41.6	2.7	44.9	2.9	47.7	2.8	50.2	3.4	52.6	3.0	55.0	3.9
	1	19.6	1.3	22.0	1.2	24.1	1.6	26.7	1.6	29.0	1.7	30.9	1.8	32.7	2.1	34.4	2.1	36.3	2.3
								Females											
Distal	5	7.8	0.6	8.4	0.6	9.1	0.7	9.9	0.7	10.6	0.8	11.4	0.9	12.1	1.0	12.7	1.1	13.5	1.2
	4	9.1	0.7	9.9	0.7	10.6	0.8	11.5	0.9	12.4	1.0	13.2	1.1	14.0	1.1	14.4	1.2	15.5	1.4
	3	8.8	0.7	9.9	0.8	10.2	0.7	11.1	0.9	12.2	1.3	12.7	1.1	13.5	1.1	14.1	1.1	15.0	1.4
	2	8.0	0.8	8.6	0.7	9.4	0.7	10.1	0.8	10.9	0.9	11.7	1.0	12.3	1.1	13.1	1.1	13.8	1.4
	1	11.3	0.8	12.5	0.8	13.2	0.8	14.4	1.0	15.4	1.1	16.3	1.2	17.3	1.3	17.8	1.3	19.0	1.6
Middle	5	9.0	1.2	9.8	1.1	10.5	1.1	11.2	1.1	12.2	1.2	12.9	1.3	13.6	1.4	14.2	1.4	15.2	1.6
	4	13.5	0.9	14.9	1.0	15.8	1.1	16.9	1.2	18.1	1.3	19.1	1.4	20.1	1.4	20.9	1.5	22.2	1.7
	3	14.2	0.9	15.6	1.1	16.6	1.2	17.9	1.2	19.2	1.3	20.3	1.4	21.4	1.4	22.1	1.6	23.6	1.8
	2	11.6	0.9	12.8	1.0	13.6	1.1	14.8	1.1	16.0	1.2	16.8	1.3	17.8	1.4	18.1	1.5	19.6	1.7
Proximal	5	16.3	1.0	17.9	1.1	19.1	1.1	20.6	1.1	22.0	1.4	23.1	1.6	24.4	1.6	25.2	1.6	27.1	2.0
	4	20.7	1.1	22.9	1.3	24.6	1.3	26.3	1.5	28.2	1.7	29.7	1.9	31.2	2.0	32.4	2.0	34.5	2.4
	3	22.2	1.2	24.5	1.3	26.4	1.4	28.3	1.8	30.4	1.8	32.1	2.0	33.7	2.2	35.0	2.2	37.3	2.6
	2	20.1	1.2	22.3	1.3	24.0	1.8	25.8	1.7	27.7	1.7	29.2	1.9	30.7	2.0	31.5	2.4	34.0	2.4
	1	14.9	1.0	16.3	1.1	17.2	1.3	18.8	1.3	20.2	1.3	21.4	1.5	22.7	1.6	23.5	2.0	25.5	2.1
Metacarpal	5	23.7	1.5	26.9	2.1	29.4	1.8	32.6	2.0	35.1	2.1	37.2	2.4	39.4	2.5	40.8	2.5	43.8	2.8
	4	26.0	1.9	29.6	2.7	32.2	2.0	35.6	2.5	38.4	2.7	40.5	2.8	43.1	3.0	44.3	2.8	47.5	3.5
	3	29.4	2.1	33.4	2.9	36.3	2.2	40.3	2.7	43.3	3.1	45.8	3.1	48.7	3.2	49.9	3.2	53.6	3.8
	2	31.3	1.9	35.2	2.7	38.2	2.3	42.2	2.7	45.6	3.2	48.1	3.3	51.2	3.3	52.6	3.4	56.6	4.1
	1	19.9	1.6	22.7	1.6	24.8	1.7	27.3	1.8	29.6	1.9	31.5	2.0	33.5	2.1	34.8	2.4	37.4	2.6

For each sex *N* = 150 at age 4, 124 at age 9, 78 in adulthood, and 30 to 85 at intermediate ages. All values are in millimeters.

TABLE 8. *Standards for metacarpal and phalangeal lengths and variability (age 11–adult)*

BONES		11 MEAN	11 S.D.	12 MEAN	12 S.D.	13 MEAN	13 S.D.	14 MEAN	14 S.D.	15 MEAN	15 S.D.	16 MEAN	16 S.D.	17 MEAN	17 S.D.	18 MEAN	18 S.D.	ADULTS MEAN	ADULTS S.D.
								Males											
Distal	5	14.2	0.9	15.0	0.9	15.8	0.9	16.8	1.0	17.6	1.1	17.9	1.0	18.1	1.0	18.1	1.2	18.7	1.3
	4	16.1	1.2	17.0	1.3	17.8	1.4	18.8	1.3	19.6	1.4	20.0	1.3	20.3	1.3	20.0	1.3	20.5	1.2
	3	15.6	1.2	16.4	1.2	17.1	1.3	18.2	1.3	19.0	1.4	19.3	1.4	19.5	1.3	19.4	1.3	20.1	1.2
	2	14.3	1.1	15.0	1.0	15.7	1.4	16.7	1.2	17.5	1.2	17.8	1.3	18.2	1.3	18.1	1.3	18.8	1.4
	1	19.7	1.2	20.6	1.3	21.7	1.4	22.8	1.3	24.1	1.4	24.5	1.4	24.9	1.4	24.8	1.5	25.2	1.4
Middle	5	15.7	1.4	16.5	1.5	17.5	1.5	18.9	1.6	19.9	1.4	20.5	1.4	20.6	1.4	21.0	1.4	21.6	1.6
	4	22.6	1.5	23.6	1.5	24.8	1.7	26.5	1.6	27.7	1.5	28.4	1.5	28.7	1.4	29.1	1.5	29.6	1.6
	3	24.0	1.4	24.9	1.4	26.3	1.6	28.0	1.5	29.2	1.5	30.0	1.6	30.2	1.6	30.6	1.8	31.1	1.8
	2	19.8	1.8	20.4	1.3	21.6	1.6	23.2	1.5	24.3	1.5	25.0	1.5	25.3	1.4	25.6	1.7	26.1	1.6
Proximal	5	27.6	1.7	28.9	2.0	30.5	2.4	32.9	2.4	34.7	2.0	35.6	1.8	36.1	1.8	35.9	2.0	36.3	2.0
	4	35.3	2.0	37.0	2.4	38.8	2.8	41.6	2.8	43.7	2.6	44.9	2.3	45.4	2.2	45.2	2.5	45.5	2.3
	3	37.8	2.3	39.5	2.6	41.5	2.9	44.4	2.8	46.6	2.5	47.8	2.4	48.3	2.3	48.2	2.7	48.5	2.6
	2	33.9	2.1	35.5	2.4	37.2	2.6	39.8	2.6	41.8	2.2	42.8	2.0	43.3	2.1	43.4	2.4	43.7	2.2
	1	25.4	1.6	26.7	2.0	28.5	2.2	30.9	2.2	32.9	1.8	33.8	1.5	34.6	2.6	34.7	1.8	35.0	1.9
Metacarpal	5	44.6	2.8	47.1	3.2	49.1	4.0	52.2	3.9	55.4	3.6	57.1	2.8	57.9	2.5	57.5	2.9	58.0	3.0
	4	48.4	3.1	51.0	3.7	53.1	4.6	56.4	4.5	59.5	4.1	62.6	3.7	63.2	2.9	62.5	3.4	63.0	3.5
	3	54.6	3.4	57.3	4.0	59.5	5.1	63.1	4.9	66.7	4.4	68.7	4.1	69.7	3.3	69.0	3.7	69.0	3.8
	2	57.3	3.5	60.6	3.9	63.3	5.1	67.1	4.8	70.6	4.3	73.2	3.8	74.2	2.9	73.9	3.5	73.7	3.8
	1	38.2	2.4	40.2	2.7	42.5	3.0	45.1	2.8	47.6	2.6	48.8	2.3	49.5	2.1	49.4	2.7	49.6	2.9
								Females											
Distal	5	14.2	1.3	15.0	1.3	15.4	1.3	15.6	1.3	15.9	1.4	15.9	1.4	16.2	1.3	16.0	1.2	16.2	1.2
	4	16.2	1.4	17.1	1.4	17.6	1.2	17.9	1.3	18.0	1.4	18.0	1.3	18.1	1.4	17.9	1.3	18.0	1.3
	3	15.8	1.3	16.6	1.4	17.1	1.4	17.3	1.3	17.6	1.5	17.5	1.4	17.6	1.4	17.7	1.3	18.0	1.3
	2	14.4	1.3	15.2	1.5	15.7	1.5	15.8	1.5	16.1	1.6	16.0	1.6	16.3	1.5	16.2	1.3	16.6	1.3
	1	20.0	1.7	20.9	1.7	21.4	1.6	21.7	1.6	22.0	1.7	22.0	1.7	22.1	1.8	22.0	1.6	22.1	1.6
Middle	5	16.2	1.7	17.2	1.7	17.9	1.8	18.1	1.6	18.4	1.7	18.5	1.7	18.5	1.9	18.6	1.7	18.7	1.7
	4	23.4	1.8	24.7	1.8	25.7	1.9	25.9	1.6	26.3	1.8	26.4	1.8	26.5	1.9	26.3	1.8	26.4	1.7
	3	24.9	1.9	26.2	1.9	27.2	2.0	27.5	1.7	28.1	1.8	28.0	1.9	28.0	1.8	27.8	1.8	27.9	1.7
	2	20.6	1.8	21.8	1.9	22.7	1.8	23.0	1.8	23.5	1.8	23.3	1.9	23.4	1.9	23.1	1.6	23.2	1.6
Proximal	5	28.7	2.1	30.5	2.2	31.9	2.2	32.3	2.1	32.9	2.2	32.8	2.3	32.8	2.3	32.5	2.0	32.5	1.9
	4	36.5	2.5	38.8	2.6	40.3	2.5	40.9	2.3	41.5	2.5	41.6	2.6	41.7	2.6	41.1	2.2	40.8	2.4
	3	39.5	2.7	41.7	2.8	43.5	2.8	44.1	2.4	44.8	2.6	44.8	2.7	44.8	2.5	44.2	2.4	44.0	2.3
	2	35.9	2.6	38.0	2.6	39.5	2.6	39.9	2.4	40.6	2.6	40.6	2.6	40.7	2.6	44.2	2.4	44.0	2.3
	1	27.2	2.3	29.2	2.4	30.6	2.2	31.1	1.9	31.8	2.0	31.7	2.1	31.9	2.2	31.3	1.9	31.4	2.0
Metacarpal	5	46.3	2.9	48.7	2.9	50.8	2.8	52.1	2.8	52.6	3.0	52.8	3.0	53.0	2.7	52.0	2.7	51.9	3.6
	4	50.2	3.8	52.8	3.7	55.1	3.6	56.2	3.6	56.9	3.6	57.2	3.9	57.2	3.5	56.1	2.9	56.0	3.5
	3	56.5	4.0	59.5	4.2	62.1	4.0	63.4	3.9	63.9	3.9	64.3	4.0	64.5	4.0	63.2	2.9	62.6	4.0
	2	59.9	4.3	63.2	4.4	66.2	4.2	67.4	3.9	68.1	4.2	68.6	4.3	68.9	4.1	67.5	3.4	66.9	4.3
	1	39.7	3.0	42.0	3.0	43.8	2.7	44.4	2.5	45.3	2.4	45.0	2.8	45.0	2.6	44.6	2.2	44.2	2.6

For each sex *N* = 150 at age 4, 124 at age 9, 78 in adulthood, and 30 to 85 at intermediate ages. All values are in millimeters.

Source: Garn SM, Hertzog KP, Poznanski AK, Nagy JM. Metacarpophalangeal length in the evaluation of skeletal malformation. *Radiology* 1972;105:375–81.

Metacarpal Index of Infants

The index is calculated by measuring the 2nd, 3rd, 4th, and 5th metacarpals. The sum of the lengths is divided by the sum of the breadth, as measured at the midpoint of each metacarpal.

TABLE 9. *Metacarpal index of 50 normal children during the first 2 years of life*

Age (mo)	Sex	Metacarpal index	
		Mean	SD
6	M	5.23	0.46
	F	5.60	0.37
12	M	5.30	0.41
	F	5.75	0.41
18	M	5.28	0.40
	F	5.82	0.45
24	M	5.40	0.43
	F	5.84	0.43

Data were obtained from X-rays of hands of normal children who had been observed in a longitudinal study of growth at Oxford.

TABLE 10. *Metacarpal index of seven children with abnormally long fingers compared to normal children of the same age*

Diagnosis	Age (mo)	Sex	Metacarpal index	Normal index $\pm$ SD
Marfan syndrome	24	F	7.4	5.84 $\pm$ 0.43
Marfan syndrome	12	F	8.4	5.75 $\pm$ 0.41
Marfan syndrome	6	M	7.0	5.23 $\pm$ 0.46
Arachnodactyly	12	F	8.6	5.75 $\pm$ 0.41
Arachnodactyly	6	F	7.5	5.60 $\pm$ 0.37
Arachnodactyly	6	M	6.1	5.23 $\pm$ 0.46
Arachnodactyly	6	F	7.2	5.60 $\pm$ 0.37

TABLE 11. *Comparison of metacarpal indices of normal and abnormal children*

Diagnosis	No. of children	Mean $\pm$ SD (% of normal)	Significance of difference from normal mean
Normal children	50	100 $\pm$ 13	
Marfan syndrome	3	136 $\pm$ 8	$p < 0.003$
Arachnodactyly	4	132 $\pm$ 12	$p < 0.006$
Mongolism	43	98 $\pm$ 10	$p > 0.4$

Source: Joseph MC, Meadow SR. The metacarpal index of infants. *Arch Dis Child* 1969;4:515–16.

Bones of the Thumb

The normative values of the ratio of the lengths of each bone to the others as well as to the second metacarpal (MET-2) are tabulated. These ratios are useful for objective evaluation of relative lengthening or shortening of the thumb bones. Anomalies of the thumb may be associated with congenital malformation syndromes, including enlargement, duplication, and hypoplasia. The thumb may also be absent, have abnormal ossification centers, or be abnormal in position. Measurements of the bones were taken along the longitudinal axis of each bone. The length was defined as the maximal distance between the perpendiculars drawn to each end of the bone. In the adult the entire bone, including the epiphysis, was measured for the 9-year or 4-year standards. For the 1-year standards, only the diaphysis was measured.

TABLE 12. *Relative proportions of the bones of the thumb*

| | | Males | | | | Females | | | |
| | | Diaphysis and Epiphysis | | | Diaphysis | Diaphysis and Epiphysis | | | Diaphysis |
		Adult	9 yr	4 yr	1 yr	Adult	9 yr	4 yr	1 yr
MET 2/MET 1	Mean	1.49	1.53	1.57	1.64	1.52	1.52	1.55	1.60
	S.D.	0.05	0.05	0.06	0.06	0.07	0.06	0.07	0.09
MET 2/P1	Mean	2.10	2.28	2.22	2.13	2.13	2.25	2.22	2.15
	S.D.	0.10	0.12	0.11	0.11	0.12	0.13	0.11	0.13
MET 2/D1	Mean	2.93	2.93	2.88	2.85	3.02	2.96	2.90	2.89
	S.D.	0.16	0.15	0.16	0.18	0.20	0.16	0.14	0.19
MET 1/MET 2	Mean	0.67	0.66	0.64	0.61	0.66	0.66	0.65	0.63
	S.D.	0.02	0.02	0.02	0.02	0.04	0.03	0.03	0.04
MET 1/P1	Mean	1.41	1.49	1.41	1.31	1.41	1.49	1.44	1.34
	S.D.	0.06	0.06	0.06	0.06	0.05	0.07	0.06	0.07
MET 1/D1	Mean	1.97	1.92	1.82	1.74	1.99	1.95	1.88	1.81
	S.D.	0.12	0.10	0.10	0.10	0.12	0.11	0.11	0.14
P1/MET 2	Mean	0.48	0.44	0.45	0.47	0.47	0.45	0.45	0.47
	S.D.	0.02	0.02	0.02	0.02	0.03	0.02	0.02	0.03
P1/MET 1	Mean	0.71	0.67	0.71	0.77	0.71	0.67	0.70	0.75
	S.D.	0.03	0.03	0.03	0.04	0.03	0.03	0.03	0.04
P1/D1	Mean	1.40	1.29	1.30	1.34	1.42	1.32	1.31	1.35
	S.D.	0.08	0.07	0.07	0.08	0.09	0.08	0.07	0.09
D1/MET 2	Mean	0.34	0.34	0.35	0.35	0.33	0.34	0.35	0.35
	S.D.	0.02	0.02	0.02	0.02	0.02	0.02	0.02	0.02
D1/MET 1	Mean	0.51	0.52	0.55	0.58	0.50	0.51	0.53	0.56
	S.D.	0.03	0.03	0.03	0.03	0.03	0.03	0.03	0.04
D1/P1	Mean	0.72	0.78	0.77	0.75	0.71	0.76	0.77	0.75
	S.D.	0.04	0.04	0.04	0.04	0.04	0.05	0.04	0.05

MET 1 = metacarpal of the thumb. P1 = proximal phalanx of the thumb. D1 = distal phalanx of the thumb.

Source: Poznanski AK, Garn SM, Holt JF. The thumb in the congenital malformation syndrome. *Radiology* 1971;100:115–29.

Carpal Length in Children

The distance between the midpoint of the distal radial epiphyseal growth plate and the proximal end of the third metacarpal offers a useful measure for determining wrist size. The sample consists of 539 hand radiographs selected using a stratified random sampling strategy from a large collection of radiographs assembled as part of a 10-state nutritional survey of 1967. The sample was composed of 280 boys ranging in age from 1.5 to 15.4 years and 259 girls ranging in age from 1.5 to 14.5 years. The sample was selected so that the age distribution would be approximately uniform within the chosen age range.

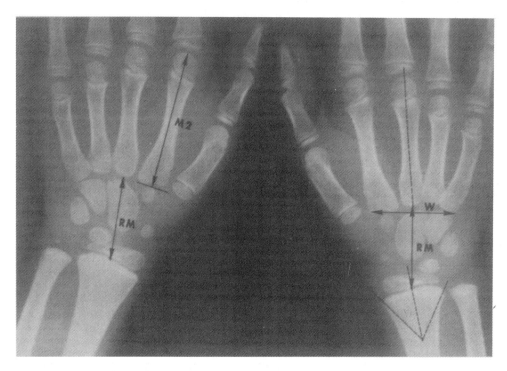

FIG. 8. Measures used in evaluating carpal size. RM is the measurement used to indicate carpal size. It can be related to the size of the hand by comparing it to the length of the second metacarpal (M2), or to the width of the proximal metacarpals (W). The dashed, bisected triangle in the right side of the radiograph is used to find the center of the distal radial growth plate. This can be done by using an overlay, or the center of the radial growth plate can be determined by simple examination.

To determine how deviant a specific child is from the mean, a ruler is placed between the two points on the scales that correspond to these measures in the child in question. The intersection of the line with the central scales gives the number of standard deviations this relationship deviates from the mean. Note that there are separate scales for males and females.

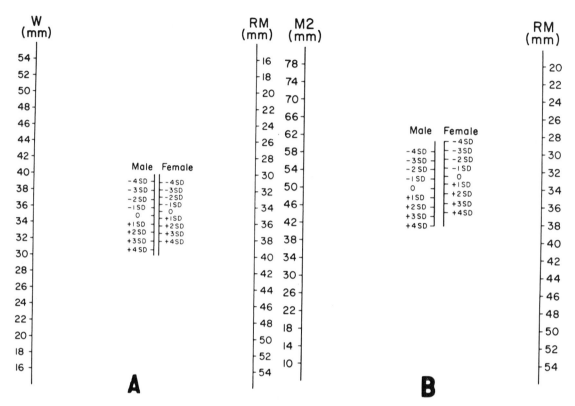

FIG. 9. Nomograms for determining the relationships between W versus RM and MS versus RM. RM is the measurement used to indicate carpal size. It can be related to the size of the hand by comparing it to the length of the second metacarpal (M2), or to the width of the proximal metacarpals (W).

Source: Poznanski AK, Hernandez RJ, Guire KE, Bereza JL, Garn SM. Carpal length in children—a useful measurement in the diagnosis of rheumatoid arthritis and some congenital malformation syndromes. *Radiology* 1978;129:661–8.

Carpal Angle

Kosowicz defined the carpal angle as the angle between two lines, one tangential to the scaphoid and lunate, and the other tangential to the lunate and the triquetrium. The carpal angles were measured in a normal population of 928 well individuals from the 10-state nutritional survey.

TABLE 13. *Carpal angle in 928 well individuals from the ten-state nutrition survey*

AGE	WHITE MALE		WHITE FEMALE		BLACK MALE		BLACK FEMALE	
	Mean	*S.D.*	*Mean*	*S.D.*	*Mean*	*S.D.*	*Mean*	*S.D.*
4–6	123.1	5.6	127.1	6.3	130.6	6.1	131.3	7.1
6–8	127.0	11.5	130.0	10.0	131.0	8.9	133.7	8.6
8–10	133.0	7.7	124.5	7.6	139.6	7.7	138.9	8.1
10–12	132.7	7.1	135.8	8.2	138.5	11.1	138.6	8.3
12–14	131.6	8.1	129.4	8.5	141.7	8.5	141.2	9.2
14–above	133.8	9.8	129.6	8.7	141.7	9.5	138.6	8.7

Sources: Harper HAS, Poznanski AP, Garn SM. Carpal angle in American populations. *Investigative Radiology* 1974;9:217–21.

Poznanski AK, *The hand in radiologic diagnosis*. Philadelphia: W. B. Saunders Co., 1974.

Accessory Bones of the Carpus

In addition to the eight carpal bones, there are many accessory ossicles in the region of the carpus. O'Rahilly compiled an extensive list from his own work and accounts from previous publications. The definition he used was for the foot, but it is satisfactory for the hand: "Accessory bones are all inconsistent, independent well-defined bones in an otherwise normally developed foot, the existence of which is not due to recent minor fracture or other definitely pathologic conditions, no matter whether these bones bear no, less or more intimate relationship to the constant bones or entirely replace them because of a division of the latter into several segments."

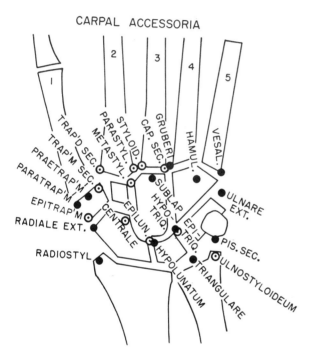

CARPAL ACCESSORIA

FIG. 10.   Name and location of the accessoria.

TABLE 14. *Terminology of the accessoria*

Os capitatum secundarium
   (carpometacarpale V)[a]
Os centrale (centrale dorsale, episcaphoid)[a]
Os epilunatum (centrale II)[a]
Os epitrapezium[a]
Os epitrapezoideum (trapezoideum dorsale)
Os epitriquetrum (epipyramis, centrale IV)[a]
Os gruberi (carpometacarpale VI)[a]
Os hamulare basale (carpometacarpale VII)
Os hamuli proprium[a]
Os hypolunatum (centrale III)[a]
Os hypotriquetrum
Os metastyloideum
Os parastyloideum (carpometacarpale III)
Os paratrapezium[a]
Os pisiforme secundarium (ulnare
   antebrachii, metapisoid)[a]?
Os praetrapezium (carpometacarpale I)
Os radiale externum (parascaphoid)[a]
Os radiostyloideum[a]
Os styloideum (carpometacarpale IV)[a,b]
Os subcapitatum
Os trapezium secundarium (multangulum
   majus secundarium, carpometacarpale II)[a]
Os trapezoideum secundarium (multangulum
   minus secundarium)[a]
Os triangulare (intermedium antebrachii,
   triquetrum secundarium)
Os ulnare externum[a]
Os ulnostyloideum
Os vesalianum manus (vesalii,
   carpometacarpale VIII)[a]

Synonyms are in parentheses for reference purposes.
[a]From Kohler, A. (rev. by E. A. Zimmer and ed. by J. T. Case): *Borderlands of the Normal and Early Pathologic in Skeletal Roentgenology*, ed. 10. New York, Grune, 1956.
[b]From Werthemann, A.: *Die Entwicklungsstorungen der Extremitaten*, vol. 9, part 6, of Lubarsch, Henke and Rossle's *Handbuch der speziellen pathologischen Anatomie und Histologie*. Berlin, Springer, 1952.

Source: O'Rahilly R. Developmental deviations in the carpus and tarsus. *Clin Orthop* 1957;10:9–18.

Hand Breadth and Length in Infants

The infant's hand is fully extended, palm up, thumb abducted from the hand. The automatic sliding caliper measures the maximum width across the metacarpophalangeal joints 2 to 5. An assistant is required to ensure that the infant is in the correct position.

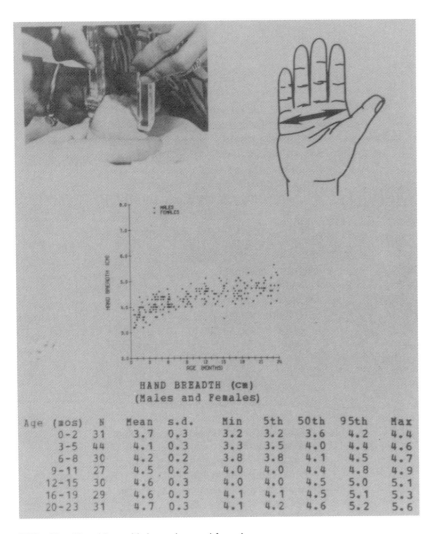

HAND BREADTH (cm)
(Males and Females)

Age (mos)	N	Mean	s.d.	Min	5th	50th	95th	Max
0-2	31	3.7	0.3	3.2	3.2	3.6	4.2	4.4
3-5	44	4.1	0.3	3.3	3.5	4.0	4.4	4.6
6-8	30	4.2	0.2	3.8	3.8	4.1	4.5	4.7
9-11	27	4.5	0.2	4.0	4.0	4.4	4.8	4.9
12-15	30	4.6	0.3	4.0	4.0	4.5	5.0	5.1
16-19	29	4.6	0.3	4.1	4.1	4.5	5.1	5.3
20-23	31	4.7	0.3	4.1	4.2	4.6	5.2	5.6

FIG. 11. Hand breadth in males and females.

The length is measured using the sliding caliper to measure distance from the right wrist crease to the tip of the middle finger parallel to the fingers. An assistant is required to ensure that the infant is in the correct position.

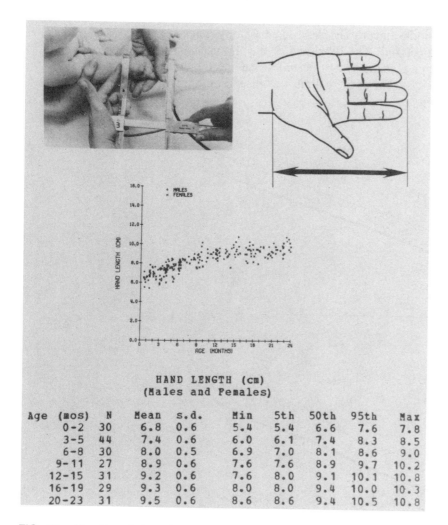

HAND LENGTH (cm)
(Males and Females)

Age (mos)	N	Mean	s.d.	Min	5th	50th	95th	Max
0-2	30	6.8	0.6	5.4	5.4	6.6	7.6	7.8
3-5	44	7.4	0.6	6.0	6.1	7.4	8.3	8.5
6-8	30	8.0	0.5	6.9	7.0	8.1	8.6	9.0
9-11	27	8.9	0.6	7.6	7.6	8.9	9.7	10.2
12-15	31	9.2	0.6	7.6	8.0	9.1	10.1	10.8
16-19	29	9.3	0.6	8.0	8.0	9.4	10.0	10.3
20-23	31	9.5	0.6	8.6	8.6	9.4	10.5	10.8

FIG. 12. Hand length in males and females.

Source: Snyder RB, Schneider LW, Owings CL, Reynolds HM, Golomg BH, Schork MA. *Anthropometry of infants and children and youths to age 18, for product safety design.* Highway Safety Research Institute, University of Michigan, publishers. The Society for Automotive Engineers, Warrendale, PA, 1977.

Mean Hand Length of White and Black Children by Sex and Age

Hand length was measured as the distance from the wrist (midpoint of the most distal crease or groove) to the tip of the middle finger. The right hand is fully extended and supinated, and the thumb straight but relaxed. The fixed end of the sliding caliper was placed at the midpoint of the distal crease at the wrist (located by having the child flex the hand at the wrist) and the movable crossbar of the caliper was placed in light contact with the distal tip of the middle finger.

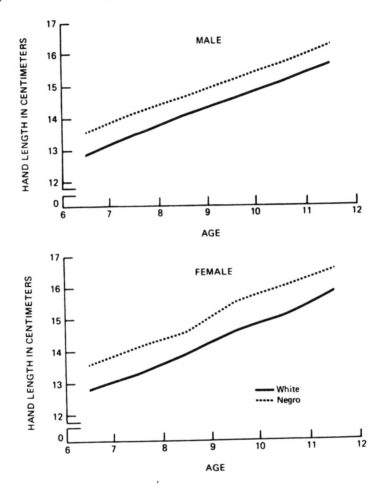

FIG. 13.   Hand length, male/female, black/white children, 6 to 12 years of age.

TABLE 15. *Hand length of children by race, sex, and age at last birthday; sample size, mean, standard deviation, standard error of the mean, and selected percentiles, United States, 1963–65*

Race, sex, and age	n	N	$\overline{X}$	s	$s_{\overline{x}}$	Percentile (cm)						
						5th	10th	25th	50th	75th	90th	95th
White: Boys						In centimeters						
6 years	489	1,787	12.9	0.68	0.04	11.7	12.1	12.4	13.1	13.6	13.9	16.5
7 years	551	1,781	13.5	0.71	0.04	12.2	12.4	13.1	13.5	14.0	14.6	14.3
8 years	537	1,739	14.1	0.81	0.04	12.5	13.1	13.5	14.2	14.7	15.3	14.8
9 years	525	1,730	14.6	0.78	0.04	13.2	13.5	14.2	14.6	15.2	15.7	15.6
10 years	509	1,692	15.1	0.82	0.04	13.7	14.1	14.5	15.1	15.7	16.3	15.9
11 years	542	1,662	15.7	0.87	0.03	14.2	14.4	15.1	15.6	16.3	16.8	17.3
Girls												
6 years	461	1,722	12.8	0.70	0.04	11.4	11.8	12.2	12.7	13.4	13.8	14.2
7 years	512	1,716	13.3	0.76	0.03	12.1	12.3	12.8	13.4	13.8	14.4	14.7
8 years	498	1,674	13.9	0.76	0.05	12.4	13.0	13.3	13.8	14.5	15.1	15.4
9 years	494	1,663	14.6	0.77	0.04	13.2	13.4	14.1	14.5	15.1	15.7	16.0
10 years	505	1,632	15.1	0.86	0.04	13.5	14.0	14.4	15.2	15.7	16.4	16.7
11 years	477	1,605	15.9	0.91	0.04	14.3	14.6	15.2	15.8	16.6	17.2	17.6
Black: Boys												
6 years	84	289	13.6	0.66	0.09	12.3	12.6	13.1	13.6	14.1	14.6	14.8
7 years	79	286	14.2	0.71	0.09	13.1	13.2	13.6	14.2	14.7	15.3	15.7
8 years	79	279	14.7	0.73	0.10	13.5	13.7	14.2	14.7	15.4	15.7	15.8
9 years	74	269	15.2	0.83	0.07	13.8	14.1	14.5	15.2	15.7	16.5	16.9
10 years	65	264	15.7	0.84	0.11	14.2	14.4	15.1	15.7	16.4	16.8	17.0
11 years	83	255	16.3	0.76	0.07	14.9	15.2	15.8	16.4	16.8	17.4	17.7
Girls												
6 years	72	281	13.6	0.85	0.09	12.1	12.3	13.0	13.6	14.3	14.7	14.8
7 years	93	284	14.1	0.72	0.09	13.0	13.1	13.5	14.2	14.6	15.2	15.5
8 years	113	281	14.6	0.89	0.08	13.1	13.3	13.8	14.5	15.3	15.9	16.4
9 years	84	265	15.5	1.01	0.08	13.9	14.2	14.6	15.4	16.2	16.8	17.3
10 years	77	266	16.0	1.00	0.08	14.3	15.0	15.3	15.8	16.6	17.3	17.8
11 years	84	253	16.6	1.06	0.12	15.0	15.2	15.8	16.6	17.5	18.3	18.5

n = sample size; N = estimated number of children in population in thousands; $\overline{X}$ = mean; s = standard deviation; $s_{\overline{x}}$ = standard error of the mean.

Source: Malina RM, Hamill PVV, Lemeshow S. Body dimensions and proportions of white and negro children, six to eleven years. Washington, D.C.: U.S. Government Printing Office, 1974; DHEW Publication no. (HRA)75-1625.

Hand Length and Breadth in Males

The hand is extended and the thumb abducted. The width across the metacarpal heads is then measured. Length is measured as the distance from the wrist crease to the tip of the middle finger, parallel to the fingers.

TABLE 16. *Hand length in males*

Age (yrs)	No.	Hand length (cm)						
		Mean	SD	Min.	5th	50th	95th	Max.
2.0–3.5	114	10.7	0.8	8.6	9.3	10.7	11.9	12.6
3.5–4.5	118	11.4	0.7	9.7	10.3	11.3	12.5	13.9
4.5–5.5	142	12.0	0.9	5.5	10.9	12.0	13.0	13.8
5.5–6.5	108	12.9	0.8	11.0	11.6	12.8	14.4	15.4
6.5–7.5	104	13.4	0.9	11.1	11.8	13.3	14.8	15.9
7.5–8.5	98	13.9	0.8	11.5	12.6	13.8	15.2	16.1
8.5–9.5	114	14.5	0.9	12.8	13.0	14.3	15.9	16.9
9.5–10.5	123	15.1	0.9	12.9	13.6	14.9	16.4	17.1
10.5–11.5	141	15.5	0.9	13.5	14.0	15.4	17.0	18.1
11.5–12.5	154	16.2	1.0	13.7	14.5	16.0	17.8	20.0
12.5–13.5	152	16.9	1.1	14.5	15.1	16.7	18.7	19.6
13.5–14.5	153	17.8	1.2	14.9	15.9	17.7	19.4	21.7
14.5–15.5	130	18.2	1.0	15.6	16.3	18.2	19.7	20.4
15.5–16.5	99	18.9	1.0	15.1	17.3	18.9	20.4	21.6
16.5–17.5	104	18.9	0.9	16.5	17.2	18.8	20.1	21.7
17.5–19.0	88	19.2	0.9	17.0	17.4	19.1	20.5	21.6

TABLE 17. *Hand breadth in males*

Age (yrs)	No.	Hand breadth (cm)						
		Mean	SD	Min.	5th	50th	95th	Max.
2.0–3.5	114	5.2	0.4	4.2	4.4	5.1	5.9	6.1
3.5–4.5	118	5.4	0.3	4.7	4.9	5.4	6.1	6.5
4.5–5.5	142	5.7	0.4	4.9	5.1	5.6	6.3	6.6
5.5–6.5	108	6.0	0.4	5.2	5.3	6.0	6.6	7.1
6.5–7.5	104	6.3	0.4	5.4	5.6	6.2	7.0	7.4
7.5–8.5	98	6.5	0.4	5.6	5.9	6.5	7.2	7.6
8.5–9.5	114	6.7	0.4	5.7	6.1	6.7	7.4	7.9
9.5–10.5	123	7.0	0.4	6.1	6.3	6.9	7.6	7.9
10.5–11.5	141	7.2	0.4	6.1	6.5	7.1	7.8	8.2
11.5–12.5	154	7.4	0.5	6.4	6.7	7.3	8.4	9.0
12.5–13.5	151	7.8	0.5	6.8	7.0	7.6	8.8	9.3
13.5–14.5	154	8.3	0.6	6.7	7.1	8.2	9.1	9.7
14.5–15.5	131	8.5	0.5	7.3	7.5	8.5	9.3	9.8
15.5–16.5	99	8.8	0.5	7.0	7.7	8.8	9.5	10.0
16.5–17.5	104	8.8	0.4	7.8	8.2	8.8	9.5	9.9
17.5–19.0	88	9.0	0.5	7.6	8.2	8.9	9.8	10.2

Source: Snyder RB, Schneider LW, Owings CL, Reynolds HM, Golomg BH, Schork MA. *Anthropometry of infants and children and youths to age 18, for product safety design.* Highway Safety Research Institute, University of Michigan, publishers. The Society for Automotive Engineers, Warrendale, PA, 1977.

Hand Length and Breadth in Females

The hand is extended and the thumb abducted. The width across the metacarpal heads is then measured. Length is measured as the distance from the wrist crease to the tip of the middle finger, parallel to the fingers.

TABLE 18. *Hand length in females*

Age (yrs)	No.	Hand length (cm)						
		Mean	SD	Min.	5th	50th	95th	Max.
2.0–3.5	98	10.3	0.6	9.0	9.3	10.2	11.4	11.8
3.5–4.5	109	11.5	0.8	9.4	10.2	11.4	12.7	13.9
4.5–5.5	118	12.0	0.7	10.3	10.7	11.9	13.0	13.6
5.5–6.5	111	12.6	0.7	10.8	11.4	12.5	13.8	14.2
6.5–7.5	120	13.1	0.8	11.5	11.8	13.1	14.5	15.0
7.5–8.5	94	13.7	0.7	12.2	12.6	13.6	14.8	15.2
8.5–9.5	137	14.4	0.9	11.8	12.9	14.2	15.9	18.1
9.5–10.5	128	15.0	0.9	12.6	13.5	14.9	16.5	17.4
10.5–11.5	140	15.7	1.1	13.2	14.0	15.6	17.4	18.8
11.5–12.5	133	16.3	1.0	14.1	14.6	16.2	17.7	19.7
12.5–13.5	160	16.9	1.0	14.7	15.1	16.9	18.4	20.1
13.5–14.5	116	17.0	0.9	14.6	15.6	16.9	18.4	19.6
14.5–15.5	132	17.3	0.9	15.2	15.8	17.2	18.8	19.7
15.5–16.5	98	17.2	0.9	15.2	15.6	17.1	18.6	20.9
16.5–17.5	117	17.1	0.9	14.4	15.6	17.1	18.4	18.8
17.5–19.0	68	17.3	0.8	15.5	15.7	17.3	18.5	19.0

TABLE 19. *Hand breadth in females*

Age (yrs)	No.	Hand breadth (cm)						
		Mean	SD	Min.	5th	50th	95th	Max.
2.0–3.5	98	5.0	0.3	4.0	4.4	4.9	5.5	5.8
3.5–4.5	109	5.4	0.4	4.5	4.6	5.3	5.9	6.3
4.5–5.5	118	5.5	0.3	4.8	4.9	5.5	6.1	6.7
5.5–6.5	111	5.8	0.4	5.1	5.2	5.8	6.4	7.0
6.5–7.5	121	6.0	0.4	5.2	5.4	6.0	6.6	6.9
7.5–8.5	94	6.3	0.4	5.1	5.6	6.2	6.8	7.6
8.5–9.5	137	6.5	0.4	5.7	5.8	6.4	7.1	7.8
9.5–10.5	128	6.7	0.4	5.6	5.9	6.6	7.3	7.5
10.5–11.5	140	7.0	0.5	5.9	6.1	6.9	7.8	8.6
11.5–12.5	132	7.2	0.4	6.0	6.4	7.2	7.8	8.2
12.5–13.5	160	7.5	0.4	6.3	6.6	7.5	8.1	8.4
13.5–14.5	116	7.5	0.4	6.6	6.8	7.4	8.1	8.2
14.5–15.5	132	7.5	0.4	6.6	6.9	7.4	8.0	8.6
15.5–16.5	98	7.6	0.4	6.6	6.8	7.5	8.2	8.7
16.5–17.5	117	7.5	0.4	6.7	6.8	7.4	8.3	8.8
17.5–19.0	68	7.6	0.4	6.6	6.8	7.6	8.1	8.4

Source: Snyder RB, Schneider LW, Owings CL, Reynolds HM, Golomg BH, Schork MA. *Anthropometry of infants and children and youths to age 18, for product safety design.* Highway Safety Research Institute, University of Michigan, publishers. The Society for Automotive Engineers, Warrendale, PA, 1977.

LOWER EXTREMITY

Ultrasound Measurement of Fetal Limb Bones

A study was made of 41 patients who underwent serial examination of fetal limb lengths every one to three weeks starting an 8-week-gestation (humerus, femur, radius and ulna, and tibia and fibula). The values are expressed as mean ± 2 SD for each week of gestation.

The growth of the fetal limb bones was linear from 12 to 20 weeks gestation, but the various bones appeared to grow at different rates. The femur was the first to be well defined and easiest to measure with reproducibility. All the limb bone lengths correlate with gestational age and may serve as indicators of skeletal dysplasia. To substantiate the validity of the technique, ultrasound measurements were compared with X-ray measurements taken at the nearest millimeter of the limb lengths in four aborted fetuses. The differences were within 2 mm.

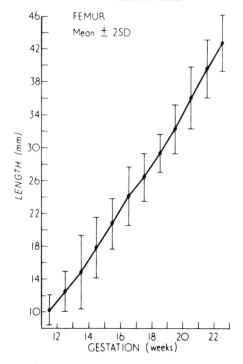

FIG. 1. Graph illustrating length of femur in millimeters versus gestational age in weeks.

FIG. 2. Length of humerus in millimeters versus gestational age in weeks.

TABLE 1. *Data from which the graph in Fig. 1 was constructed*

Weeks' gestation	Arithmetic mean (mm)	±2 SD (mm)	No. of determinations
11	10.2	1.8	9
12	12.5	2.4	15
13	14.8	4.5	17
14	17.9	3.7	15
15	20.8	3.1	20
16	24.1	3.6	16
17	26.4	2.9	18
18	29.4	2.3	15
19	32.3	3.0	21
20	36.1	3.8	17
21	39.7	3.5	14
22	42.8	3.4	12

TABLE 2. *Data from which the graph in Fig. 2 was constructed*

Weeks' gestation	Arithmetic mean (mm)	±2 SD (mm)	No. of determinations
11	9.7	1.5	10
12	12.0	3.1	14
13	15.1	5.9	17
14	18.0	3.4	13
15	20.6	4.2	17
16	24.0	3.2	12
17	26.0	3.5	11
18	28.7	2.0	13
19	31.0	3.9	17
20	34.9	3.9	14
21	36.4	4.3	12
22	40.4	3.6	9

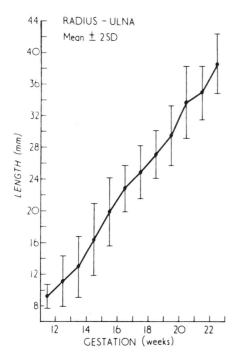

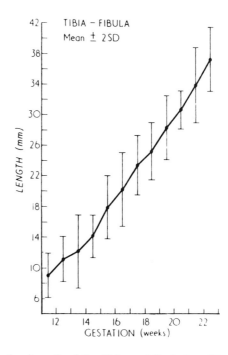

FIG. 3. Length of radius and ulna in millimeters versus gestational age in weeks.

FIG. 4. Length of the tibia and fibula in millimeters versus gestational age in weeks.

TABLE 3. *Data from which the graph in Fig. 3 was constructed*

Weeks' gestation	Arithmetic mean (mm)	±2 SD (mm)	No. of determinations
11	9.2	1.5	9
12	11.1	3.2	15
13	12.9	3.8	16
14	16.4	4.5	13
15	19.8	4.3	18
16	22.8	2.9	15
17	24.9	3.4	12
18	27.1	3.0	14
19	29.5	3.8	19
20	33.8	4.6	13
21	35.0	3.4	10
22	38.7	3.8	10

TABLE 4. *Data from which the graph in Fig. 4 was constructed*

Weeks' gestation	Arithmetic mean (mm)	±2 SD (mm)	No. of determinations
11	9.0	2.9	6
12	11.1	2.9	10
13	12.1	4.8	12
14	14.1	2.8	10
15	17.8	4.1	15
16	20.2	4.8	11
17	23.4	3.9	13
18	25.2	3.7	9
19	28.3	4.2	13
20	30.7	2.5	11
21	33.9	4.9	14
22	37.3	4.2	12

Source: Queenan JI, O'Brien GD, Campbell S. Ultrasound measurement of fetal limb bones. *Am J Obstet Gynecol* 1980;138:297–302.

Ossification of the Bones of the Lower Extremity

TABLE 5. *Time of ossification of the bones of the lower extremity*

No	C	263,c	A	56	333	B	202	274	263,b,2	266	263,b,1	272	J	I	282	K	L	284	288,b	M	N	300	O	S	Q	306,a	306,b	P	R
Length	18	19	..	24	..	29	30	31	32	33	34	34	36	41	42	53	54	54	57	69	70	73	73	75	81	100	105	105	110
Age	42	44	..	49	..	54	55	56	56	57	58	58	60	64	65	72	73	73	75	83	83	85	85	88	90	100	105	105	110

The first horizontal column indicates the number of embryos; the second, their crown/rump length in mm; the third, their probable age in days.

*, bone given in first column is ossified. ?, ossification is uncertain. 0, specimen was injured.

Source: Mall FP. On ossification centers in human embryos less than 100 days old. *Am J Anat* 1906;5:433.

Primary Ossification Centers of the Lower Extremity

TABLE 6. *Time of appearance of the primary ossification centers of the lower extremity in the first five prenatal months*

1 CENTERS	2 SMALLEST SPECIMEN(S) WITH CENTER PRESENT (mm CR)[1]	3 SPECIMEN(S) OF A CR LENGTH AFTER WHICH CENTER ALWAYS OBSERVED	4 SPECIMENS BETWEEN THOSE LISTED IN COLUMNS 2 AND 3 WITH THE BONE OSSIFIED	5 DATA IN LITERATURE[2] IN MM CR
Ilium	29(2)	38(1,3,4)	34(2), 35(2,4), 37	31(M), 35(O), 30–35(Ad)
Ischium	105(1,2)	124(1,2)	106, 108, 112, 113(1,2,3), 115(1), 116(1), 120(1,2)	88–93(Ad), 105(M), 120–155(O)
Pubis	161	161		150–170(Ad), 160–220(O)
Femur	23	35(2,3,4)	24(2,3), 27, 28(3), 29(1,2), 30(2), 31, 32, 34(1,2)	18(M)
Tibia	23	35(2,3,4)	24(2,3), 27, 28(3), 29(1,2), 31, 32, 34(1,2)	19(M)
Fibula	29(1,2)	35(2,3,4)	31, 34(1,2)	30(M)
Metatarsal 1	49	60(1,2)	52, 56(1,2), 57	34(M)
Metatarsal 2	38(4)	49	40(3), 44(1,2), 45(2,3,4), 48(1)	34(M)
Metatarsal 3	38(4)	49	40(3), 44(1,2), 45(2,4), 48(1)	34(M)
Metatarsal 4	40(3)	51	44(1,2), 45(4), 48(1), 49	34(M)
Metatarsal 5	45(4)	60(1,2)	48(1), 50, 52, 56(1,2), 57	34(M)
Prox. phalanges 1	69(1)	78		69(M)
Prox. phalanges 2	69(1)	76		70(M)
Prox. phalanges 3	88	91		70(M)
Prox. phalanges 4	91	91		70(M)
Prox. phalanges 5	91	115(2)	all present except 112, 113	70(M)
Middle phalanges 2	116(1)	147(2)	120(3), 127(2), 133, 134, 135, 138, 139(2), 140, 141, 143, 145	
Middle phalanges 3	140	after 235	141, 145, 148, 153, 161, 163(2), 173, 175	
Middle phalanges 4		after 235		
Middle phalanges 5		after 235		
Distal phalanges 1	38(4)	49	40(3,4), 44, 45(1,2,3,4)	34(M)
Distal phalanges 2	45(4)	56(1,2)	49, 51, 52, 53	34(M)
Distal phalanges 3	45(4)	56(1,2)	49, 51, 52, 53	34(M)
Distal phalanges 4	45(4)	68	49, 52, 53, 56, 60(2), 61(2), 65(3), 67	34(M)
Distal phalanges 5	60(1)	147(2)	65(1), 70, 71(after 71 mm, 37 specimens have this center), [45(4)][3]	69(M)
Calcaneus			120(2,3), 140, 173, 175, 235	
Talus		235	235	42(M, Ad)

The data are from 136 human embryos ranging in crown/rump length from 14 to 235 mm. The chart notes the bone, the smallest specimen with an ossification center present. The number refers to the crown/rump length in millimeters. When there was more than one specimen at that crown/rump length which also had the ossification present, its number was indicated in parentheses. Also shown are the specimen of a crown/rump length in which the ossification center was always observed; specimens between those listed in columns 2 and 3, with the bone ossified; and reviews of the previous literature pertaining to those specific bones. (Ad) = Adair, *Am J Obst Dis Women & Child* 1918;78:175–199. (M) = Mall, *Am J Anat* 1906;5:433–458. (O) = Obata, *Ztschet F Geburtsh & Gynak* 1912;22:533–574.

Source: Noback C, Robertson GG. Sequences of appearance of ossification centers in the human skeleton during the first five prenatal months. *Am J Anat* 1951;89:1–27.

Primary Ossification Centers in Shafts of Long Bones

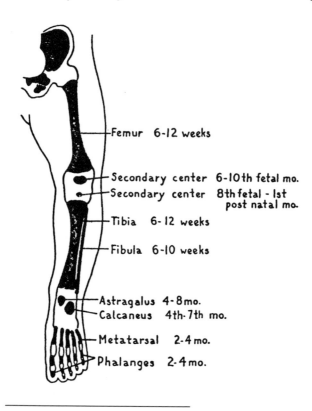

Femur 6-12 weeks

Secondary center 6-10th fetal mo.
Secondary center 8th fetal - 1st post natal mo.
Tibia 6-12 weeks
Fibula 6-10 weeks

Astragalus 4-8mo.
Calcaneus 4th-7th mo.
Metatarsal 2-4 mo.
Phalanges 2-4 mo.

FIG. 5. Time schedule for the appearance of the primary ossification centers in the shafts of long bones in the lower extremity and the foot during fetal life. (From J. Caffey et al., with permission.)

Source: Caffey J. et al. *Pediatric x-ray diagnosis*. 7th ed. Chicago: Yearbook Medical Publishers, Inc., 1978.

Secondary Epiphyseal Ossification Centers

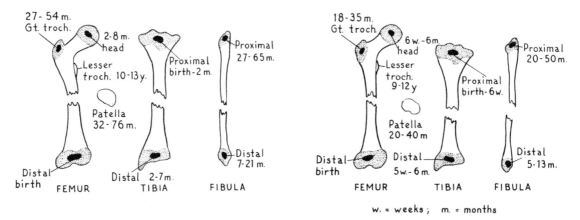

27-54 m. Gt. troch.
2-8 m. head
Lesser troch. 10-13 y.
Proximal birth-2 m.
Proximal 27-65 m.
Patella 32-76 m.
Distal birth FEMUR
Distal 2-7 m. TIBIA
Distal 7-21 m. FIBULA

18-35 m. Gt. troch.
6 w.-6 m. head
Lesser troch. 9-12 y
Proximal birth-6 w.
Proximal 20-50 m.
Patella 20-40 m
Distal birth
Distal 5 w.-6 m. FEMUR
Distal 5-13 m. FIBULA
TIBIA

w. = weeks ; m. = months

FIG. 6. Time schedule for appearance of secondary epiphyseal ossification centers in the lower extremity of boys **(left)** and girls **(right)**. (From J. Caffey et al., with permission.)

For a more detailed review of time of ossification, the reader is referred to the Chapter on Growth and Maturation, *this volume.*

Source: Caffey J. et al. *Pediatric x-ray diagnosis* 7th ed. Chicago: Yearbook Medical Publishers, Inc., 1978. (Modified from Voght EC and Vickers VE. Osseous Growth and Development. *Radiology* 1938;31:411–444.)

Femur in the Fetus

TABLE 7. *Development of the femur in the fetus*

C.-R. length	Overall length of femur	Total length of shaft	Length of ossified shaft	Percentage of overall length occupied by ossified shaft	Percentage of total length occupied by ossified shaft
37	9	7	1.5	17	21
57	15	14	6	40	43
61	17	16	6	35	37
63	17	16	8	47	50
64	15	14	5	33	36
69	17	16	7	41	44
73	19.5	18	9	46	50
77	22	21	10	45	48
85	26	25	14	54	56
86	26	25	13	50	52
92	26	25	13	50	52
93	26	26	14	54	54
97	26	25	14	54	56
103	28	27	16	57	60
105	26.5	25.5	14	53	55
110	32	31	19	60	61
111	30	29	17	57	59
113	36.5	35	23	63	66
118	36	35	23	64	66
125	38	38	24	63	63
127	37	36	23	62	64
130	41.5	40.5	26	63	64
135	41	40	27	66	67
138	45	43	30	67	70
146	45	43	30	67	70
148	44	43	29	66	67
151	44	43	29	66	67
165	59	58	42	71	72
180	52	50	36	69	72
185	53.5	52	37	69	71
185	55	54	37	67	69
211	61	59	42	70	71
277	78	76	55	70	72
302	83.5	83	61	73	73
316	84	81	59	70	73
342	87	84	64	73	77
342	95	94	71	75	76

This study included 40 pairs of femurs from a series of embryos and fetuses ranging from 26 to 342 mm in crown/rump length. They were measured, radiographed, and sectioned for microscopic study. The crown/rump (C.R.) lengths of the specimens in which enchondral ossification appeared, the overall lengths of the femur, the total lengths of the shaft, the length of the parts of the shaft occupied by enchondral bone, the percentage of overall lengths of the femurs occupied by ossified shaft, and the percentage of the total length of the femurs occupied by ossified shaft were recorded. The various lengths are given in millimeters.

Source: Gardner E, Gray D. The prenatal development of the human femur. *Am J Anat* 1971;129:121–40.

Linear Growth of Long Bones of the Lower Extremity from Infancy to Adolescence

TABLE 8. *Linear growth of long bones of the lower extremity from infancy through adolescence*

Yr.—Mo.	FEMUR 10%	25%	50%	75%	90%	Range	TIBIA 10%	25%	50%	75%	90%	Range	FIBULA 10%	25%	50%	75%	90%	Range
Boys																		
							Measurements Between Epiphyseal Plates											
0—2	7.76	8.18	8.58	8.85	9.20	7.2- 9.6	6.28	6.65	6.90	7.25	7.67	6.0- 8.3	5.94	6.36	6.65	7.04	7.44	5.6- 8.0
0—4	9.15	9.60	10.00	10.25	10.65	8.8-10.9	7.46	7.75	7.98	8.32	8.73	7.1- 8.8	7.16	7.46	7.70	8.00	8.33	6.8- 8.6
0—6	10.45	10.87	11.21	11.46	11.72	10.2-12.3	8.44	8.70	8.91	9.22	9.63	8.1-10.1	8.03	8.30	8.54	8.84	9.13	7.8- 9.8
0—9	12.75	13.19	13.66	13.96	14.28	12.8-14.9	10.32	10.63	10.87	11.20	11.62	9.9-12.2	9.90	10.21	10.57	10.92	11.26	9.6-11.7
1—0	14.62	15.08	15.50	15.92	16.30	14.5-16.8	11.92	12.26	12.55	12.90	13.34	11.5-13.7	11.48	11.84	12.24	12.61	13.04	11.3-13.5
1—6	16.24	16.78	17.17	17.61	18.03	15.8-18.5	13.22	13.60	13.97	14.35	14.82	13.0-15.1	12.86	13.24	13.68	14.08	14.55	12.7-15.1
2—0	17.66	18.21	18.67	19.13	19.62	16.9-20.0	14.37	14.80	15.22	15.61	16.12	14.0-16.5	14.09	14.50	14.97	15.39	15.88	13.8-16.4
2—6	18.98	19.52	20.00	20.50	21.06	18.2-21.3	15.43	15.87	16.32	16.73	17.26	14.8-17.7	15.22	15.66	16.14	16.58	17.07	14.8-17.6
3—0	20.09	20.70	21.20	21.75	22.35	19.2-22.8	16.43	16.88	17.35	17.78	18.32	16.1-18.9	16.26	16.71	17.20	17.64	18.14	15.9-18.7
3—6	21.23	21.86	22.36	22.97	23.64	19.9-24.8	17.37	17.84	18.33	18.78	19.34	16.8-20.9	17.18	17.65	18.15	18.62	19.15	16.5-20.9
4—0	22.34	22.98	23.51	24.16	24.92	21.0-25.3	18.28	18.77	19.28	19.74	20.31	17.6-21.0	18.08	18.57	19.08	19.58	20.12	17.4-20.7
4—6	23.44	24.10	24.65	25.34	26.18	21.9-27.6	19.15	19.65	20.18	20.66	21.25	18.2-23.0	18.96	19.46	19.98	20.52	21.06	17.9-23.0
5—0	24.52	25.20	25.77	26.51	27.42	23.9-28.3	19.99	20.51	21.06	21.57	22.18	19.6-24.2	19.80	20.31	20.84	21.44	22.03	19.6-24.0
5—6	25.58	26.27	26.87	27.66	28.62	24.7-29.6	20.79	21.34	21.92	22.46	23.10	20.4-25.0	20.62	21.14	21.68	22.33	22.98	20.4-25.0
6—0	26.62	27.38	27.98	28.79	29.78	26.0-30.7	21.57	22.14	22.75	23.35	24.01	21.1-26.4	21.42	21.95	22.50	23.21	23.87	21.0-26.1
6—6	27.64	28.37	29.02	29.90	30.92	26.9-32.9	22.33	22.94	23.57	24.23	24.91	21.6-27.5	22.19	22.74	23.30	24.07	24.77	21.4-27.3
7—0	28.62	29.37	30.06	30.98	32.08	28.2-33.5	23.06	23.73	24.39	25.10	25.81	22.0-28.6	22.94	23.52	24.09	24.92	25.67	22.0-28.4
7—6	29.56	30.35	31.09	32.08	33.10	29.4-35.1	23.88	24.52	25.20	25.96	26.71	23.0-29.6	23.67	24.28	24.87	25.75	26.56	22.8-29.3
8—0	30.52	31.31	32.06	33.08	34.14	30.4-34.6	24.57	25.30	26.01	26.82	27.61	24.1-28.1	24.38	25.02	25.63	26.57	27.44	23.9-29.1
8—6	31.42	32.23	33.02	34.02	35.16	31.3-37.3	25.31	26.06	26.80	27.67	28.50	24.6-31.6	25.07	25.74	26.38	27.37	28.32	24.6-31.0
9—0	32.30	33.12	33.96	35.00	36.14	31.6-38.5	26.08	26.78	27.59	28.50	29.38	24.6-32.5	25.74	26.44	27.13	28.17	29.19	24.8-31.9
9—6	33.16	33.99	34.86	35.96	37.11	33.1-39.2	26.74	27.51	28.23	29.31	30.26	26.2-33.3	26.38	27.13	27.86	28.95	30.06	26.0-32.5
10—0	34.00	34.85	35.76	36.91	38.07	33.3-40.2	27.45	28.23	29.14	30.10	31.13	26.0-34.0	27.01	27.82	28.59	29.75	30.92	26.2-33.8
10—6	34.84	35.76	36.64	37.85	39.08	34.6-41.0	28.16	28.96	29.90	30.89	32.00	27.6-35.2	27.64	28.51	29.31	30.53	31.77	27.1-34.2
11—0	35.67	36.56	37.53	38.79	39.96	33.0-42.0	28.84	29.66	30.65	31.67	32.85	27.0-35.9	28.27	29.19	30.02	31.30	32.61	27.1-35.0
11—6	36.50	37.40	38.40	39.73	40.98	38.7-43.3	29.52	30.37	31.42	32.45	33.70	28.4-36.4	28.90	29.86	30.73	32.05	33.44	27.9-35.3
							Measurements Include Epiphyses											
10—0	37.10	37.70	38.63	39.73	40.96	35.3-43.8	30.28	31.06	32.10	33.11	34.35	29.2-37.9	29.42	30.15	31.06	32.22	33.66	28.8-35.9
10—6	37.85	38.58	39.44	40.67	41.94	36.9-45.3	30.95	31.80	32.92	34.01	35.33	29.6-38.6	30.08	30.80	31.68	32.90	34.38	29.0-36.7
11—0	38.64	39.46	40.39	41.67	43.00	38.0-46.7	31.70	32.59	33.80	34.96	36.34	30.8-39.3	30.65	31.50	32.44	33.68	35.16	30.2-37.6
11—6	39.46	40.85	41.87	42.70	44.10	36.5-45.8	32.50	33.45	34.73	35.95	37.37	31.0-40.6	31.34	32.25	33.27	34.53	36.08	30.0-38.7
12—0	40.32	41.26	42.40	43.80	45.26	37.2-48.0	33.35	34.38	35.70	36.99	38.42	32.2-41.3	32.06	33.05	34.16	35.44	36.97	30.7-38.9
12—6	41.23	42.19	43.44	44.95	46.45	40.7-48.8	34.27	35.35	36.73	38.04	39.50	33.3-42.0	32.87	33.91	35.10	36.43	38.00	32.1-39.7
13—0	42.15	43.16	44.50	46.18	47.67	41.0-49.3	35.25	36.33	37.90	39.18	40.64	34.1-42.7	33.73	34.58	36.10	37.51	39.15	33.0-40.7
13—6	43.12	44.18	45.60	47.45	48.97	40.5-50.9	36.36	37.57	39.00	40.40	41.98	34.5-43.5	34.64	35.51	37.25	38.73	40.43	31.1-41.3
14—0	44.10	45.27	46.77	48.70	50.23	41.3-51.9	37.55	38.70	39.95	41.37	43.08	36.5-44.5	35.70	36.59	38.25	39.79	41.57	35.1-43.6
14—6	45.18	46.43	47.95	49.90	51.36	41.9-52.5	38.53	39.57	40.80	42.25	43.96	35.9-45.3	36.70	37.89	39.15	40.74	41.57	34.5-43.1
15—0	46.30	47.60	49.00	50.65	52.23	44.9-53.7	39.17	40.25	41.50	42.98	44.78	38.5-45.9	37.55	38.65	39.94	41.56	43.43	36.5-44.3
15—6	47.25	48.45	49.98	51.52	52.90	46.4-54.2	39.61	40.75	42.10	43.62	45.39	37.9-47.0	38.08	39.20	40.54	42.20	44.11	37.0-45.6
16—0	47.67	48.83	50.51	51.98	53.58	45.3-54.9	39.82	41.07	42.50	44.05	45.90	38.6-48.3	38.36	39.50	40.95	42.66	44.63	38.1-46.3
16—6	47.96	49.07	50.40	52.16	53.76	47.1-56.5	39.96	41.20	42.75	44.33	46.51	39.1-48.7	38.43	39.63	41.23	42.99	45.08	38.3-46.3
17—0	48.10	49.14	50.45	52.35	54.03	47.0-57.0	40.04	41.27	42.90	44.51	46.43	39.1-49.1	38.47	39.66	41.37	43.32	45.33	37.9-46.8
17—6	48.17	49.19	50.48	52.52	54.20	47.0-57.0	40.08	41.30	42.96	44.60	46.51	39.1-49.1	38.49	39.69	41.45	43.38	45.54	37.9-46.8
18—0	48.20	49.22	50.50	52.60	54.30	48.1-57.4	40.10	41.33	43.08	44.65	46.60	39.0-49.6	38.50	39.70	41.50	43.45	45.68	37.9-47.5

Girls

Measurements Between Epiphyseal Plates

Age																		
0-2	8.20	8.50	8.72	9.00	9.28	7.8-9.7	6.32	6.67	7.00	7.28	7.58	6.0-8.0	6.06	6.30	6.55	6.86	7.16	5.7-7.5
0-4	9.43	9.78	10.00	10.25	10.50	9.4-10.9	7.35	7.69	8.03	8.30	8.60	7.0-8.8	7.02	7.36	7.67	7.90	8.21	6.7-8.4
0-6	10.57	10.91	11.15	11.36	11.58	9.8-12.0	8.20	8.60	8.87	9.17	9.48	7.3-9.8	7.74	8.16	8.52	8.78	9.06	6.9-9.4
1-0	12.67	13.06	13.36	13.80	14.18	12.3-14.8	10.12	10.50	10.77	11.10	11.51	9.6-12.0	9.67	10.13	10.52	10.86	11.15	9.3-11.6
1-6	14.44	14.88	15.26	15.80	16.30	14.2-16.7	11.64	12.05	12.37	12.73	13.20	11.2-13.5	11.23	11.73	12.17	12.56	12.90	10.6-13.4
2-0	16.00	16.47	16.89	17.48	18.02	15.8-18.7	12.92	13.39	13.75	14.14	14.65	12.4-15.2	12.55	13.06	13.54	13.96	14.36	12.0-15.1
2-6	17.39	17.89	18.37	19.00	19.58	17.0-20.1	14.03	14.54	15.00	15.42	15.95	13.7-16.4	13.74	14.29	14.78	15.22	15.67	13.3-16.3
3-0	18.64	19.19	19.74	20.40	21.02	17.8-21.4	14.99	15.56	16.10	16.57	17.15	14.0-17.8	14.82	15.40	15.93	16.40	16.85	14.1-17.7
3-6	19.80	20.39	21.01	21.73	22.41	19.1-22.9	15.87	16.52	17.14	17.67	18.30	15.0-19.1	15.83	16.45	17.02	17.51	18.02	15.1-18.8
4-0	20.90	21.54	22.24	23.02	23.76	20.1-24.2	16.71	17.46	18.15	18.73	19.43	15.7-20.0	16.76	17.42	18.03	18.58	19.12	15.8-19.8
4-6	21.96	22.66	23.44	24.27	25.07	21.2-25.8	17.55	18.38	19.12	19.75	20.54	16.7-21.1	17.58	18.30	18.96	19.62	20.20	16.6-21.0
5-0	23.00	23.76	24.68	25.50	26.35	22.4-27.1	18.38	19.28	20.06	20.74	21.62	17.5-22.6	18.35	19.15	19.85	20.62	21.26	17.4-22.4
5-6	24.02	24.84	25.79	26.71	27.60	23.3-28.2	19.20	20.16	20.96	21.71	22.63	18.3-23.5	19.12	19.97	20.73	21.59	22.29	18.3-23.1
6-0	25.02	25.92	26.94	27.89	28.81	24.2-30.0	20.00	21.01	21.83	22.67	23.61	19.3-24.3	19.88	20.78	21.60	22.52	23.27	19.6-24.0
6-6	26.02	26.96	28.07	29.04	29.98	25.2-30.8	20.77	21.84	22.70	23.60	24.57	20.7-26.7	20.64	21.59	22.46	23.41	24.21	19.9-25.3
7-0	27.01	28.08	29.16	30.15	31.10	26.0-32.2	21.54	22.67	23.56	24.51	25.51	20.7-26.7	21.39	22.39	23.32	24.27	25.09	20.6-26.3
7-6	27.99	29.11	30.22	31.22	32.18	26.8-34.0	22.31	23.50	24.41	25.42	26.45	21.5-27.5	22.13	23.19	24.18	25.10	25.91	21.3-27.2
8-0	28.94	30.11	31.25	32.25	33.21	27.8-34.3	23.07	24.32	25.25	26.32	27.38	22.3-29.4	22.87	23.98	25.04	25.91	26.74	22.1-27.9
8-6	29.84	31.06	32.25	33.26	34.24	28.8-34.9	23.80	25.12	26.08	27.22	28.28	23.1-29.2	23.58	24.76	25.88	26.74	27.58	22.7-28.6
9-0	30.69	31.96	33.22	34.24	35.26	29.6-36.2	24.50	25.91	26.98	28.12	29.18	23.7-30.1	24.26	25.52	26.70	27.62	28.52	23.4-29.5
9-6	31.50	32.80	34.14	35.18	36.28	30.5-38.1	25.19	26.67	27.77	29.02	30.10	24.4-31.3	24.92	26.25	27.48	28.60	29.60	24.1-30.7
10-0	32.28	33.62	35.02	36.17	37.30	31.3-38.3	25.87	27.42	28.59	29.98	31.06	25.9-33.8	25.61	26.99	28.28	29.54	30.65	24.8-31.4
10-6	33.03	34.47	35.96	37.20	38.35	32.2-41.6	26.54	28.17	29.40	30.86	32.01	26.5-35.0	26.31	27.77	29.12	30.46	31.67	25.4-33.0
11-0	33.78	35.38	36.95	38.28	39.45	33.3-43.2	27.28	28.95	30.28	31.80	32.98	27.8-35.6	27.02	28.56	29.90	31.31	32.61	25.9-33.9
11-6	34.60	36.29	38.06	39.40	40.60	34.0-44.1	28.10	29.77	31.18	32.77	33.99	28.1-36.6	27.72	29.32	30.60	32.08	33.45	26.7-35.0
12-0	35.50	37.35	39.32	40.56	41.85	35.3-44.9	29.02	30.71	32.18	33.80	35.10	28.1-36.6	28.40	30.02	31.26	32.80	34.30	27.3-35.7

Measurements Include Epiphyses

Age																		
10-0	35.57	37.06	39.03	40.15	41.50	34.6-42.0	29.51	31.10	32.55	34.12	35.22	28.4-35.9	28.47	30.12	31.55	32.70	33.75	27.6-34.6
10-6	36.39	37.93	40.02	41.50	43.15	35.5-46.3	30.34	32.00	33.64	35.30	36.60	29.2-37.8	29.13	30.82	32.28	33.88	35.12	28.3-36.1
11-0	37.32	38.90	41.02	42.72	44.41	36.6-47.8	31.18	32.92	34.64	36.35	37.76	30.3-39.0	29.87	31.58	33.04	34.86	36.12	28.9-37.3
11-6	38.33	40.04	42.08	43.85	45.49	37.5-48.7	32.08	33.86	35.52	37.28	38.70	31.1-40.4	30.68	32.42	33.90	35.74	37.08	29.7-38.4
12-0	39.40	41.21	43.30	44.90	46.48	38.9-49.3	32.91	34.80	36.30	38.13	39.49	32.7-41.0	31.47	33.26	34.75	36.53	37.83	30.4-39.2
12-6	40.34	42.22	44.37	45.83	47.35	39.8-48.4	33.74	35.66	37.00	38.88	40.14	32.7-41.0	32.25	34.08	35.55	37.22	38.56	31.2-39.4
13-0	41.18	43.10	45.27	46.62	48.09	39.9-51.0	34.50	36.39	37.66	39.47	40.67	33.6-42.1	33.01	34.83	36.28	37.80	39.18	32.0-40.6
13-6	41.95	43.90	46.03	47.24	48.67	41.5-49.1	35.21	37.02	38.28	39.93	41.08	34.3-42.8	33.63	35.46	36.87	38.26	39.65	32.6-41.3
14-0	42.65	44.58	46.65	47.69	49.10	41.7-52.1	35.90	37.55	38.78	40.28	41.39	34.6-43.4	34.13	35.94	37.33	38.61	39.98	33.1-41.8
14-6	43.31	45.09	47.06	48.03	49.42	42.3-50.1	36.21	37.92	39.17	40.51	41.58	34.9-43.3	34.51	36.30	37.70	38.86	40.20	33.3-41.7
15-0	43.96	45.41	47.22	48.27	49.58	42.2-52.0	36.50	38.15	39.36	40.66	41.67	34.8-41.9	34.82	36.60	37.94	39.00	40.82	33.5-40.6
15-6	44.17	45.60	47.28	48.37	49.65	42.2-52.0	36.69	38.30	39.45	40.75	41.70	34.8-42.0	35.05	36.83	38.06	39.07	40.36	33.4-40.7
16-0	44.35	45.66	47.28	48.40	49.65	42.2-52.0	36.78	38.37	39.50	40.78	41.70	34.8-42.0	35.20	36.98	38.10	39.10	40.36	33.4-40.7

The data are comprised from several groups. The first 55 children whose bone lengths were measured were 2 months through 3 to 4 years of age. The second group (59 children) were 3 to 4 years through 9 to 11 years; and the third group of 59 young adults were measured from childhood or early adolescence to the completion of growth. In the younger children the measurement was made between the epiphyseal plates, and in the older children the measurement includes the epiphyses. Included are the percentiles and the observed range of roentgenographic bone lengths.

Related references:
Maresh MM. Growth of major long bones in healthy children—a preliminary report in successive roentgenographs of the extremities from early infancy to twelve years of age. *Am J Dis Child* 1943;66:227–257.
Source: Maresh MM. Linear growth of long bones of the extremities. *Am J Dis Child* 1955;89:725–42.

Distribution of Lengths of Normal Femur and Tibia in Children 1 to 18 Years of Age

A group of 67 boys and 67 girls were followed longitudinally. These children had regular repeated roentgenograms of the lower extremities. It is a part of the recorded observations in a comprehensive longitudinal study of child health and development in the Harvard School of Public Health.

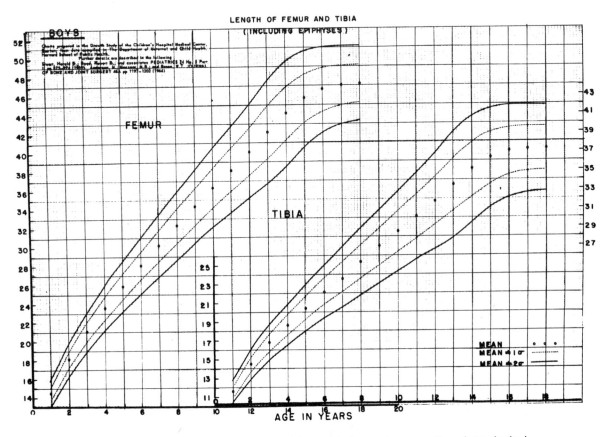

FIG. 7. Length of femur and tibia (including the epiphyses) in boys at consecutive chronological ages from 1 to 18.

Source: Tachdijian MO. *Pediatric Orthopedics* W. B. Saunders Co., 1972. (Modified from Anderson MS, Messner MB, and Green WT. Distributions of lengths of the normal femur and tibia in children from 1 to 18 years of age. *J Bone Joint Surg* 1964;46(A):1197–1202.)

Table 9 consists of orthoroentgenographic measurements of the longitudinal series of 67 children. The data were used to construct the graphs in Fig. 7.

TABLE 9. *Length of the long bones including epiphyses in 67 boys*

Femur

No.	Age	Mean	σ_d	σ_m	Distribution			
					$+2\sigma_d$	$+1\sigma_d$	$-1\sigma_d$	$-2\sigma_d$
21	1	14.48	0.628	0.077	15.74	15.11	13.85	13.22
57	2	18.15	0.874	0.107	19.90	19.02	17.28	16.40
65	3	21.09	1.031	0.126	23.15	22.12	20.06	19.03
66	4	23.65	1.197	0.146	26.04	24.85	22.45	21.26
66	5	25.92	1.342	0.164	28.60	27.26	24.58	23.24
67	6	28.09	1.506	0.184	31.10	29.60	26.58	25.08
67	7	30.25	1.682	0.205	33.61	31.93	28.57	26.89
67	8	32.28	1.807	0.221	35.89	34.09	30.47	28.67
67	9	34.36	1.933	0.236	38.23	36.29	32.43	30.49
67	10	36.29	2.057	0.251	40.40	38.35	34.23	32.18
67	11	38.16	2.237	0.276	42.63	40.40	35.92	33.69
67	12	40.12	2.447	0.299	45.01	42.57	37.67	35.23
67	13	42.17	2.765	0.338	47.70	44.95	39.40	36.64
67	14	44.18	2.809	0.343	49.80	46.99	41.37	38.56
67	15	45.69	2.512	0.307	50.71	48.20	43.19	40.67
67	16	46.66	2.244	0.274	51.15	48.90	44.42	42.17
67	17	47.07	2.051	0.251	51.17	49.12	45.02	42.97
67	18	47.23	1.958	0.239	51.15	49.19	45.27	43.31

Tibia

No.	Age	Mean	σ_d	σ_m	Distribution			
					$+2\sigma_d$	$+1\sigma_d$	$-1\sigma_d$	$-2\sigma_d$
61	1	11.60	0.620	0.074	12.84	12.22	10.98	10.36
67	2	14.54	0.809	0.099	16.16	15.35	13.73	12.92
67	3	16.79	0.935	0.114	18.66	17.72	15.86	14.92
67	4	18.67	1.091	0.133	20.85	19.76	17.58	16.49
67	5	20.46	1.247	0.152	22.95	21.71	19.21	17.97
67	6	22.12	1.418	0.173	24.96	23.54	20.87	19.46
67	7	23.76	1.632	0.199	27.02	25.39	22.13	20.50
67	8	25.38	1.778	0.217	28.94	27.16	23.60	21.82
67	9	26.99	1.961	0.240	30.91	28.95	25.02	23.06
67	10	28.53	2.113	0.258	32.76	30.64	26.42	24.30
67	11	30.10	2.301	0.281	34.70	32.40	27.80	25.50
67	12	31.75	2.536	0.310	36.82	34.29	29.21	26.68
67	13	33.49	2.833	0.346	39.16	36.32	30.66	27.82
67	14	35.18	2.865	0.350	40.91	38.04	32.32	29.45
67	15	36.38	2.616	0.320	41.61	39.00	33.76	31.15
67	16	37.04	2.412	0.295	41.86	39.45	34.63	32.22
67	17	37.22	2.316	0.283	41.85	39.54	34.90	32.59
67	18	37.29	2.254	0.275	41.80	39.54	35.04	32.78

Source: Anderson MS, Messner MB, Green WT. Distribution of lengths of the normal femur and tibia in children from 1 to 18 years of age. *J Bone Joint Surg* 1964;46(A):1197–1202.

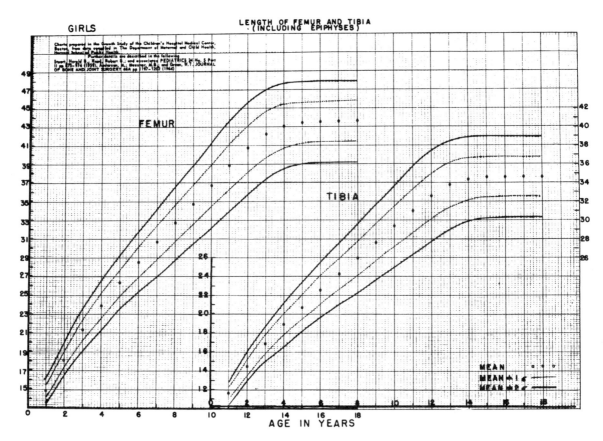

FIG. 8. Length of femur and tibia (including the epiphyses) in girls at consecutive chronological ages from 1 through 18.

Source: Tachdijian MO. *Pediatric Orthopedics* W. B. Saunders Co., 1972. (Modified from Anderson MS, Messner MB, and Green WT. Distributions of lengths of the normal femur and tibia in children from 1 to 18 years of age. *J Bone Joint Surg* 1964;46(A):1197–1202.)

Table 10 consists of orthoroentgenographic measurements from longitudinal series of 67 children. The data were used to construct the graphs in Fig. 8.

TABLE 10. *Length of the long bones including epiphyses in 67 girls*

Femur

No.	Age	Mean	σ_d	σ_m	Distribution			
					$+2\sigma_d$	$+1\sigma_d$	$-1\sigma_d$	$-2\sigma_d$
30	1	14.81	0.673	0.082	16.16	15.48	14.14	13.46
52	2	18.23	0.888	0.109	20.01	19.12	17.34	16.45
63	3	21.29	1.100	0.134	23.49	22.39	20.19	19.09
66	4	23.92	1.339	0.164	26.60	25.26	22.58	21.24
66	5	26.32	1.437	0.176	29.19	27.76	24.88	23.45
66	6	28.52	1.616	0.197	31.75	30.14	26.90	25.29
67	7	30.60	1.827	0.223	34.25	32.43	28.77	26.95
67	8	32.72	1.936	0.236	36.59	34.66	30.78	28.85
67	9	34.71	2.117	0.259	38.94	36.83	32.59	30.48
67	10	36.72	2.300	0.281	41.32	39.02	34.42	32.12
67	11	38.81	2.468	0.302	43.75	41.28	36.34	33.87
67	12	40.74	2.507	0.306	45.75	43.25	38.23	35.73
67	13	42.31	2.428	0.310	47.17	44.74	39.88	37.45
67	14	43.14	2.269	0.277	47.68	45.41	40.87	38.60
67	15	43.47	2.197	0.277	47.86	45.67	41.27	39.08
67	16	43.58	2.193	0.268	47.97	45.77	41.39	39.19
67	17	43.60	2.192	0.268	47.98	45.79	41.41	39.22
67	18	43.63	2.195	0.269	48.02	45.82	41.44	39.24

Tibia

No.	Age	Mean	σ_d	σ_m	Distribution			
					$+2\sigma_d$	$+1\sigma_d$	$-1\sigma_d$	$-2\sigma_d$
61	1	11.57	0.646	0.082	12.86	12.22	10.92	10.28
67	2	14.51	0.739	0.090	15.99	15.25	13.77	13.03
67	3	16.81	0.893	0.109	18.60	17.70	15.92	15.02
67	4	18.86	1.144	0.140	21.15	20.00	17.72	16.57
67	5	20.77	1.300	0.159	23.37	22.07	19.47	18.17
67	6	22.53	1.458	0.178	25.45	23.99	21.07	19.61
67	7	24.22	1.640	0.200	27.50	25.86	22.58	20.94
67	8	25.89	1.786	0.218	29.46	27.68	24.10	22.32
67	9	27.56	1.993	0.243	31.55	29.55	25.57	23.57
67	10	29.28	2.193	0.259	33.67	31.47	27.09	24.89
67	11	31.00	2.384	0.291	35.77	33.38	28.62	26.23
67	12	32.61	2.424	0.296	37.46	35.03	30.19	27.76
67	13	33.83	2.374	0.290	38.58	36.20	31.46	29.08
67	14	34.43	2.228	0.272	38.89	36.66	32.20	29.97
67	15	34.59	2.173	0.265	38.94	36.76	32.42	30.24
67	16	34.63	2.151	0.263	38.93	36.78	32.48	30.33
67	17	34.65	2.158	0.264	38.97	36.81	32.49	30.33
67	18	34.65	2.161	0.264	38.97	36.81	32.49	30.33

Source: Anderson MS, Messner MB, and Green WT. Distributions of lengths of the normal femur and tibia in children from 1 to 18 years of age. *J Bone Joint Surg* 1964;46(A):1197–1202.

Growth Predictions in the Lower Extremity

One hundred children, 50 girls and 50 boys, were measured at least once a year over the 8 years before growth terminated in their lower extremities. Of this number, 51 children were normal (25 girls, 26 boys) and 49 children (25 girls, 24 boys) had paralytic poliomyelitis which affected only the lower extremity opposite the one included here. Each child, in order to be included in the group, had to have a continuous record which covered the years from the age of 8 in girls and age of 10 in boys until all growth had ceased in the lower extremities and epiphyseal fusion was complete. The femur and tibia were measured from orthoroentgenograms, and each length, including both the proximal and distal epiphysis was recorded. Maturity was regularly evaluated using the hand and wrist and the Greulich and Pyle Atlas as a standard reference.

TABLE 11. *Variation in size and relative maturity at consecutive chronological ages from a completely longitudinal series of 50 boys*

Age	Stature (cm)		Femur (cm)		Tibia (cm)		Skeletal Age (Years)	
	Mean	σ	Mean	σ	Mean	σ	Mean	σ
8	127.6	5.94	(32.8)	(1.53)	(25.9)	(1.55)	(7.8)	(1.00)
9	133.3	6.15	(34.6)	(1.78)	(27.1)	(1.86)	(8.8)	(1.04)
10	138.5	6.58	36.4	1.87	28.6	1.89	9.9	0.96
11	143.5	6.94	38.2	2.07	30.1	2.07	11.0	0.88
12	149.4	7.72	40.2	2.23	31.8	2.27	12.1	0.76
13	156.3	9.13	42.3	2.52	33.6	2.49	13.1	0.80
14	163.7	9.54	44.3	2.58	35.3	2.54	14.1	0.93
15	169.8	8.68	45.8	2.38	36.4	2.34	15.1	1.14
16	173.2	7.74	46.6	2.27	36.9	2.21	16.3	1.20
17	175.0	7.41	46.9	2.30	37.1	2.21	17.3	1.10
18	175.9	7.37	47.0	2.35	37.1	2.22	(18.0)	(0.89)

Bone lengths, measured from orthoroentgenograms, include both proximal and distal epiphyses. Skeletal ages read according to Greulich and Pyle Atlas (1950). (See Chapter on the Hand, *this volume*.)

Figures in parentheses are based on 31 to 49 boys only, as data were not available on all subjects at these ages.

TABLE 12. *Variation in size and relative maturity at consecutive chronological ages from a completely longitudinal series of 50 girls*

Age	Stature (cm)		Femur (cm)		Tibia (cm)		Skeletal Age (Years)	
	Mean	σ	Mean	σ	Mean	σ	Mean	σ
8	128.1	4.78	33.1	1.63	26.3	1.39	7.6	1.02
9	133.8	4.78	35.0	1.71	28.0	1.50	8.7	1.02
10	139.9	5.24	37.0	1.82	29.8	1.67	9.9	1.03
11	146.6	5.93	39.2	2.00	31.6	1.84	11.1	1.07
12	153.2	6.36	41.1	2.12	33.2	1.95	12.5	1.12
13	158.3	6.14	42.4	2.12	34.2	1.94	13.8	1.06
14	160.8	6.16	43.1	2.15	34.5	1.97	14.8	1.05
15	162.3	6.02	43.2	2.18	34.6	1.98	15.8	1.00
16	162.9	6.10	43.3	2.20	34.6	2.00	16.4	0.92
17	(163.8)	(6.37)	(43.3)	(2.21)	(34.7)	(2.00)	(17.1)	(0.85)
18	(164.9)	(6.10)	(43.3)	(2.21)	(34.7)	(2.00)	(17.8)	(0.46)

Bone lengths, measured from orthoroentgenograms, include both proximal and distal epiphyses. Skeletal ages read according to Greulich and Pyle Atlas (1950). (See chapter on the Hand, *this volume*.)

Figures in parentheses are based on 21 to 24 girls only, as data were not available on all subjects at these ages.

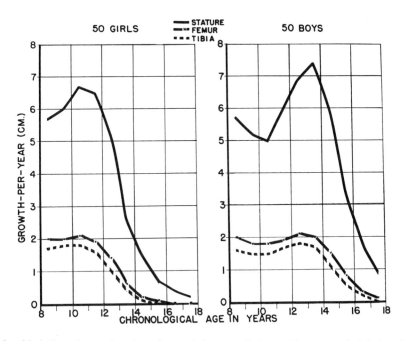

FIG. 9. Variations in yearly rates of growth (average) derived from completely longitudinal series of 50 girls and 50 boys.

Source: Anderson M. Growth and predictions of growth in the lower extremities. *J Bone Joint Surg* 1963;45(A).

TABLE 13. *Variations in yearly rates of growth at consecutive chronological ages from a completely longitudinal series of 50 girls and 50 boys.*

50 Girls						Age Interval in Years	50 Boys					
Stature		Femur		Tibia			Stature		Femur		Tibia	
Mean	σ	Mean	σ	Mean	σ		Mean	σ	Mean	σ	Mean	σ
5.7	0.77	2.0	0.28	1.7	0.29	8– 9	5.7	0.88	(2.0)	(0.27)	(1.6)	(0.22)
6.0	1.39	2.0	0.32	1.8	0.36	9–10	5.2	0.91	(1.8)	(0.32)	(1.5)	(0.27)
6.7	1.70	2.1	0.35	1.8	0.38	10–11	5.0	0.80	1.8	0.34	1.5	0.28
6.5	1.91	1.9	0.52	1.6	0.56	11–12	5.9	1.60	1.9	0.42	1.7	0.42
5.2	**2.20**	1.4	**0.67**	1.0	**0.63**	12–13	6.9	2.16	2.1	0.50	1.8	0 49
2.5	1.50	0.6	0.50	0.4	0.41	13–14	7.4	2.02	2.0	0.52	1.7	0.58
1.4	1.15	0.2	0.30	0.1	0.24	14–15	6.0	**2.56**	1.5	**0.79**	1.1	0.68
0.7	0.79	0.1	0.20	0.0	0.14	15–16	3.5	2.37	0.8	0.73	0.5	**0.77**
(0.4)	(0.58)	(0.0)	(0.06)	(0.0)	(0.04)	16–17	1.8	1.74	0.3	0.38	0.2	0.25
(0.2)	(0.46)	(0.0)	(0.00)	(0.0)	(0.00)	17–18	0.9	1.04	0.1	0.17	0.0	0.08

All values in centimeters.

Figures in parentheses are based on 35 to 44 children only, as data were not available on every subject at these ages. Maximum variation shown by boldface figures.

These data were used to construct the graph in Fig. 9.

TABLE 14. *Variation in total growth remaining (entire bone) before epiphyseal fusion, by consecutive chronological ages*

50 Girls						Age in Years	50 Boys					
Stature		Femur		Tibia			Stature		Femur		Tibia	
Mean	σ	Mean	σ	Mean	σ		Mean	σ	Mean	σ	Mean	σ
34.8	3.88	10.2	1.54	8.4	1.32	8	48.2	4.03	(14.2)	(1.44)	(11.4)	(1.20)
29.1	3.87	8.3	1.55	6.6	1.29	9	42.6	3.93	(12.2)	(1.50)	(9.9)	(1.17)
23.0	4.54	6.3	1.61	4.8	1.38	10	37.4	4.01	10.5	1.46	8.5	1.17
16.3	**5.28**	4.2	**1.71**	3.0	**1.45**	11	32.3	4.21	8.7	1.48	7.0	1.18
9.8	4.57	2.3	1.42	1.4	1.15	12	26.5	5.10	6.8	1.66	5.3	1.40
4.6	2.95	0.9	0.91	0.5	0.71	13	19.6	**6.48**	4.7	**1.90**	3.5	**1.63**
2.1	1.77	0.2	0.53	0.1	0.40	14	12.1	6.38	2.7	1.78	1.8	1.42
0.7	0.79	0.1	0.24	0.0	0.17	15	6.1	4.63	1.2	1.21	0.7	0.88
						16	2.6	2.58	0.4	0.54	0.2	0.33
						17	0.9	1.05	0.1	0.19	0.0	0.10

Figures in parentheses are based on 35 to 44 children only, as data were not available on every subject at these ages. Maximum variation shown by boldface figures.

Source: Anderson M. Growth and predictions of growth in the lower extremities. *J Bone Joint Surg* 1963;45(A).

Growth Remaining in Normal Distal Femur and Proximal Tibia, by Skeletal Age

These data were derived from the same longitudinal series of 50 girls and 50 boys as in Figs. 11 and 12. The emphasis here however, is on the remaining growth in the distal femur and proximal tibia. The latter data were directed toward the entire bone.

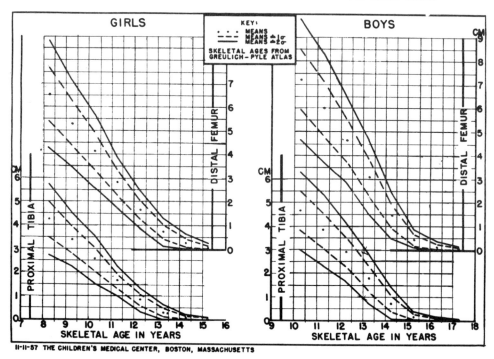

11-11-57 THE CHILDREN'S MEDICAL CENTER, BOSTON, MASSACHUSETTS

FIG. 10. Growth remaining in normal distal femur and proximal tibia following consecutive skeletal age levels.

Source: Anderson MS, Messner MB, Green WT. Distribution of lengths of the normal femur and tibia in children from 1 to 18 years of age. *J Bone Joint Surg* 1964;46(A):1197–1202.

TABLE 15. *Growth in the distal end of the normal femur and proximal end of the normal tibia in a longitudinal series, by given skeletal ages*

	50 Girls								50 Boys							
	8^3*	9^3	10^3	11^3	12^3	13^3	14^3	15^3	10^3	11^3	12^3	13^3	14^3	15^3	16^3	17^3
Distal End of the Femur (Total Growth Femur × 71%)																
Mean	6.54	5.30	4.15	2.82	1.66	0.75	0.27	0.05	7.21	6.01	4.65	3.09	1.48	0.45	0.15	0.04
σ	1.14	0.92	0.78	0.53	0.40	0.30	0.18	0.08	1.28	1.14	0.91	0.78	0.50	0.23	0.12	0.06
Extreme	9.8	8.6	7.2	4.7	2.8	1.5	0.7	0.4	9.7	8.4	7.2	5.7	3.0	1.0	0.6	0.2
90th	8.4	6.7	5.0	3.4	2.1	1.1	0.6	0.1	8.9	7.8	5.7	4.2	2.2	0.8	0.3	0.1
Percentiles 75th	7.2	5.8	4.6	3.2	1.9	1.0	0.4	0.1	8.3	6.7	5.2	3.5	1.8	0.6	0.2	0.1
Percentiles 50th	6.5	5.2	4.1	2.8	1.7	0.7	0.3	0.0	7.2	6.1	4.8	2.9	1.4	0.4	0.1	0.0
Percentiles 25th	5.8	4.8	3.7	2.4	1.4	0.6	0.1	0.0	6.3	5.2	4.1	2.6	1.2	0.3	0.1	0.0
10th	5.0	4.3	3.3	2.2	1.1	0.4	0.0	0.0	5.3	4.4	3.4	2.3	1.0	0.2	0.0	0.0
Extreme	4.1	3.1	2.2	1.6	0.7	0.1	0.0	0.0	4.8	3.8	2.8	1.6	0.4	0.1	0.0	0.0
Proximal End of the Tibia (Total Growth Tibia × 57%)																
Mean	4.25	3.39	2.58	1.65	0.86	0.32	0.09	0.02	4.65	3.83	2.92	1.80	0.74	0.16	0.04	0.01
σ	0.74	0.58	0.50	0.32	0.26	0.17	0.06	0.03	0.83	0.75	0.62	0.53	0.35	0.12	0.06	0.02
Extreme	6.0	5.1	4.3	2.8	1.5	0.8	0.3	0.1	6.7	5.6	4.7	3.4	2.2	0.7	0.3	0.1
90th	5.5	4.2	3.2	1.9	1.2	0.6	0.2	0.1	5.8	4.8	3.6	2.5	1.1	0.3	0.1	0.0
Percentiles 75th	4.6	3.7	2.7	1.8	1.0	0.4	0.1	0.1	5.3	4.3	3.3	2.0	0.8	0.2	0.0	0.0
Percentiles 50th	4.1	3.3	2.6	1.6	0.8	0.3	0.0	0.0	4.6	3.8	3.0	1.8	0.7	0.2	0.0	0.0
Percentiles 25th	3.8	3.0	2.3	1.5	0.7	0.2	0.0	0.0	4.0	3.2	2.6	1.4	0.5	0.0	0.0	0.0
10th	3.3	2.8	2.0	1.2	0.6	0.1	0.0	0.0	3.4	2.7	2.0	1.1	0.3	0.0	0.0	0.0
Extreme	2.5	1.9	1.1	0.9	0.3	0.0	0.0	0.0	3.0	2.3	1.6	1.0	0.1	0.0	0.0	0.0

These data were used to construct the graphs in Fig. 10. (Growth recorded in centimeters; skeletal ages assessed from Greulich and Pyle Atlas)

Source: Anderson MS, Messner MB, Green WT. Distribution of lengths of the normal femur and tibia in children from 1 to 18 years of age. *J Bone Joint Surg* 1964;46(A):1197–1202.

Related reference:

Green WT, Anderson M. Experiences with epiphyseal arrest in correcting discrepencies in length of the lower extremities in infantile paralysis: a method of predicting effect. *J Bone Joint Surg(A)* 1947;29:659–675.

Moseley's Straight Line Graph for Leg Length Discrepancies

Moseley's straight line graph facilitates the recording and interpretation of data in cases of leg length discrepancy. This chart provides a mechanism for predicting future growth that automatically takes into account the child's growth percentile in addition to the short leg. The straight line graph method is believed to be significantly more accurate than the growth remaining (see Fig. 10), particularly in cases of growth inhibition.

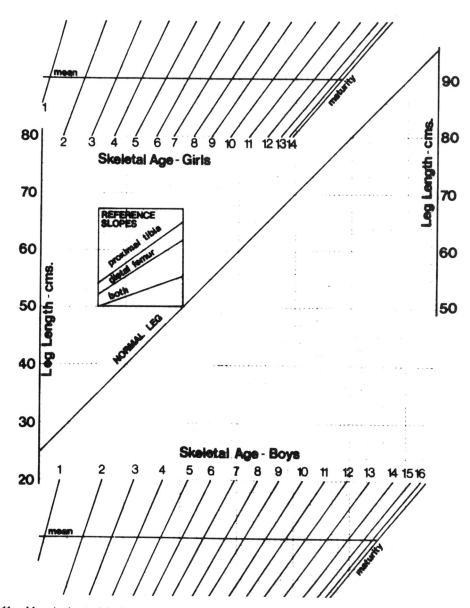

FIG. 11. Moseley's straight line graph.

Source: Moseley CF. A straight line graph for leg length discrepancies. *J Bone Joint Surg* 1977;59A:174–9.

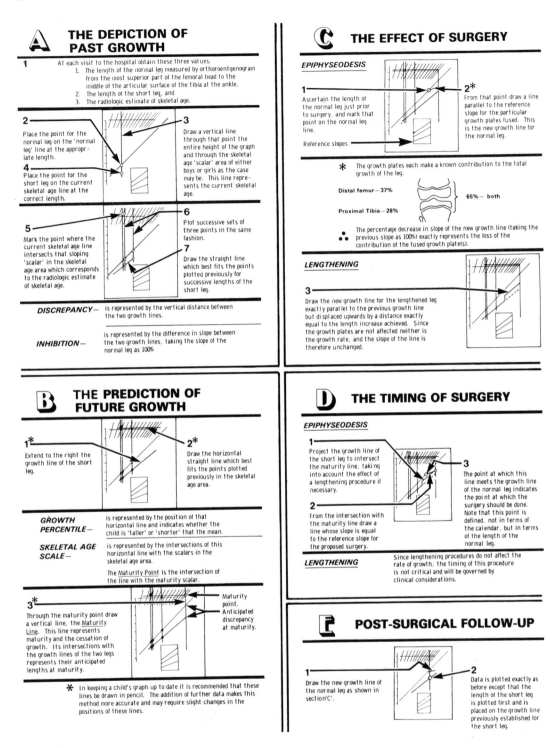

A **THE DEPICTION OF PAST GROWTH**

1 At each visit to the hospital obtain these three values:
1. The length of the normal leg measured by orthoroentgenogram from the most superior part of the femoral head to the middle of the articular surface of the tibia at the ankle,
2. The length of the short leg, and
3. The radiologic estimate of skeletal age.

2 Place the point for the normal leg on the 'normal leg' line at the appropriate length.

4 Place the point for the short leg on the current skeletal age line at the correct length.

3 Draw a vertical line through that point the entire height of the graph and through the skeletal age 'scalar' area of either boys or girls as the case may be. This line represents the current skeletal age.

5 Mark the point where the current skeletal age line intersects that sloping 'scalar' in the skeletal age area which corresponds to the radiologic estimate of skeletal age.

6 Plot successive sets of three points in the same fashion.

7 Draw the straight line which best fits the points plotted previously for successive lengths of the short leg.

DISCREPANCY — is represented by the vertical distance between the two growth lines.

INHIBITION — is represented by the difference in slope between the two growth lines, taking the slope of the normal leg as 100%

B **THE PREDICTION OF FUTURE GROWTH**

1* Extend to the right the growth line of the short leg.

2* Draw the horizontal straight line which best fits the points plotted previously in the skeletal age area.

GROWTH PERCENTILE — is represented by the position of that horizontal line and indicates whether the child is 'taller' or 'shorter' that the mean.

SKELETAL AGE SCALE — is represented by the intersections of this horizontal line with the scalars in the skeletal age area.

The Maturity Point is the intersection of the line with the maturity scalar.

3* Through the maturity point draw a vertical line, the Maturity Line. This line represents maturity and the cessation of growth. Its intersections with the growth lines of the two legs represents their anticipated lengths at maturity.

Maturity point.
Anticipated discrepancy at maturity.

* In keeping a child's graph up to date it is recommended that these lines be drawn in pencil. The addition of further data makes this method more accurate and may require slight changes in the positions of these lines.

C **THE EFFECT OF SURGERY**

EPIPHYSEODESIS

1 Ascertain the length of the normal leg just prior to surgery, and mark that point on the normal leg line.

Reference slopes

2* From that point draw a line parallel to the reference slope for the particular growth plates fused. This is the new growth line for the normal leg.

* The growth plates each make a known contribution to the total growth of the leg.

Distal femur — 37%

Proximal Tibia — 28%

65% — both

∴ The percentage decrease in slope of the new growth line (taking the previous slope as 100%) exactly represents the loss of the contribution of the fused growth plate(s).

LENGTHENING

3 Draw the new growth line for the lengthened leg exactly parallel to the previous growth line but displaced upwards by a distance exactly equal to the length increase achieved. Since the growth plates are not affected neither is the growth rate, and the slope of the line is therefore unchanged.

D **THE TIMING OF SURGERY**

EPIPHYSEODESIS

1 Project the growth line of the short leg to intersect the maturity line, taking into account the effect of a lengthening procedure if necessary.

2 From the intersection with the maturity line draw a line whose slope is equal to the reference slope for the proposed surgery.

3 The point at which this line meets the growth line of the normal leg indicates the point at which the surgery should be done. Note that this point is defined, not in terms of the calendar, but in terms of the length of the normal leg.

LENGTHENING Since lengthening procedures do not affect the rate of growth, the timing of this procedure is not critical and will be governed by clinical considerations.

E **POST-SURGICAL FOLLOW-UP**

1 Draw the new growth line of the normal leg as shown in section 'C'.

2 Data is plotted exactly as before except that the length of the short leg is plotted first and is placed on the growth line previously established for the short leg.

FIG. 12. Detailed explanation of how to use Moseley's graph and its role in the depiction of past growth **(A)**; the prediction of future growth **(B)**; the effect of surgery **(C)**; the timing of surgery **(D)**; and postsurgical follow-up **(E)**.

Source: Moseley CF. A straight line graph for leg length discrepancies. *J Bone Joint Surg* 1977;59A:174–9.

Iliocristale Height

Illiocristale height (in centimeters) is measured from the highest point of the right iliac crest to the standing surface. Data represents a total of 4,000 randomly selected children.

TABLE 16. *Ilocristale height (cm)*

Age (yrs)	No.	Mean	SD	Min.	5th	50th	95th	Max.
Males								
2.0–3.5	37	51.3	3.7	46.1	46.4	50.2	58.9	59.0
3.5–4.5	44	55.0	3.5	49.5	50.6	54.3	60.1	64.3
4.5–5.5	35	61.2	3.5	54.5	54.8	61.3	66.1	67.1
5.5–6.5	43	66.3	3.6	61.2	61.3	65.6	72.6	77.2
6.5–7.5	34	71.8	4.4	63.0	63.9	71.9	78.7	82.5
7.5–8.5	32	75.1	3.5	68.4	69.3	75.0	80.9	81.5
8.5–9.5	33	79.8	3.8	71.7	71.8	80.9	84.2	84.9
9.5–10.5	37	83.1	4.7	72.9	74.9	83.1	89.4	94.4
10.5–11.5	49	85.3	4.9	75.4	76.0	85.1	94.6	97.6
11.5–12.5	52	91.5	6.3	80.3	81.9	89.9	104.4	107.5
12.5–13.5	50	95.1	5.6	85.7	86.4	94.5	104.6	110.4
13.5–14.5	51	97.8	5.3	87.2	90.7	97.2	105.3	110.4
14.5–15.5	39	100.4	3.7	90.4	84.1	100.5	105.5	106.0
15.5–16.5	31	104.5	5.6	92.5	93.5	104.8	111.8	113.1
16.5–17.5	38	104.9	4.8	94.8	95.3	105.0	110.4	114.7
17.5–19.0	23	106.9	4.9	99.2	99.3	106.1	115.7	117.9
Females								
2.0–3.5	30	51.6	3.6	43.4	45.1	51.1	58.1	60.0
3.5–4.5	35	57.6	3.4	51.0	52.0	57.8	62.8	65.8
4.5–5.5	41	61.6	2.9	55.4	56.8	61.3	65.7	68.2
5.5–6.5	34	66.5	3.3	57.6	60.0	66.5	71.5	72.2
6.5–7.5	41	71.4	4.0	64.0	64.8	71.1	78.0	79.1
7.5–8.5	32	74.8	4.2	65.7	66.9	74.2	81.2	83.9
8.5–9.5	48	79.6	4.6	71.5	72.3	79.7	86.1	93.1
9.5–10.5	38	84.2	4.4	77.7	77.8	83.6	91.6	94.7
10.5–11.5	48	89.0	5.6	77.9	79.9	89.1	97.8	99.0
11.5–12.5	43	91.0	5.1	78.3	82.5	91.9	97.5	101.5
12.5–13.5	50	94.5	4.8	82.5	85.2	94.6	101.9	105.0
13.5–14.5	31	96.3	6.1	78.8	83.0	95.6	104.9	106.3
14.5–15.5	48	98.3	4.8	89.5	90.2	97.3	106.9	108.2
15.5–16.5	32	98.7	5.2	90.1	90.5	98.2	107.2	108.1
16.5–17.5	36	98.4	4.0	88.5	90.3	98.7	105.2	107.5
17.5–19.0	23	98.1	4.3	91.6	91.8	96.7	104.3	110.6

Source: Snyder RG, Schneider LW, Owings CL, Reynolds HM. Golomb DH, Schork, MA. *Anthropometry of Infants, Children and Youths to Age Eighteen.* Product Safety Design, SP450. Highway Safety Research Institute, University of Michigan. Published by Society of Automotive Engineers, Inc., Warrendale, PA, 1977.

Buttock-Knee Length

Data are from 7,119 children aged 6 to 11 years who constituted a nationally representative sample. Buttock-knee length was measured as the distance from the rearmost projection of the buttock to the front of the right kneecap. The subject was seated, and the fixed crossbar of the anthropometer was placed in light contact with the rearmost projection of the buttock; the movable crossbar was then brought into light contact with the front surface of the right patella.

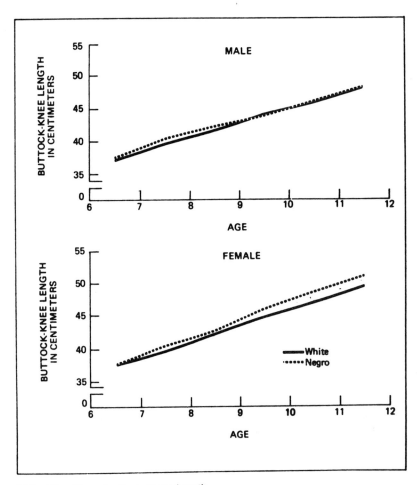

FIG. 13.   Mean buttock–knee length.

Source: Malina RM, Hamill PVV, Lemeschow S. Selected body measurements of children 6 to 11 years, United States. Washington, D.C.: U.S. Government Printing Office, 1973; DHEW publication no. (HSM)73-1605 (series 11, no 143).

Data in Table 17 consist of a population sample of 4,000 children randomly selected to be representative of a national sample, ages 2 to 19 years. This was measured by the same method as used in Fig. 13.

TABLE 17. *Buttock-knee length (cm)*

Age (yrs)	No.	Mean	SD	Min.	5th	50th	95th	Max.
Males
2.0–3.5	113	28.5	1.9	24.2	25.1	28.5	31.4	32.9
3.5–4.5	117	31.0	1.9	26.9	29.4	30.8	34.3	37.2
4.5–5.5	141	33.6	1.9	28.4	30.7	33.5	36.6	39.0
5.5–6.5	117	36.1	2.2	31.1	32.8	35.8	39.6	42.1
6.5–7.5	105	39.0	2.2	33.5	35.7	38.8	42.6	44.2
7.5–8.5	102	41.2	2.5	35.3	37.7	40.9	45.9	47.1
8.5–9.5	117	43.6	2.4	37.2	39.9	43.3	47.2	51.0
9.5–10.5	123	45.7	2.7	40.0	41.3	45.4	50.1	54.3
10.5–11.5	140	47.6	2.5	41.8	43.8	47.4	52.1	54.1
11.5–12.5	153	49.8	3.1	41.7	45.0	49.5	54.5	60.7
12.5–13.5	154	51.9	3.3	45.0	46.3	51.4	57.6	60.8
13.5–14.5	154	54.5	3.3	45.1	48.7	54.4	59.7	61.9
14.5–15.5	131	56.1	3.2	47.3	50.7	56.3	60.9	63.7
15.5–16.5	99	58.5	3.1	49.2	52.6	58.7	62.8	66.6
16.5–17.5	104	58.8	2.8	53.2	53.9	58.8	63.6	66.7
17.5–19.0	88	59.5	3.0	52.2	54.2	59.4	64.4	69.7
Females
2.0–3.5	98	28.4	1.9	24.6	25.6	28.4	31.4	33.5
3.5–4.5	108	31.9	2.1	28.4	28.8	31.7	35.5	38.9
4.5–5.5	126	34.2	1.9	29.7	31.2	34.1	37.1	41.2
5.5–6.5	124	36.1	2.3	27.5	31.8	36.0	39.0	42.3
6.5–7.5	124	39.2	2.6	33.1	34.8	38.8	43.6	48.1
7.5–8.5	94	41.3	2.4	35.7	37.4	41.0	45.3	48.2
8.5–9.5	140	44.0	2.6	39.7	40.2	43.3	48.9	51.6
9.5–10.5	134	46.1	2.9	39.3	41.6	46.0	51.2	53.4
10.5–11.5	138	48.8	3.5	40.3	43.2	48.5	54.8	59.8
11.5–12.5	133	50.8	3.3	43.6	45.5	51.0	55.9	60.8
12.5–13.5	160	52.9	3.0	45.6	48.0	52.6	57.6	62.1
13.5–14.5	116	54.1	3.0	46.5	49.3	53.8	59.0	62.5
14.5–15.5	132	55.5	2.8	48.9	51.5	55.1	60.7	63.0
15.5–16.5	97	55.2	2.7	48.6	51.1	54.5	59.8	61.0
16.5–17.5	116	55.3	2.6	49.4	50.9	55.1	59.6	61.8
17.5–19.0	68	55.4	2.6	49.4	51.3	55.0	59.9	61.8

Source: Snyder RG, Schneider LW, Owings CL, Reynolds HM, Golomb DH, Schork, MA. *Anthropometry of Infants, Children and Youths to Age Eighteen.* Product Safety Design, SP450. Highway Safety Research Institute, University of Michigan. Published by Society of Automotive Engineers, Inc., Warrendale, PA, 1977.

Popliteal Height

Data from 7,119 children 6 to 11 years of age constituted a nationally representative sample. Popliteal height was measured as the distance from the standing surface to the underside of the right knee. With the subject seated, the anthropometer with its attached base was placed on the footrest adjacent to the right foot, and the movable arm was brought to the level of the table surface on which the child was seated. This is the level of the underside of the right thigh where the tendon of the biceps femoris muscle comes into contact with the table surface.

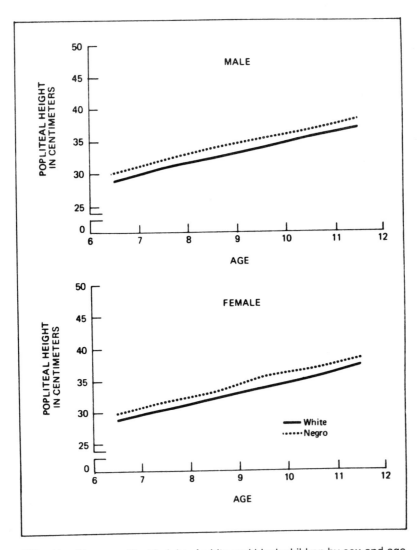

FIG. 14.   Mean popliteal height of white and black children by sex and age.

Source: Malina RM, Hamill PVV, Lemeschow S. Selected body measurements in children 6 to 11 years, United States. Washington, D.C.: U.S. Government Printing Office, 1973; DHEW publication no. (HSM)73-1605 (series 11, no 143).

Knee Height

Knee height was measured at the top of the thigh at the patella to the floor, with the patient in the seated position.

TABLE 18. *Knee height (cm)*

Age (yrs)	No.	Mean	SD	Min.	5th	50th	95th	Max.
Males								
2.0–3.5	111	27.4	2.0	22.5	24.2	27.3	30.8	31.8
3.5–4.5	109	29.7	2.0	22.0	26.7	29.7	33.0	35.8
4.5–5.5	135	32.4	2.0	28.1	29.1	32.2	35.5	37.8
5.5–6.5	107	35.3	2.2	30.3	31.4	35.2	38.8	40.6
6.5–7.5	104	37.7	2.2	32.4	33.8	37.9	40.9	42.2
7.5–8.5	96	39.9	2.4	33.1	36.6	39.5	44.1	45.7
8.5–9.5	114	42.0	2.5	34.5	38.2	42.0	45.9	48.5
9.5–10.5	122	43.8	2.8	37.7	39.1	43.6	48.8	53.4
10.5–11.5	140	45.4	2.2	40.1	41.8	45.4	48.9	51.7
11.5–12.5	144	47.8	2.8	40.9	43.8	47.3	52.7	59.3
12.5–13.5	137	49.7	3.3	42.1	44.7	49.8	55.7	59.8
13.5–14.5	137	51.8	3.3	45.2	46.9	51.6	57.4	60.3
14.5–15.5	127	53.1	3.1	46.4	47.6	52.9	58.3	60.2
15.5–16.5	87	55.2	3.0	46.2	49.9	55.2	59.7	61.6
16.5–17.5	95	55.2	2.9	48.8	49.4	55.5	59.4	62.0
17.5–19.0	83	55.6	3.0	48.1	51.0	55.3	60.6	62.8
Females								
2.0–3.5	92	26.6	1.9	22.5	23.4	26.4	29.5	32.3
3.5–4.5	97	30.0	2.0	25.5	26.7	30.0	33.0	35.2
4.5–5.5	106	32.3	2.0	28.2	29.1	32.2	35.7	38.2
5.5–6.5	107	34.6	1.9	29.6	31.6	34.4	37.7	39.2
6.5–7.5	115	36.9	2.2	31.0	33.1	36.6	40.7	43.6
7.5–8.5	92	38.8	2.2	34.7	35.3	38.8	42.4	46.4
8.5–9.5	135	41.5	2.4	36.3	37.8	41.1	45.5	48.7
9.5–10.5	128	43.3	2.4	37.6	39.5	43.3	47.6	51.1
10.5–11.5	139	45.7	3.0	37.9	41.2	45.5	50.6	53.3
11.5–12.5	133	47.2	2.6	41.8	43.1	47.2	51.3	56.7
12.5–13.5	160	48.5	2.5	41.2	44.4	48.4	52.4	54.8
13.5–14.5	115	49.3	2.7	42.1	44.9	49.5	53.6	56.3
14.5–15.5	132	50.0	2.7	43.6	45.9	49.6	55.0	57.3
15.5–16.5	98	49.8	2.6	44.3	46.0	49.3	54.6	56.8
16.5–17.5	117	49.6	2.6	41.6	45.1	49.6	53.8	55.2
17.5–19.0	68	49.8	2.4	44.4	46.1	49.5	53.8	56.5

Source: Snyder RG, Schneider LW, Owings CL, Reynolds HM, Golomb DH, Schork MA. *Anthropometry of Infants, Children and Youths to Age Eighteen.* Product Safety Design, SP450. Highway Safety Research Institute, University of Michigan. Published by Society of Automotive Engineers, Inc., Warrendale, PA, 1977.

Tibiale Height

Tibiale height was measured with the child standing. The distance to the right tibial plateau was determined from the standing surface.

TABLE 19. *Tibiale height (cm)*

Age (yrs)	No.	Mean	SD	Min.	5th	50th	95th	Max.
Males								
2.0–3.5	37	21.9	1.8	17.7	19.0	21.9	25.1	25.6
3.5–4.5	44	23.6	1.8	20.4	20.6	23.3	26.8	27.5
4.5–5.5	35	26.4	1.9	22.7	22.7	26.3	29.0	29.7
5.5–6.5	43	29.2	1.8	25.9	26.5	28.6	31.8	34.9
6.5–7.5	34	31.3	2.4	26.1	26.2	31.3	34.5	37.1
7.5–8.5	32	33.7	1.9	30.5	30.6	33.8	36.4	37.8
8.5–9.5	33	35.2	1.8	30.1	30.9	35.3	37.7	38.0
9.5–10.5	37	36.7	2.4	31.8	32.5	36.8	40.1	43.0
10.5–11.5	49	37.9	2.4	32.7	34.1	37.5	41.8	43.4
11.5–12.5	52	40.5	2.9	35.0	36.1	39.8	45.7	47.0
12.5–13.5	50	42.3	2.8	37.1	37.8	41.9	46.1	50.2
13.5–14.5	51	42.7	2.6	37.5	37.7	42.8	46.3	48.0
14.5–15.5	39	44.1	2.3	38.5	39.3	44.3	47.3	47.9
15.5–16.5	31	46.1	3.0	40.2	40.4	46.0	50.0	52.4
16.5–17.5	37	46.1	2.2	40.8	41.6	46.6	49.4	49.9
17.5–19.0	23	46.7	3.3	42.5	42.5	45.2	51.8	55.5
Females								
2.0–3.5	30	22.7	1.9	18.1	18.6	23.0	24.7	27.1
3.5–4.5	35	24.6	1.8	21.8	21.9	24.2	27.8	28.1
4.5–5.5	41	26.4	1.8	22.5	22.6	26.2	29.0	30.2
5.5–6.5	34	28.5	2.0	23.7	24.9	28.6	31.4	31.8
6.5–7.5	42	31.0	1.9	27.5	27.9	30.7	34.9	35.7
7.5–8.5	32	31.5	1.7	26.5	28.1	31.4	34.1	34.4
8.5–9.5	48	34.5	2.1	29.0	30.8	34.2	37.8	39.4
9.5–10.5	37	36.1	2.1	32.4	32.7	35.8	39.5	40.0
10.5–11.5	48	38.2	2.6	31.6	33.2	38.2	42.5	42.7
11.5–12.5	43	39.3	2.4	32.8	34.7	39.6	42.7	44.6
12.5–13.5	50	40.4	2.6	34.0	35.6	40.3	44.2	47.5
13.5–14.5	31	41.1	3.0	33.0	34.1	41.3	45.3	46.7
14.5–15.5	48	41.9	2.4	36.0	37.9	42.1	45.2	47.6
15.5–16.5	32	42.2	2.7	37.5	37.9	41.6	46.5	48.6
16.5–17.5	36	41.8	2.2	37.4	37.7	42.2	44.6	45.0
17.5–19.0	23	41.8	2.7	37.4	37.5	41.1	45.4	50.8

Source: Snyder RG, Schneider LW, Owings CL, Reynolds HM, Golomb DH, Schork MA. *Anthropometry of Infants, Children and Youths to Age Eighteen.* Product Safety Design, SP450. Highway Safety Research Institute, University of Michigan. Published by Society of Automotive Engineers, Inc., Warrendale, PA, 1977.

Tibiofemoral Angle

This study includes 978 patients from the pediatric clinic at the University of Helsinki. The knees and legs were roentgenographically examined for reasons unrelated to their illness. The study also includes 300 patients from the Orthopaedic Hospital Invalid Foundation, Helsinki, 59 of whom were examined roentgenographically twice and 52 examined three or more times at intervals of 6 months. The entire series comprises 1,480 examinations of the tibiofemoral angle done roentgenographically and clinically. The extremity was positioned with the patella straight ahead. The angle was measured on the roentgenogram by drawing a longitudinal axis midway between the femoral and tibial diaphyseal cortices and measuring the angle in degrees. If there was torsion or bowing of the tibia, a longitudinal axis was estimated between the patella and the midpoint of the ankle. If there was a divergence between the angles in both legs, the mean was taken as the representative figure. The study was divided into groups according to age, with each group containing an average of 40 patients, using 6 month intervals from birth to 16 years.

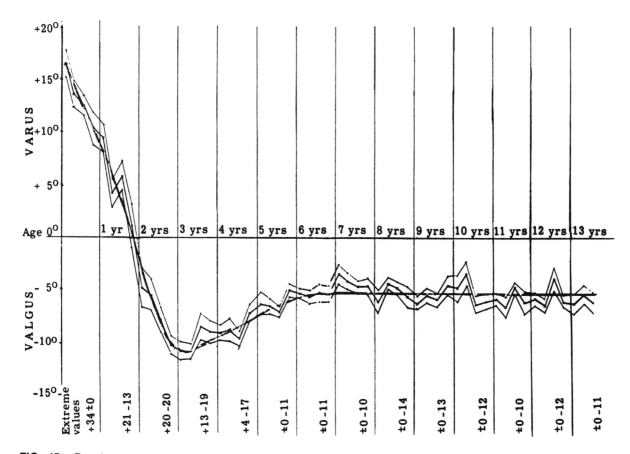

FIG. 15. Development of the tibiofemoral angle in children during growth. The mean of the measurements is in the middle; on both sides of this is the error of the mean, which was an average of ±4.4°. SD = ±8°.

Source: Salenius P, Vanka E. The development of tibiofemoral angle in children. *J Bone Joint Surg* 1975;57(A):259–61.

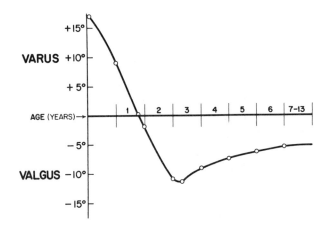

FIG. 16. Graph constructed by the editor from the material in Fig. 15 showing only the mean. The standard errors have been eliminated.

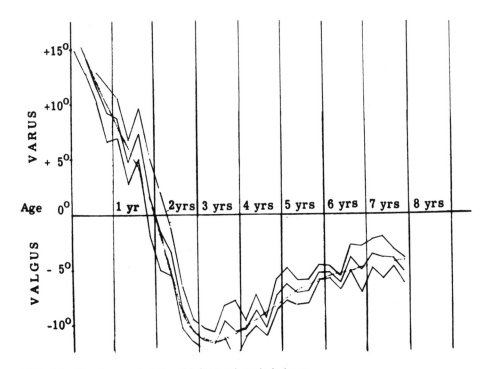

FIG. 17. Development of the tibiofemoral angle in boys.

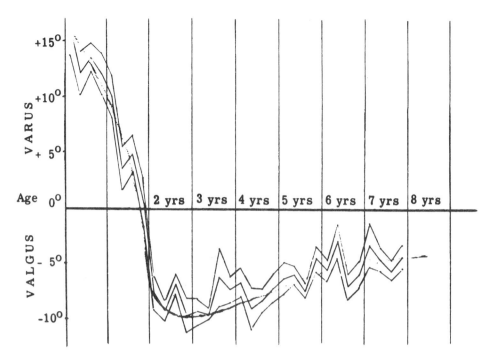

FIG. 18. Development of the tibiofemoral angle in girls.

Source: Salenius P, Vanka E. The development of tibiofemoral angle in children. *J Bone Joint Surg* 1975;57(A):259–61.

FOOT

Various Stages in the Early Development of the Lower Extremity

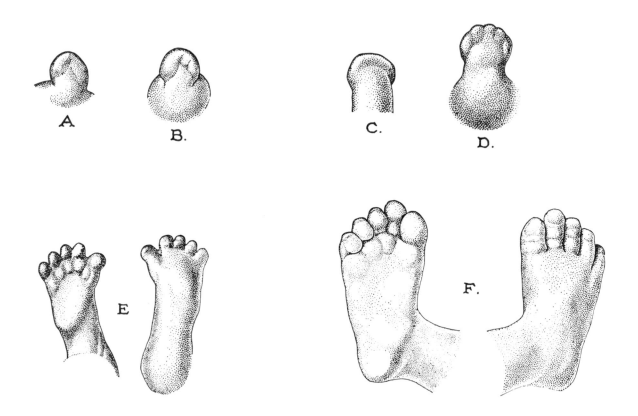

FIG. 1.   A: Posterior limb bud of an embryo 12 mm long.   **B:** Posterior limb bud of an embryo 15 mm long.   **C:** Posterior limb bud of an embryo 17 mm long.   **D:** Foot and calf of an embryo 19 mm long.   **E:** Two views of the foot and ankle of an embryo 25 mm long.   **F:** Two views of the foot of a fetus 55 mm long. (From Retzius G. Zur kenntnis der entwicklung der koperformendesmenschen wahrend der fotalen lebensstuben. *Biol Untersch M F*, 1904;11:33–76.)

Source: Morris H. *Human anatomy, a complete systematic treatise*. 11th Ed. New York: McGraw-Hill Book Co., 1953.

Appearance of Ossification Centers

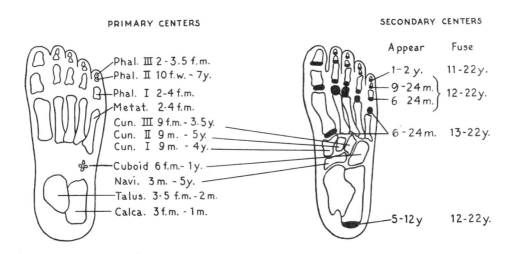

PRIMARY CENTERS

Phal. III 2 - 3.5 f.m.
Phal. II 10 f.w. - 7y.
Phal. I 2-4 f.m.
Metat. 2-4 f.m.
Cun. III 9 f.m. - 3.5y.
Cun. II 9 m. - 5y.
Cun. I 9 m. - 4y.
Cuboid 6 f.m.- 1y.
Navi. 3 m. - 5y.
Talus. 3.5 f.m. - 2 m.
Calca. 3 f.m. - 1m.

SECONDARY CENTERS

Appear   Fuse

1 - 2 y.   11 - 22 y.
9 - 24 m. ⎫ 12 - 22 y.
6 24 m. ⎭
6 - 24 m.   13 - 22 y.

5 - 12 y   12 - 22 y.

FIG. 2. Time schedule for appearance of the primary and secondary ossification centers and fusion of secondary centers with the shafts in the feet. f.m. = Fetal months; m = postnatal months; y = year.

Source: Caffey J. *Pediatric x-ray diagnosis.* 7th ed. Chicago: Yearbook Medical Publishers Inc., 1978.

Average Osseous Growth and Development of the Feet

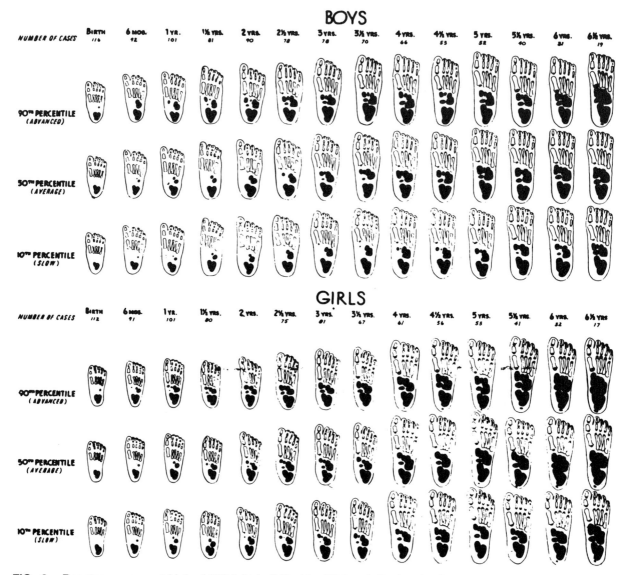

FIG. 3. Roentgenograms at birth of 228 infants (112 girls, 116 boys). During the first year, roentgenograms were repeated at 3 month intervals, and thereafter at 6 month intervals.

Source: Voght EC, Vickers VS. Osseous growth and development. *Radiology* 1938; 31:441–4.

Age and Order of Onset of Ossification

TABLE 1. *Mean chronologic age and order of onset of ossification in the hindfoot, midfoot, and forefoot*

Ossification center	Mean Age (Months) 50 boys	182–235 boys	Mean Age (Months) 50 girls	156–236 girls
Hindfoot				
Calcaneus, Body	before birth	*	before birth	*
Talus	before birth	*	before birth	*
Tibia, Distal epiphysis	3.9	4.4	3.4	4.0
Fibula, Distal epiphysis	·12.5	12.6	9.3	9.0
Calcaneus, Epiphysis	89.6	90.3	63.7	68.3
Midfoot				
Cuboid	0.5	*	0.4	*
Lateral cuneiform	4.4	*	3.8	*
Medial cuneiform	21.9	24.1	16.7	15.7
Intermediate cuneiform	28.4	29.3	21.3	20.0
Navicular	33.4	33.8	25.8	23.3
Forefoot				
Toe I, Distal phal. epiphysis	16.8	15.5	10.6	9.4
Toe III, Prox. phal. epiphysis	19.5	18.1	12.2	11.5
Toe IV, Prox. phal. epiphysis	21.0	20.0	13.6	12.7
Toe II, Prox. phal. epiphysis	22.2	20.7	14.1	13.6
Metatarsal 1, Epiphysis	27.7	28.5	20.1	19.9
Toe I, Prox. phal. epiphysis	29.9	27.7	20.3	18.8
Toe V, Prox. phal. epiphysis	32.0	30.5	21.3	20.9
Metatarsal 2, Epiphysis	33.4	35.3	25.8	24.3
Metatarsal 3, Epiphysis	41.5	42.1	29.1	28.6
Metatarsal 4, Epiphysis	48.7	47.8	34.0	33.4
Toe IV, Distal phal. epiphysis	51.2	52.2	30.7	30.3
Toe III, Distal phal. epiphysis	53.5	53.7	43.8	34.0
Metatarsal 5, Epiphysis	53.6	53.6	38.6	38.9
Toe II, Distal phal. epiphysis	57.0	58.5	35.5	36.2

Because the children were X-rayed approximately every 6 months, these are approximate dates of ossifications. Note that the addition of a larger group of children changes the mean age. The large group of children was X-rayed initially at age 3 months, the small group at birth.

Source: Hoerr NL, Pyle, SI, Francis CC. *Radiographic atlas of skeletal development of the foot and ankle. A standard reference.* Springfield, IL; Charles C Thomas, 1962.

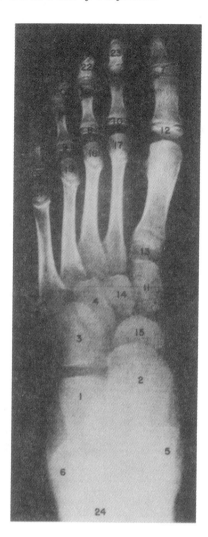

FIG. 4. Dorsoplantar, radiograph of the foot showing the order of appearance of centers of ossification in the region as a whole. The numbers indicate the order of onset of ossification most frequently seen in boys: 1, Calcaneus, body; 2, Talus; 3, Cuboid; 4, Lateral cuneiform; 5, Tibia, distal epiphysis; 6, Toe I, distal phal. epiphysis; 7, Toe III, prox. phal. epiphysis; 8, Toe IV, prox. phal. epiphysis; 9, Toe II, prox. phal. epiphysis; 10, Medial cuneiform; 11, Toe I, prox. phal. epiphysis; 12, Metatarsal 1, epiphysis; 13, Intermediate cuneiform; 14, Navicular; 15, Toe V, prox. phal. epiphysis; 16, Metatarsal 2, epiphysis; 17, Metatarsal 3, epiphysis; 18, Metatarsal 4, epiphysis; 19, Toe IV, distal phal. epiphysis; 20, Metatarsal 5, epiphysis; 21, Toe III, distal phal. epiphysis; 22, Toe II, distal phal. epiphysis; 23, Calcaneus, epiphysis.

Source: Hoerr NL, Pyle SI, Francis CC. *Radiographic atlas of skeletal development of the foot and ankle. A standard reference.* Springfield, IL: Charles C Thomas, 1962.

TABLE 2. *Approximate boundaries for early and late appearance of the initial osseous nodule in the bone growth centers of the foot and ankle in boys*

Bone growth centers grouped according to "sheaf" method[a]	Early Average for 80th percentile bones[a]	Moderate rate		Late Slutsker-Whittaker mean plus 1 SD
		50% range[c]	50th percent average[b]	
Cuboid	at birth	0.5– 1.5	2	*
Lateral cuneiform	2	2.5– 7	5.0	*
Tibia, Distal epiphysis	3	4 – 6	5.7	6
Fibula, Distal epiphysis	6	11 – 18	10.8	17
Toe I, Distal phal. epiphysis	11	13 – 18	14.0	21
Toe III, Prox. phal. epiphysis	13	15 – 23	20.8	23
Medial cuneiform	13	17 – 33	25.5	35
Toe IV, Prox. phal. epiphysis	14	16 – 24	21.8	25
Toe II, Prox. phal. epiphysis	14	16 – 27	21.9	26
Toe I, Prox. phal. epiphysis	20	25 – 34	28.8	33
Intermediate cuneiform	20	24 – 38	31.4	38
Navicular	21	25 – 58	38.1	48
Toe V, Prox. phal. epiphysis	21	24 – 36	28.8	37
Metatarsal 1, Epiphysis	22	23 – 34	31.9	34
Metatarsal 2, Epiphysis	26	29 – 32	39.0	42
Metatarsal 3, Epiphysis	35	37 – 49	39.5	50
Metatarsal 4, Epiphysis	39	42 – 58	47.5	56
Toe III, Distal phal. epiphysis	43	46 – 61	41.5	66
Toe IV, Distal phal. epiphysis	43	46 – 61	41.7	64
Metatarsal 5, Epiphysis	44	48 – 62	48.2	63
Toe II, Distal phal. epiphysis	44	50 – 68	39.5	61
Calcaneus, Epiphysis	74	87 –103	—	103

Because Brush Foundation children were not filmed until age 3 months, the SD could not be properly derived for these centers. Ages are given in months.

[a]From Francis CC, Werle PP, Behm A. The appearance of centers of ossification from birth to 5 years. *Am J Phys Anthrop* 1939;24:273–99.

[b]From Elgenmark O. The normal development of the ossific centers during infancy and childhood. *Acta Paed* 1946;33(suppl. I):1–79.

[c]From Harding VV. Time schedule for the appearance and fusion of a second accessory center of ossification of the calcaneus. *Child Develop* 1952;23:181–4.

TABLE 3. Approximate boundaries for early and late appearance of the initial oseous nodule in the bone growth centers of the foot and ankle in girls

Bone growth centers grouped according to "sheaf" method[a]	Early Average for 80th percentile bones[a]	Moderate rate		Late Slutsker-Whittaker mean plus 1 S.D.
		50% range[c]	50th per cent average[b]	
Cuboid	at birth	birth – 0.7	1.7	*
Lateral cuneiform	2	2 – 6	4.2	*
Tibia, Distal epiphysis	3	4 – 5	5.6	6
Fibula, Distal epiphysis	6	8 – 12	8.8	12
Toe I, Distal phal. epiphysis	7	7 – 11	10.2	12
Toe III, Prox. phal. epiphysis	8	10 – 14	12.3	15
Toe IV, Prox. phal. epiphysis	9	10 – 15	13.3	17
Medial cuneiform	9	16 – 25	20.6	23
Toe II, Prox. phal. epiphysis	10	11 – 17	14.9	18
Toe I, Prox. phal. epiphysis	14	15 – 22	19.6	24
Toe V, Prox. phal. epiphysis	14	15 – 26	21.0	24
Intermediate cuneiform	14	16 – 25	22.5	27
Navicular	14	17 – 31	25.9	34
Metatarsal 1, Epiphysis	14	16 – 22	20.0	24
Metatarsal 2, Epiphysis	19	20 – 30	25.9	29
Metatarsal 3, Epiphysis	22	25 – 34	29.1	34
Toe III, Distal phal. epiphysis	24	27 – 40	29.3	43
Toe IV, Distal phal. epiphysis	24	25 – 36	29.5	38
Toe II, Distal phal. epiphysis	26	29 – 43	29.1	45
Metatarsal 4, Epiphysis	26	28 – 39	32.0	41
Metatarsal 5, Epiphysis	29	33 – 45	35.0	48
Calcaneus, Epiphysis	54	56 – 71	—	74

Because Brush Foundation children were not filmed until age 3 months, the SD could not be properly derived for these centers. Ages are given in months.

[a]From Francis CC, Werle PP, Behm A. The appearance of centers of ossification from birth to 5 years. *Am J Phys Anthrop* 1939;24:273–99.

[b]From Elgenmark O. The normal development of the ossific centers during infancy and childhood. *Acta Paed* 1946;33(Suppl. I):33:1–79.

[c]From Harding VV. Time schedule for the appearance and fusion of a second accessory center of ossification of the calcaneus. *Child Develop* 1952;23:181–4.

Source: Hoerr NL, Pyle, SI, Francis, CC. *Radiographic atlas of skeletal development of the foot and ankle. A standard reference.* Springfield, IL: Charles C Thomas, 1962.

Age of Appearance of the Separate Centers of Ossification of the Tip of the Medial Malleolus

Table 4 is from the Fels Research Institute longitudinal study and consisted of 151 children from 75 families, 88 boys and 63 girls. The top section of the table represents the age of the child when the extra center first appeared in boys and girls. The lower portion of the table indicates the age at which the extra center joined the tibia.

TABLE 4. *Separate centers of ossification of the tip of the medial malleolus*

AGE OF APPEARANCE OF EXTRA CENTERS

Age (yr.)	6.0	6.5	7.0	7.5	8.0	8.5	9.0	9.5	10.0	10.5	11.0	Combined Total
Boys	1	—	1	1	1	2	5	1	2	—	1	15
Girls	—	6	1	11	3	6	3	—	—	—	—	30
Total	1	6	2	12	4	8	8	1	2	—	1	45

AGE AT WHICH THE EXTRA CENTER JOINED TIBIA

Age (yr.)	6.0	7.5	8.0	8.5	9.0	9.5	10.0	10.5	11.0	11.5	12.0	Combined Total
Boys		1	—	1	1	—	4	—	4	—	1	12
Girls		3	3	10	6	2	4	—	—	1	—	29
Total		4	3	11	7	2	8	—	4	1	1	41

Source: Selby S. Separate centers of ossification of the tip of the internal malleolus. *AJR* 1961;86:496–501.

Developmental Deviations in the Tarsal Accessoria

TABLE 5. *Ossa tarsalia accessoria*

Calcaneus accessorius (os trochleae)[a]

Calcaneus secundarius (calcaneus bifidus, calcaneum surnuméraire, secondary os calcis) [a–c]

Os aponeurosis plantaris[c]

Os cuboideum secundarium[a]

Os cuneometatarsale I dorsale fibulare

Os cuneometatarsale I plantare (pars peronaea metatarsalis I, praehallux)

Os cuneometatarsale I tibiale (praehallux)[c]

Os cuneometatarsale II dorsale[a,c]

Os cuneonaviculare I dorsale (naviculocuneiforme I dorsale, infranaviculare, paracuneiforme I)[a,c,d]

Os infranaviculare. *See* Os cuneonaviculare I dorsale

Os in sinus tarsi

Os intercuneiforme

Os intermetatarsale I (intermetatarseum gruberi)[a–c]

Os intermetatarsale IV[a,c]

Os naviculocuneiforme I dorsale. *See* Os cuneonaviculare I dorsale

Os paracuneiforme (praecuneiforme, praehallux, ossicle of Cameron and Carlier)[c]

Os peronaeum. *See* Os sesamoideum peronaeum

Os retinaculi (patella malleoli?)[c]

Os sesamoideum peronaeum (peroneale, sesamum peronaeum, cuboideum accessorium)[a–d]

Os sesamoideum tibialis anterior[a]

Os sesamoideum tibialis posterior

Os subfibulare (talus secundarius, patella malleoli?)[a–c]

Os subtibiale (talus accessorius, talus secundarius, astragalus accessorius, astragalus secundarius, tibiale inferius, os malleoli)[a,c,d]

Os supranaviculare. *See* Os talonaviculare dorsale

Os supratalare (supertalare, talus secundarius, astragalus secundarius, sometimes incorrectly called Pirie's ossicle)[a,c]

Os sustentaculi (sustentaculi proprium, subtibiale)[a,c]

Os talocalcaneare laterale (talocalcaneus). *See* Calcaneus accessorius

Os talocalcaneare posterior[c]

Os talonaviculare dorsale (supranaviculare, dorsal astragaloscaphoid ossicle, intertaloscaphoid, taloscaphoid, processus trochlearis of scaphoid or of talus, Pirie's ossicle)[a,d]

Os talotibiale dorsale (talotibiale)[c]

Os tendinis calcanei (tendinis achillis)[c]

Os tibiale externum (naviculare accessorius, naviculare secundarius, accessory tarsal scphoid, tibiale anterior, tibiale, praehallux)[a–c]

Os trigonum (talus accessorius, talus secundarius, astragalus accessorius, astragalus secundaris, intermedium tarsi)[a–c]

Os trochleae. This term has also been used for the calcaneus accessorius and for the os supratalare

Os uncinatum (unci, processus uncinatus of lateral cuneiform)

Os vesalianum pedis (vesalii)[a–c]

Subcalcaneus (os subcalcis, os tuberis calcanei)[a]

Supracalcaneus (os accessorium supracalcaneum)[a]

Articles in which items have appeared in the past:

[a]Kohler A (rev. by E. A. Zimmer and ed. by J. T. Case): *Borderlands of the Normal and Early Pathologic in Skeletal Roentgenology*, ed. 10. New York, Grune, 1956.

[b]Marti T. Die Skelettvarietaten des Fusses, Part 2 of Debrunner and Francillon's *Praktische Beitrage zur Orthopaedie*. Berne, Huber, 1947.

[c]Trolle D (trans. by E. Aagesen): *Accessory Bones of the Human Foot*. Copenhagen, Munksgaard, 1948.

[d]Werthemann A. Die Entwicklungsstorungen der Extremitaten, vol. 9, part 6, of Lubarsch, Henke and Rossle's *Handbuch der Speziellen Pathologischen Anatomie und Histologie*. Berlin, Springer, 1952.

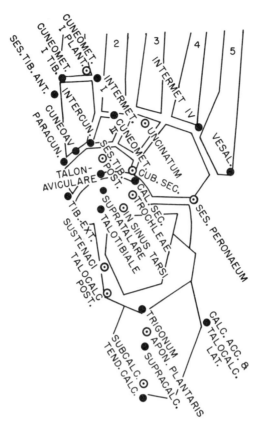

FIG. 5.   Scheme of the tarsus to show the sites of the various accessoria. Scheme was developed by O'Rahilly after an extensive review of the literature.

Source: O'Rahilly R. Development deviations in the carpus and the tarsus. *Clin Orthop* 1975;10:9–18.

Roentgenographic Evaluation of Weightbearing Views of the Pediatric Foot

Anteroposterior and lateral roentgenograms of the weightbearing foot were obtained in normal children ages 12 days to 12 years. The normal range of the commonly employed talo-calcaneal, calcaneo-fifth metatarsal, and mid-talar-calcaneal angles were determined.

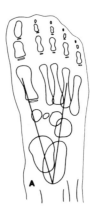
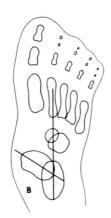
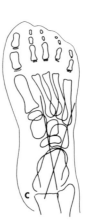

FIG. 6. A: Normal talo-calcaneal angle. At this age and in older children a line drawn through the long central axis of the talus usually passes just medial to the base of the first metatarsal. A line through the long mid-axis of the calcaneus tends to pass through the medial aspect of the base of the fourth metatarsal. In infants and young children, the long central axis of the talus is shifted medially. **B:** Same angle measured in a 2-year-old with severe valgus. The angle is 58°. **C:** The hindfoot varus is demonstrated in an 8-year-old. The talo-calcaneal angle measures 29°.

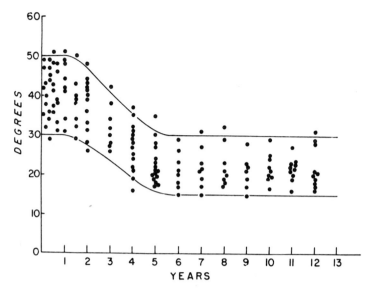

FIG. 7. Talo-calcaneal angle. The normal variation for the talo-calcaneal angle is seen to be age-dependent up to the age of 5 years.

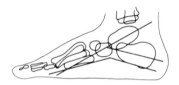

FIG. 8. On the lateral view the line drawn through the long axis of the calcaneus forms an acute angle with a line through the mid-axis of the talus. This mid-talar/mid-calcaneal angle was found to vary normally from 25° to 50°. A line drawn through the inferior cortex of the body of the calcaneus makes an obtuse angle with a line drawn through the inferior cortex of the fifth metatarsal. The normal range for this calcaneal-fifth metatarsal angle was 150°. The normal range of these angles as seen in lateral view did not vary with the age of the child, as did the talo-calcaneal angle.

Source: Templeton AW, McAlister WH, Zim ID. Standards of terminology and evaluation of osseous relationships in congenitally abnormal feet. *AJR* 1965;93:374–81.

Lateral Roentgenographic Evaluation of Weightbearing Feet in Normal Children

Roentgenograms of the left foot in normal children were obtained at intervals of 6 months. The ages of these children ranged from 2.5 to 13 years. Each child had one to nine X-rays. Over 800 X-rays have been studied. The marks used were: (1) the lowest point of the head of the talus; (2) the lowest point of the calcaneus; (3) the lowest point of the head of the first metatarsal; (4) the lowest point of the base of the first metatarsal; (5) the lowest point of the calcaneus at the calcaneocuboid articulation; and (6) the lowest point of the head of the fifth metatarsal. The angles a and c in Figs. 9 and 10 measure the height of the medial and lateral aspects, respectively, of the longitudinal arch. Angle b measures the anterior medial part of the arch, and angle d measures the inclination of the calcaneus with the horizontal.

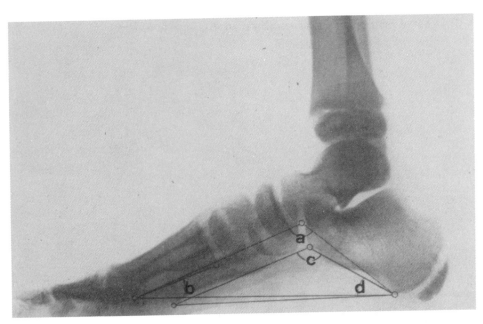

FIG. 9. Reproduction of an X-ray illustrating a high arch with angle a, 119.0°, b, 20.5°, c, 129.0°, d, 31.0°.

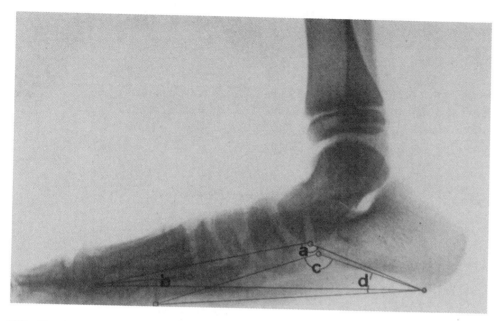

FIG. 10. Reproduction of an X-ray with angles marked illustrating a low arch. *a*, 147.5°, *b*, 6.0°, *c*, 144.0°, *d*, 21.0°.

TABLE 6. *Normal range of foot angles for 683 children (mean ± 1 SD)*

NUM-BER OF CASES	AGE YR.	ANGLE			
		A	B	C	D
24	2½	121.5 to 133.5	14.5 to 20.5	137.5 to 149.5	20.0 to 28.0
40	3	121.5 to 135.5	15.5 to 22.5	137.0 to 149.0	20.0 to 28.0
44	3½	121.0 to 134.0	16.0 to 23.0	138.0 to 149.0	20.0 to 28.0
43	4	120.5 to 133.5	16.0 to 24.0	136.5 to 147.5	20.5 to 28.5
39	4½	120.5 to 133.5	15.5 to 21.5	133.5 to 146.5	21.0 to 30.0
43	5	121.0 to 133.0	16.0 to 22.0	135.5 to 146.5	21.5 to 29.5
50	5½	120.5 to 131.5	14.5 to 21.5	133.0 to 146.0	21.5 to 30.5
52	6	121.5 to 131.5	14.5 to 21.5	133.0 to 145.0	22.5 to 30.5
40	6½	121.5 to 131.5	14.0 to 22.0	133.5 to 144.5	22.5 to 29.5
42	7	121.0 to 133.0	13.5 to 20.5	133.5 to 144.5	22.0 to 30.0
36	7½	122.5 to 133.5	13.5 to 20.5	134.0 to 146.0	21.5 to 29.5
60	8	121.5 to 132.5	13.5 to 20.5	133.0 to 145.0	22.0 to 30.0
38	8½	121.5 to 132.5	13.0 to 19.0	134.0 to 147.0	21.5 to 29.5
35	9	121.0 to 133.0	12.5 to 18.5	135.0 to 145.0	22.0 to 29.0
29	9½	122.0 to 133.0	12.0 to 18.0	135.5 to 147.5	20.5 to 28.5
29	10	121.0 to 131.0	12.5 to 18.5	136.0 to 146.0	22.0 to 28.0
23	10½	121.5 to 132.5	11.5 to 17.5	135.5 to 146.5	22.0 to 29.0
16	11	120.0 to 132.0	11.0 to 18.0	138.0 to 148.0	21.0 to 27.0
683	All Ages	121.5 to 132.5	13.5 to 20.5	135.0 to 147.0	21.0 to 29.0

Source: Robinow M, Johnston M, Anderson M. Feet of normal children. A study of lateral x-rays of the weightbearing foot. *J Pediatr* 1943;23:141–9.

Length of the Normal Foot

Serial measurements of normal feet of 227 girls and 285 boys with poliomyelitis in the contralateral foot provided 3,128 values, which were analyzed. The feet were measured with a simple wooden caliper, the recorded length being that from the back of the heel to the tip of the great toe with the subject in a standing position.

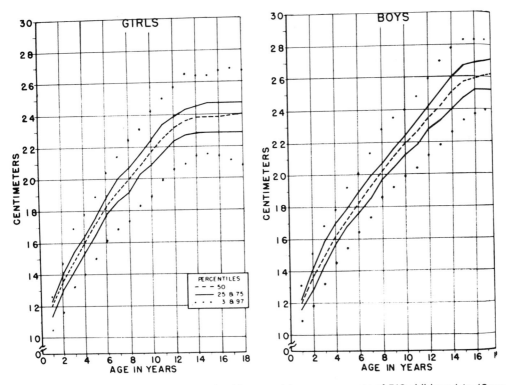

FIG. 11. Length of the normal foot derived from serial measurements of 512 children 1 to 18 years of age.

TABLE 7. *Length of the normal foot*

Girls (%)					Age	Boys (%)				
3	25	50	75	97		3	25	50	75	97
10.5	11.4	12.0	12.3	12.6	1	10.9	11.6	12.0	12.2	13.1
11.6	13.0	13.6	14.0	14.7	2	11.8	12.8	13.6	14.1	15.1
13.2	14.3	14.8	15.4	16.9	3	13.2	14.4	14.9	15.8	16.9
14.0	15.4	16.0	16.4	17.8	4	14.5	15.7	16.2	17.0	17.8
15.0	16.5	17.2	17.6	18.9	5	15.4	16.8	17.2	17.9	19.2
16.1	17.8	18.3	18.9	20.4	6	16.4	17.6	18.2	18.9	20.1
16.8	18.6	19.2	20.0	21.4	7	17.3	18.5	19.2	19.9	21.3
17.3	19.2	20.0	20.7	22.4	8	18.6	19.7	20.2	20.7	22.8
18.3	20.3	20.8	21.5	23.1	9	19.2	20.4	21.1	21.6	23.5
18.9	20.9	21.7	22.4	24.2	10	19.9	21.2	21.9	22.4	24.0
19.9	21.6	22.5	23.4	25.0	11	20.4	21.8	22.6	23.3	24.8
20.6	22.3	23.2	23.9	25.7	12	21.2	22.8	23.5	24.2	25.9
20.9	22.7	23.6	24.3	26.5	13	21.8	23.3	24.2	25.1	27.0
21.4	22.8	23.8	24.5	26.4	14	22.6	24.0	25.1	26.0	27.8
21.5	22.8	23.8	24.7	26.4	15	23.3	24.7	25.7	26.7	28.3
21.4	22.8	23.8	24.7	26.7	16	23.7	25.2	25.9	26.9	28.3
21.1	22.8	23.9	24.7	26.8	17	23.9	25.2	26.1	27.0	28.3
20.8	22.8	24.0	24.7	26.7	18	23.8	25.2	26.2	27.1	28.4

Data were used to construct the graphs in Fig. 11.

TABLE 8. *Percent of 18-year size attained at specific ages. Longitudinal series of 10 boys and 10 girls illustrating the percent of stature, femur, tibia, and foot relative to age*

Girls			Age	Boys		
Stature (%)	Femur and tibia (%)	Foot (%)		Stature (%)	Femur and tibia (%)	Foot (%)
46.1	34.8	49.9	1	42.6	31.2	45.2
53.2	41.7	57.8	2	49.7	39.2	53.0
63.6	55.1	67.8	4	58.7	49.8	62.0
77.4	73.9	82.1	8	72.4	68.7	75.8
91.3	91.6	97.0	12	84.5	85.4	91.3
99.5	100.0	100.0	16	98.6	99.6	100.0

Source: Blais MM, Green WT, Anderson M. Lengths of the growing foot. *J Bone Joint Surg (Am)* 1956;38:998–1000.

Length of Normal Weightbearing Foot

These data were developed from a group at Boston Children's Hospital examined serially from 1 to 18 years of age. The material is adapted from Anderson M, Blais M, Green WT. Growth of the foot stature and lower extremity as seen in serial records of children one to eighteen years of age. *Am J Phys Anthrop* 1956;14:287–308. Proportion of calcified os calcis, heel, cuboid, and metatarsus is expressed as percent of total foot length when measured from lateral roentgenograms in children 1 to 18 years old.

TABLE 9. *Length of foot in centimeters*

Age	No. of Boys	Foot Length	% of 15 Yr. Length	No. of Boys	Calcified Os Calcis	"Heel"	Cuboid	Metatarsus
1	17	11.90	46.2	10	21.5	32.2	13.9	15.3
2	40	13.50	52.5	10	23.9	33.1	14.3	16.1
3	61	15.07	58.6	10	25.2	33.4	14.2	15.5
4	84	16.29	63.4	10	26.4	33.7	14.2	15.9
5	80	17.27	67.2	10	27.1	34.0	14.3	15.8
6	78	18.19	70.8	10	27.2	33.6	14.2	16.0
7	76	19.23	74.8	10	27.3	33.3	14.1	16.0
8	92	20.16	78.4	10	27.4	33.1	14.0	15.8
9	83	21.08	82.0	10	27.8	33.0	13.7	15.6
10	98	21.89	85.1	10	28.2	33.1	13.5	15.4
11	112	22.58	87.8	10	28.5	33.2	13.3	15.3
12	126	23.51	91.4	10	28.9	33.2	13.1	15.2
13	138	24.22	94.2	10	29.3	33.3	12.9	15.3
14	152	25.06	97.4	10	29.7	33.7	12.7	15.6
15	147	25.71	100.0	10	30.1	33.8	12.5	16.3
16	139	26.04	101.3	10	30.1	33.5	12.5	16.6
17	128	26.11	101.6	10	30.3	33.4	12.5	16.6
18	107	26.14	101.7	10	30.2	33.4	12.5	16.6

Age	No. of Girls	Foot Length	% of 13 Yr. Length	No. of Girls	Calcified Os Calcis	"Heel"	Cuboid	Metatarsus
1	21	11.87	50.4	10	22.6	32.1	13.7	16.5
2	30	13.47	57.1	10	24.3	32.7	14.0	16.7
3	42	14.86	63.0	10	25.4	32.6	13.8	16.3
4	66	15.93	67.6	10	26.0	32.6	13.8	16.3
5	64	17.07	72.4	10	26.1	32.4	13.6	17.0
6	64	18.25	77.4	10	26.3	32.3	13.6	16.9
7	69	19.13	81.2	10	26.6	32.2	13.6	16.7
8	74	19.91	84.5	10	27.3	32.4	13.4	16.6
9	86	20.86	88.5	10	27.6	32.3	13.1	16.6
10	94	21.65	91.9	10	28.2	32.4	13.0	16.8
11	105	22.11	95.2	10	28.5	32.3	12.4	16.8
12	110	23.15	98.2	10	28.6	32.5	12.3	17.1
13	113	23.57	100.0	10	28.7	32.6	12.1	17.0
14	106	23.77	100.8	10	28.9	32.6	12.1	17.2
15	98	23.84	101.1	10	28.9	32.7	12.1	17.2
16	88	23.82	101.1	10	29.0	32.8	12.1	17.2
17	80	23.84	101.1	10	28.9	32.8	12.1	17.2
18	60	23.87	101.3	10	28.9	32.8	12.1	17.2

Foot length: From tip of great toe to back of heel, weightbearing position. Calcified os calcis: its horizontal diameter. "Heel:" from skin at back of heel to midpoint between os calcis and cuboid. Cuboid: midpoint between os calcis and cuboid to midpoint between cuboid and fourth metatarsal. Metatarsus: midpoint between cuboid and fourth metatarsal to distal epiphyseal line of fifth metatarsal.

Table 10 shows average annual change for Boston children and change at regular intervals for eight Cleveland children who were on different skeletal developmental levels at age ten years.

TABLE 10. *Percent change in foot length between ages two and ten years according to direct measurements and lengths of footprints*

Age in Years:	7th Boy:	31st Boy:	68th Boy:	100th Boy:	Boston Boys:
	Foot length ratios, according to footprint series: four Cleveland boys				direct measurements
2	62.4	60.3	57.0	—	61.7
2½	64.4	65.2	63.6	—	—
3	—	67.4	66.8	69.1	68.8
3½	68.0	70.5	70.1	—	—
4	71.6	73.2	69.2	72.4	74.4
4½	72.7	74.6	73.8	74.8	—
5	76.3	77.2	76.6	77.6	78.9
6	80.4	83.0	—	83.2	83.1
7	86.1	87.0	86.0	86.4	87.8
8	91.2	90.6	91.1	91.6	92.1
9	93.8	94.1	93.9	95.8	96.3
10	100.0	100.0	100.0	100.0	100.0
Print length at 10 years:	19.4 cm.	22.4 cm.	21.4 cm.	21.4 cm.	Average foot length at 10 years – 21.9 cm.
Boy's weight:	63.5 lbs.	76.8 lbs.	96.5 lbs.	98.0 lbs.	
Boy's height:	133.0 cm.	145.2 cm.	146.1 cm.	147.6 cm.	

Age in Years:	6th Girl:	31st Girl:	68th Girl:	98th Girl:	Boston Girls:
	Foot length ratios, according to footprint series: four Cleveland girls				direct measurements
2	—	61.0	57.9	58.7	62.2
2½	—	62.6	63.8	60.0	—
3	66.3	65.6	66.5	63.1	68.6
3½	68.9	68.2	70.6	68.9	—
4	72.4	73.8	74.2	70.7	73.6
4½	75.0	74.9	76.0	73.8	—
5	76.0	77.4	76.9	74.5	78.8
6	81.1	82.6	84.6	82.2	84.3
7	86.7	86.7	86.4	87.1	88.4
8	89.8	90.3	90.5	91.1	92.0
9	95.4	93.8	95.0	93.3	96.4
10	100.0	100.0	100.0	100.0	100.0
Print length at 10 years:	19.6 cm.	19.5 cm.	22.1 cm.	22.5 cm.	Average foot length at 10 years – 21.6 cm.
Girl's weight:	61.2 lbs.	66.8 lbs.	122.8 lbs.	56.2 lbs.	
Girl's height:	135.8 cm.	152.5 cm.	152.5 cm.	142.6 cm.	

The least mature foot in the ranked arrays of 100 films at each age was assigned number 1 and the most mature foot was assigned number 100.

Source: Hoerr NL, Pyle SI, Francis CC. *Radiographic atlas of the skeletal development of the foot and ankle. A standard reference.* Springfield, IL: Charles C Thomas, 1962.

Related reference: Meredith HV. Human foot length from embryo to adult. *Hum Biol* 1944;16:207–82.

Foot Length and Breadth in Infants

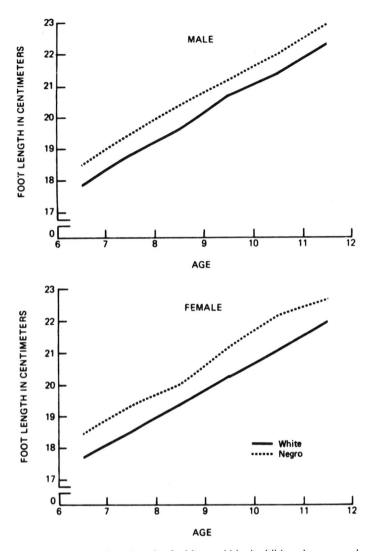

FIG. 12. Mean foot length of white and black children by sex and age.

TABLE 11. *Foot length of children by race, sex, and age at last birthday in the United States, 1963–65.*

Race, sex, and age	n	N	X̄	s	s$_\bar{x}$	Percentile (cm)						
						5th	10th	25th	50th	75th	90th	95th
White: Boys						In centimeters						
6 years	489	1,787	17.9	1.01	0.06	16.2	16.5	17.2	17.8	18.6	19.4	19.8
7 years	551	1,781	18.8	1.05	0.06	17.1	17.4	18.1	18.8	19.6	20.4	20.8
8 years	537	1,739	19.6	1.20	0.07	17.7	18.1	18.7	19.6	20.5	21.3	21.7
9 years	525	1,730	20.7	1.23	0.07	18.5	19.1	19.9	20.6	21.5	22.4	22.8
10 years	509	1,692	21.4	1.30	0.06	19.2	20.0	20.4	21.4	22.4	23.2	23.7
11 years	542	1,662	22.3	1.34	0.07	20.1	20.4	21.3	22.3	23.2	24.1	24.7
Girls												
6 years	461	1,722	17.7	1.07	0.08	15.7	16.2	17.1	17.7	18.5	19.2	19.6
7 years	512	1,716	18.5	1.06	0.04	16.6	17.1	17.7	18.5	19.3	19.9	20.5
8 years	498	1,674	19.4	1.14	0.06	17.4	18.1	18.5	19.5	20.3	21.0	21.5
9 years	494	1,663	20.3	1.20	0.06	18.2	18.6	19.5	20.4	21.1	21.9	22.5
10 years	505	1,632	21.1	1.33	0.06	19.1	19.4	20.3	21.2	22.1	22.8	23.3
11 years	477	1,605	22.0	1.27	0.06	20.0	20.3	21.1	21.9	22.9	23.7	24.2
Black: Boys												
6 years	84	289	18.5	1.07	0.17	16.7	17.1	17.7	18.5	19.2	19.9	20.5
7 years	79	286	19.5	1.02	0.12	17.5	18.0	18.7	19.5	20.2	20.8	21.3
8 years	79	279	20.4	1.06	0.14	18.8	19.1	19.6	20.4	21.2	22.0	22.4
9 years	74	269	21.2	1.30	0.12	18.9	19.4	20.3	21.2	21.9	22.8	24.1
10 years	65	264	22.0	1.22	0.15	20.1	20.3	20.9	22.1	22.9	23.6	23.9
11 years	83	255	22.9	1.20	0.12	20.7	21.2	22.1	23.1	23.6	24.3	24.8
Girls												
6 years	72	281	18.4	1.10	0.14	16.4	17.1	17.6	18.4	19.3	19.8	20.2
7 years	93	284	19.3	0.97	0.10	17.6	17.8	18.6	19.4	20.1	20.7	21.0
8 years	113	281	20.0	1.26	0.10	18.2	18.4	19.0	20.1	21.0	21.8	22.4
9 years	84	265	21.2	1.40	0.18	18.8	19.2	20.2	21.0	22.4	22.8	23.7
10 years	77	266	22.2	1.20	0.18	20.1	20.5	21.3	22.2	23.1	23.8	24.4
11 years	84	253	22.7	1.52	0.20	20.1	20.6	21.5	22.7	23.8	24.9	25.3

n = sample size; *N* = estimated number of children in population in thousands; $\overline{X}$ = mean; *s* = standard deviation; s$_\bar{x}$ = standard error of the mean.

Data were used to construct graphs in Fig. 12.

Source: Malina RM, Hamil PVV, Lemshow S. Selected body measurements of children 6–11 years. Washington, D.C.: U.S. Government Printing Office, 1973; United States DHEW Publication no. (HSM) 73-1605.

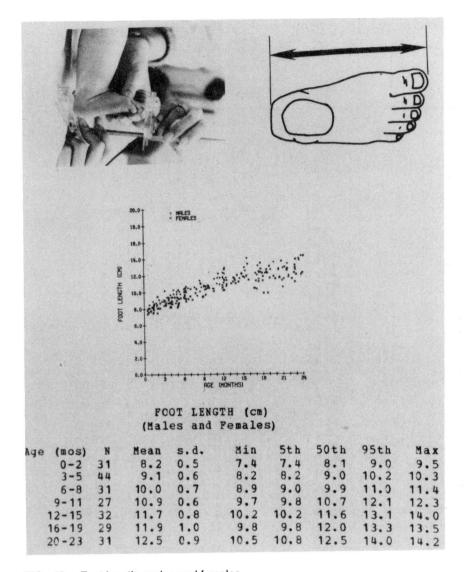

FOOT LENGTH (cm)
(Males and Females)

Age (mos)	N	Mean	s.d.	Min	5th	50th	95th	Max
0-2	31	8.2	0.5	7.4	7.4	8.1	9.0	9.5
3-5	44	9.1	0.6	8.2	8.2	9.0	10.2	10.3
6-8	31	10.0	0.7	8.9	9.0	9.9	11.0	11.4
9-11	27	10.9	0.6	9.7	9.8	10.7	12.1	12.3
12-15	32	11.7	0.8	10.2	10.2	11.6	13.1	14.0
16-19	29	11.9	1.0	9.8	9.8	12.0	13.3	13.5
20-23	31	12.5	0.9	10.5	10.8	12.5	14.0	14.2

FIG. 13. Foot length, males and females.

Foot length was measured with the infant recumbent. The paddle blades of the automated sliding caliper measured the distance from the heel to the longest toe of the right foot parallel to the long axis of the foot.

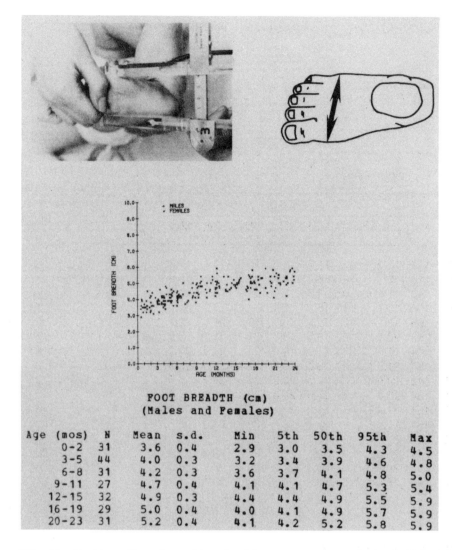

FOOT BREADTH (cm)
(Males and Females)

Age (mos)	N	Mean	s.d.	Min	5th	50th	95th	Max
0-2	31	3.6	0.4	2.9	3.0	3.5	4.3	4.5
3-5	44	4.0	0.3	3.2	3.4	3.9	4.6	4.8
6-8	31	4.2	0.3	3.6	3.7	4.1	4.8	5.0
9-11	27	4.7	0.4	4.1	4.1	4.7	5.3	5.4
12-15	32	4.9	0.3	4.4	4.4	4.9	5.5	5.9
16-19	29	5.0	0.4	4.0	4.1	4.9	5.7	5.9
20-23	31	5.2	0.4	4.1	4.2	5.2	5.8	5.9

FIG. 14. Foot breadth, males and females. Measurements were obtained with the infant recumbent. The maximum breadth across the ball of the right foot was measured with paddle blades of an automated sliding caliper.

Source: Snyder RG, Schneider LW, Owings CL, Reynolds HM, Golomb DH, Schork MA. Highway Safety Research Institute, University of Michigan. Published by Society of Automotive Engineers, Inc., Warrendale, PA, 1977.

Normal Foot Length and Breadth, by Age

Length was measured as the distance from the back of the right heel to the tip of the longest toe, the child seated, and measured to the long axis of the foot. Breadth was measured in a similar manner, using the widest portion at the ball of the foot.

TABLE 12. *Foot length in males*

Age (yrs)	No.	Foot length (cm)						
		Mean	SD	Min.	5th	50th	95th	Max.
2.0–3.5	114	15.0	1.1	11.6	13.0	15.0	16.6	17.8
3.5–4.5	118	16.1	0.9	14.2	14.7	16.0	17.7	18.9
4.5–5.5	143	17.1	1.0	14.7	15.6	17.0	18.5	20.2
5.5–6.5	108	18.1	1.1	15.3	16.4	17.8	20.2	21.5
6.5–7.5	105	19.1	1.2	15.6	16.8	18.8	20.9	22.7
7.5–8.5	98	20.0	1.0	16.8	18.3	20.0	21.6	22.9
8.5–9.5	114	21.0	1.3	17.9	19.0	20.8	23.3	23.9
9.5–10.5	124	21.8	1.4	18.8	19.6	21.6	24.0	25.3
10.5–11.5	142	22.5	1.3	19.1	20.3	22.5	24.7	25.9
11.5–12.5	154	23.4	1.4	20.0	21.3	23.4	25.6	27.1
12.5–13.5	154	24.4	1.5	21.2	22.1	24.2	27.1	28.8
13.5–14.5	154	25.4	1.6	22.4	22.9	25.3	28.0	29.5
14.5–15.5	131	25.8	1.3	22.3	23.5	25.9	27.9	29.2
15.5–16.5	99	26.5	1.2	23.5	24.3	26.6	28.2	29.3
16.5–17.5	104	26.6	1.3	23.4	24.2	26.6	28.3	30.0
17.5–19.0	88	26.9	1.6	22.9	24.5	27.0	30.1	31.1

TABLE 13. *Foot breadth in males*

Age (yrs)	No.	Foot breadth (cm)						
		Mean	SD	Min.	5th	50th	95th	Max.
2.0–3.5	114	6.3	0.4	5.3	5.5	6.2	7.0	7.2
3.5–4.5	117	6.5	0.4	5.5	5.8	6.4	7.2	7.8
4.5–5.5	143	6.9	0.4	5.9	6.1	6.9	7.6	7.9
5.5–6.5	108	7.2	0.5	5.8	6.4	7.2	7.9	8.3
6.5–7.5	105	7.6	0.5	6.7	6.8	7.5	8.5	9.2
7.5–8.5	98	7.9	0.5	6.7	7.0	7.9	8.7	9.5
8.5–9.5	114	8.2	0.5	6.9	7.2	8.1	9.1	9.6
9.5–10.5	123	8.4	0.6	7.1	7.4	8.3	9.4	10.2
10.5–11.5	142	8.7	0.6	7.4	7.8	8.7	9.7	10.5
11.5–12.5	154	9.1	0.7	7.7	7.9	9.0	10.1	10.7
12.5–13.5	154	9.5	0.7	7.8	8.4	9.4	10.6	11.3
13.5–14.5	153	9.9	0.7	8.3	8.6	9.9	11.0	12.0
14.5–15.5	131	10.1	0.7	8.3	8.9	10.1	11.1	11.6
15.5–16.5	100	10.3	0.6	8.6	9.0	10.3	11.1	11.8
16.5–17.5	104	10.4	0.6	9.1	9.4	10.4	11.2	11.9
17.5–19.0	88	10.5	0.7	9.4	9.6	10.4	11.8	12.8

Length was measured as the distance from the back of the right heel to the tip of the longest toe, the child seated, and measured to the long axis of the foot. Breadth was measured in a similar manner, using the widest portion at the ball of the foot.

TABLE 14. *Foot length in females*

| Age (yrs) | No. | Foot length (cm) | | | | | | |
		Mean	SD	Min	5th	50th	95th	Max.
2.0–3.5	98	14.5	1.0	11.9	13.0	14.5	16.0	17.1
3.5–4.5	109	16.1	1.0	13.6	14.3	16.0	17.6	20.2
4.5–5.5	120	16.9	0.9	15.0	15.4	16.8	18.3	19.7
5.5–6.5	111	17.8	1.0	14.8	16.1	17.8	19.2	20.4
6.5–7.5	120	18.8	1.1	16.2	16.9	18.8	20.4	22.4
7.5–8.5	93	19.6	1.1	17.1	17.7	19.5	21.4	23.0
8.5–9.5	137	20.7	1.3	18.0	18.9	20.5	22.9	25.4
9.5–10.5	129	21.5	1.2	17.9	19.6	21.4	23.3	24.1
10.5–11.5	140	22.3	1.4	18.2	20.0	22.2	24.8	25.6
11.5–12.5	133	23.0	1.2	19.8	21.1	23.0	24.9	27.2
12.5–13.5	161	23.4	1.2	20.7	21.4	23.4	25.5	26.6
13.5–14.5	116	23.6	1.2	20.6	21.5	23.4	25.9	27.0
14.5–15.5	133	23.8	1.3	20.3	21.9	23.6	26.2	27.5
15.5–16.5	98	23.8	1.3	21.2	21.7	23.6	26.3	27.6
16.5–17.5	117	23.6	1.1	21.5	21.9	23.4	25.7	26.3
17.5–19.0	67	23.7	1.2	20.8	21.8	23.7	25.6	27.2

TABLE 15. *Foot breadth in females*

| Age (yrs) | No. | Foot breadth (cm) | | | | | | |
		Mean	SD	Min.	5th	50th	95th	Max.
2.0–3.5	98	5.9	0.4	5.0	5.2	5.9	6.6	6.9
3.5–4.5	109	6.4	0.4	5.7	5.7	6.4	7.1	7.4
4.5–5.5	120	6.7	0.4	5.7	6.0	6.6	7.2	7.8
5.5–6.5	111	6.9	0.4	5.8	6.2	6.9	7.6	8.2
6.5–7.5	121	7.3	0.5	6.1	6.5	7.3	8.2	8.6
7.5–8.5	93	7.5	0.5	6.3	6.5	7.5	8.3	9.4
8.5–9.5	137	7.9	0.5	6.4	7.1	7.8	8.7	9.5
9.5–10.5	129	8.2	0.6	6.9	7.1	8.2	9.1	9.4
10.5–11.5	139	8.5	0.7	6.8	7.4	8.4	9.7	10.8
11.5–12.5	133	8.7	0.6	7.0	7.7	8.7	9.6	10.3
12.5–13.5	161	9.0	0.6	7.4	8.1	8.9	9.9	10.8
13.5–14.5	116	9.1	0.6	7.2	7.9	9.0	10.0	10.4
14.5–15.5	133	9.1	0.6	7.9	8.2	9.0	10.1	10.9
15.5–16.5	98	9.2	0.5	8.0	8.3	9.2	10.1	10.5
16.5–17.5	117	9.0	0.5	7.8	8.2	9.0	9.9	10.7
17.5–19.0	67	9.2	0.6	7.8	8.2	9.0	10.0	11.6

Source: Snyder RG, Schneider LW, Owings CL, Reynolds HM, Golomb DH, Schork MA. Highway Safety Research Institute, University of Michigan. Published by Society of Automotive Engineers, Inc., Warrendale, PA, 1977.

Sphyrion Height

Sphyrion height is the height from the standing surface to the tip of the right medial malleolus.

TABLE 16. *Sphyrion height in males*

Age (yrs)	No.	Sphyrion height (cm)						
		Mean	SD	Min.	5th	50th	95th	Max.
2.0–3.5	31	3.9	1.1	2.2	2.3	3.7	5.6	6.3
3.5–4.5	39	3.9	0.7	2.2	2.4	3.8	5.0	5.3
4.5–5.5	29	4.5	0.8	2.8	2.8	4.5	5.4	6.0
5.5–6.5	42	4.8	0.8	3.5	3.5	4.7	5.9	6.2
6.5–7.5	32	4.9	0.8	3.4	3.5	5.0	6.1	6.4
7.5–8.5	31	5.4	0.8	3.6	3.7	5.5	6.5	7.0
8.5–9.5	33	5.4	0.9	4.0	4.1	5.4	6.8	8.0
9.5–10.5	37	5.6	0.9	3.8	4.1	5.6	7.0	8.2
10.5–11.5	48	6.0	0.9	4.3	4.5	5.9	7.6	8.5
11.5–12.5	52	6.2	0.7	4.9	5.1	6.1	7.4	7.9
12.5–13.5	49	6.5	0.8	4.1	4.9	6.5	7.8	9.2
13.5–14.5	50	6.5	1.0	4.0	4.4	6.4	8.1	8.9
14.5–15.5	39	6.7	0.9	4.6	4.6	6.6	8.1	8.8
15.5–16.5	29	7.4	0.8	5.7	5.9	7.3	8.3	9.6
16.5–17.5	35	7.2	1.1	4.5	5.4	7.0	8.8	9.2
17.5–19.0	23	7.0	0.9	5.3	5.4	6.9	8.2	8.4

TABLE 17. *Sphyrion height in females*

Age (yrs)	No.	Sphyrion height (cm)						
		Mean	SD	Min.	5th	50th	95th	Max.
2.0–3.5	29	3.5	0.8	2.1	2.1	3.4	4.8	5.1
3.5–4.5	33	4.1	0.7	2.6	2.9	4.0	5.3	5.5
4.5–5.5	40	4.4	0.9	2.5	2.7	4.2	5.6	6.4
5.5–6.5	33	4.6	0.7	3.5	3.5	4.5	5.9	6.0
6.5–7.5	40	4.7	0.6	2.8	2.9	4.7	5.3	6.2
7.5–8.5	30	4.9	0.8	3.4	3.4	4.8	6.0	6.5
8.5–9.5	48	5.0	0.7	2.9	3.9	5.1	6.2	6.3
9.5–10.5	37	5.2	0.8	3.7	3.7	5.2	6.3	7.2
10.5–11.5	47	5.6	0.8	3.6	4.3	5.5	6.7	7.9
11.5–12.5	40	5.7	0.7	4.6	4.7	5.6	7.1	7.7
12.5–13.5	46	5.8	0.9	3.9	4.2	5.8	7.4	8.2
13.5–14.5	26	6.0	0.7	4.7	4.8	5.8	7.0	7.7
14.5–15.5	44	6.0	0.8	4.1	4.3	5.9	7.1	7.3
15.5–16.5	31	6.3	0.8	4.5	4.7	6.4	7.2	7.5
16.5–17.5	34	6.5	0.6	5.4	5.5	6.6	7.3	8.2
17.5–19.0	23	6.1	0.8	4.8	4.8	5.9	7.2	7.5

Source: Snyder RG, Schneider LW, Owings CL, Reynolds HM, Golomb DH, Schork MA. Highway Safety Research Institute, University of Michigan. Published by Society of Automotive Engineers, Inc., Warrendale, PA, 1977.

GROWTH AND MATURATION

Growth and Development of the Form of the Body

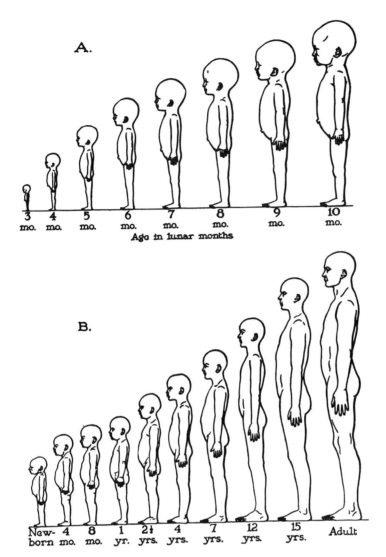

FIG. 1. Series showing growth and development of the form of the body, left lateral views. **A:** Eight fetal stages based on the empirical formula of L. A. Calkins and R. E. Scammon (Calkins LA, Scammon RE. The empirical formula for the proportionate growth of the human fetus. *Proc Soc Exp Biol* 1925;22:353–357). **B:** Ten postnatal stages.

Source: Morris H. *Human anatomy, a complete systematic treatise.* 11th ed. New York: McGraw Hill, 1953.

Fetal Maturity Based on Osseous Development

This study included 100 pregnancies in which X-rays were required of the fetus during the pregnancy. From these the weight of the fetus and number of weeks of gestation were estimated and then correlated with the weight and gestation at the time of delivery.

TABLE 1. *Roentgenograms of newborn infants in which presence of center was clear for various weight groups*

CENTER OF OSSIFICATION, RACE, AND SEX	BIRTH WEIGHT IN GRAMS					
	LESS THAN 2,000	2,000-2,499	2,500-2,999	3,000-3,499	3,500-3,999	4,000 OR MORE
	PERCENT-AGE	PERCENT-AGE	PERCENT-AGE	PERCENT-AGE	PERCENT-AGE	PERCENT-AGE
Distal epiphysis of femur.—						
White boys	9.1	75.0	85.3	100.0	100.0	100.0
White girls	50.0	91.7	98.0	100.0	100.0	100.0
Negro boys	18.2	88.5	90.7	94.0	100.0	100.0
Negro girls	50.0	93.8	99.0	100.0	100.0	100.0
Proximal epiphysis of tibia.—						
White boys	0.0	18.8	52.9	78.8	84.1	97.1
White girls	0.0	54.2	75.5	85.7	90.7	90.5
Negro boys	0.0	38.5	62.7	76.0	80.0	92.9
Negro girls	14.3	40.6	76.7	88.1	86.4	100.0

TABLE 2. *Presence or absence of distal epiphysis of femur and proximal epiphysis of tibia in relation to estimated weight and sex of fetus*

ESTIMATED WEIGHT AT TIME OF ROENTGENOGRAM* (GRAMS)	FEMUR − TIBIA −		FEMUR ± TIBIA −		FEMUR + TIBIA −		FEMUR + TIBIA ±		FEMUR + TIBIA ±	
	M	F	M	F	M	F	M	F	M	F
Under 1,000	3									
1,000-1,499		1								
1,500-1,999	4	2				4				1
2,000-2,499	5			2	3	6		1		1
2,500-2,999	2		1	1	5	5	1	2	3	3
3,000-3,499	1		1		7	4	5	1	4	3
3,500-3,999						2	1	1	6	3
4,000 and over		1			1				1	
Total	15	4	2	3	16	21	7	5	14	16
Average Weight	2,000	2,350	2,980	2,480	2,980	2,600	3,260	3,030	3,530	3,450

*Estimated from birth weight.

Source: Christie A. The estimation of fetal maturity by roentgen study of osseous development. *Am J Obstet Gynecol* 1950;60:133–9.

Prevalence and Distribution of Ossification Centers in the Newborn

A total of 1,112 newborn infants (298 white boys, 267 white girls, 271 black boys, and 276 black girls) were observed. The infants were weighed within 12 hr after birth. The roentgenograms were read for the presence or absence of centers in the calcaneus, talus, cuboid bones, third cuneiform bone, distal epiphysis of the femur, proximal epiphysis of the tibia, capitatum, hamate bone, head of the humerus, and head of the femur.

TABLE 3. *Presence of each of ten centers of ossification in roentgenograms distributed according to race, sex, and weight at birth*

| | Roentgenograms in Which Presence of Center was Clear, for Various Weight Groups (Gm.) | | | | | | | | | | | |
| | Less Than 2,000 | | 2,000 to 2,499 | | 2,500 to 2,999 | | 3,000 to 3,499 | | 3,500 to 3,999 | | 4,000 or more | |
Center of Ossification	Total Number	Percentage	Total Number	Percentage	Total Number	Percentage	Total Number	Percentage	Total Number	Percentage	Total Number	Percentage
Calcaneous												
White boys	11	100.0	15	100.0	34	100.0	113	100.0	88	100.0	35	100.0
White girls	6	100.0	24	100.0	49	100.0	111	100.0	54	100.0	21	100.0
Negro boys	11	100.0	26	100.0	75	100.0	100	100.0	45	100.0	14	100.0
Negro girls	14	100.0	32	100.0	103	100.0	101	100.0	22	100.0	4	100.0
Talus												
White boys	11	72.7	15	100.0	34	100.0	113	99.1	88	100.0	35	100.0
White girls	6	83.3	24	100.0	49	100.0	111	100.0	54	100.0	21	100.0
Negro boys	11	90.9	26	100.0	75	100.0	100	100.0	45	100.0	14	100.0
Negro girls	14	100.0	32	100.0	103	100.0	101	100.0	22	100.0	4	100.0
Distal epiphysis of femur												
White boys	11	9.1	16	75.0	34	85.3	113	100.0	88	100.0	35	100.0
White girls	6	50.0	24	91.7	49	98.0	112	100.0	54	100.0	21	100.0
Negro boys	11	18.2	26	88.5	75	90.7	100	94.0	45	100.0	14	100.0
Negro girls	14	50.0	32	93.8	103	99.0	101	100.0	22	100.0	4	100.0
Proximal epiphysis of tibia												
White boys	11	0.0	16	18.8	34	52.9	113	78.8	88	84.1	35	97.1
White girls	6	0.0	24	54.2	49	75.5	112	85.7	54	90.7	21	90.5
Negro boys	11	0.0	25	36.5	75	62.7	100	76.0	45	80.0	14	92.9
Negro girls	14	14.3	32	40.6	103	76.7	101	88.1	22	86.4	4	100.0
Cuboid bone												
White boys	11	0.0	16	6.2	34	14.7	113	39.8	88	44.3	35	60.0
White girls	6	0.0	24	37.5	49	57.1	112	65.2	54	70.4	21	76.2
Negro boys	11	0.0	26	23.1	73	43.8	100	58.0	44	68.2	14	100.0
Negro girls	14	21.4	32	37.5	103	68.0	101	78.2	22	81.8	4	75.0
Head of humerus												
White boys	11	0.0	13	7.7	29	13.8	62	41.9	51	49.0	22	59.1
White girls	4	0.0	18	5.6	31	25.8	74	41.9	36	69.4	15	86.7
Negro boys	11	0.0	23	0.0	66	15.2	76	27.6	31	48.4	11	63.6
Negro girls	13	0.0	28	10.7	88	22.7	78	52.6	18	38.9	1	100.0
Capitate bone												
White boys	11	0.0	15	0.0	33	0.0	112	8.0	88	15.9	34	17.6
White girls	6	0.0	24	0.0	47	14.9	106	15.1	53	20.8	21	38.1
Negro boys	11	0.0	26	7.7	73	16.4	96	20.8	42	26.2	13	30.8
Negro girls	14	0.0	32	12.5	101	19.8	101	41.6	22	40.9	3	100.0
Hamate bone												
White boys	11	0.0	15	6.7	32	6.2	112	6.2	87	10.3	35	11.4
White girls	6	0.0	24	0.0	47	10.6	106	13.0	53	20.8	21	33.3
Negro boys	11	0.0	26	15.4	73	16.4	96	17.7	43	44.2	14	28.6
Negro girls	14	0.0	32	9.4	101	22.5	100	41.0	22	54.5	3	66.7
Third cuneiform bone												
White boys	11	0.0	16	0.0	34	0.0	113	2.7	88	2.3	33	3.0
White girls	6	0.0	24	0.0	49	0.0	111	0.0	54	5.6	21	9.5
Negro boys	11	0.0	26	3.8	74	8.1	100	15.0	43	14.0	14	14.3
Negro girls	14	0.0	32	6.2	103	13.6	101	16.8	22	18.2	4	25.0
Head of femur												
White boys	11	0.0	16	0.0	33	0.0	107	0.0	76	0.0	30	0.0
White girls	5	0.0	21	0.0	49	0.0	105	1.0	52	0.0	20	0.0
Negro boys	11	0.0	25	0.0	75	0.0	99	0.0	43	0.0	14	0.0
Negro girls	14	0.0	31	0.0	100	0.0	96	1.0	21	0.0	4	0.0

Source: Christie A. Prevalence and distribution of ossification centers in the newborn infant. *Am J Dis Child* 1949;77:355–61.

Length of the Fibula at Birth

Thirty infants with birth weight below the 10th percentile for gestational age by the standards of L. Lubchenco et al. (Lubchenco L, Hansman C, Boyd E. Intrauterine growth in length and head circumference as estimated from live births at gestational ages from 26 to 42 weeks. *Pediatrics* 1966;37:403–8) were compared with 46 control infants whose weight was between the 10th and 90th percentiles for gestational age.

TABLE 4. *Length of the fibula at birth*

Gestational age (wk)	X-rays of infants with fetal growth retardation (group I)			X-rays of normal infants (group II)		
	No. of infants	Mean fibula length (cm)	Range	No. of infants	Mean fibula length (cm)	Range
22				1	3.65	3.65
23				—	—	—
24				3	4.17	3.80–4.50
25				1	4.72	4.72
26				—	—	—
27				—	—	—
28				3	4.39	4.20–4.70
29				—	—	—
30				5	4.88	4.50–5.20
31				4	4.95	4.33–5.35
32				7	5.12	4.45–5.63
33				2	5.30	5.10–5.50
34	2	4.65	4.30–5.00	5	5.31	5.12–5.46
35	2	4.87	4.50–5.24	3	5.61	5.58–5.66
36	4	5.22	4.90–5.79	2	5.95	5.75–6.15
37	3	5.80	5.50–6.00	1	6.31	6.31
38	5	5.50	5.31–5.76	2	6.47	6.30–6.63
39	6	5.44	4.80–5.72	2	6.17	6.02–6.32
40	5	5.61	5.35–5.84	3	6.39	6.20–6.60
41	2	5.56	5.50–5.62	1	6.52	6.52
42	1	5.23	5.23	1	6.20	6.20
Total	30			46		

Source: Wilson MG, Meyers HI, Peters AH. Postnatal bone growth of infants with fetal growth retardation. *Pediatrics* 1967;40:213.

Ossification of the Newborn

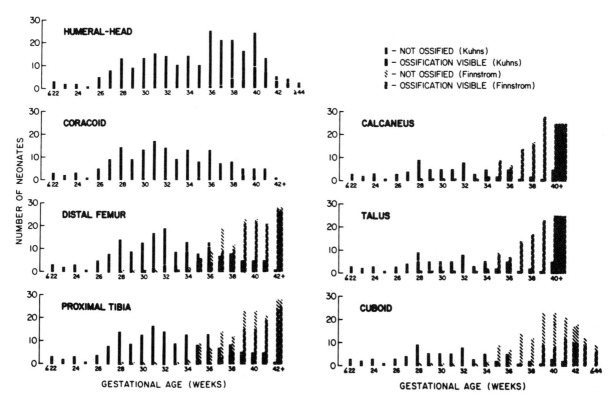

FIG. 2. Ossification of 360 white neonates of both sexes in relation to their gestational ages. The data were collected from two centers: the University of Michigan, Ann Arbor, and Umea, Sweden. The gestational age was determined by clinical history and assessed by physical and neurological examination.

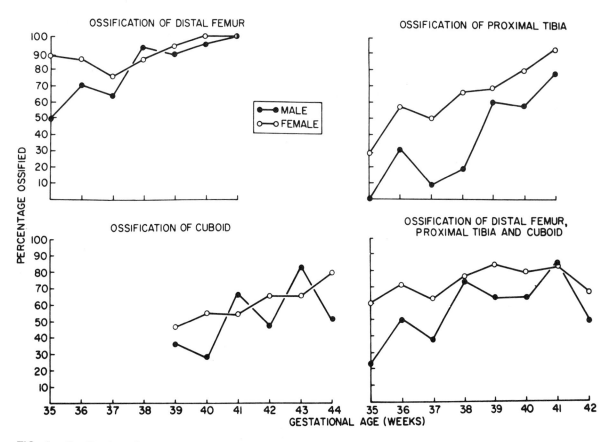

FIG. 3. Ossification of females and males in relation to gestational age where 15 or more males and females were evaluated for each week of gestation. Females had a slightly higher incidence of ossification for each epiphysis.

Source: Kuhns LR, Finnstrom O. New standards of ossification of the newborn. *Radiology* 1967;119:655–60.

Postnatal Bone Growth of Infants with Growth Retardation

Thirty infants with birth weight below the 10th percentile for gestational age by the standards of L. Lubchenco et al. (Lubchenco L, Hansman C, Boyd E. Intrauterine growth in length and head circumference as estimated from live births at gestational ages from 26 to 42 weeks. *Pediatrics* 1966;37:403–8) were compared with 46 control infants whose weight was between the 10th and 90th percentiles for gestational age.

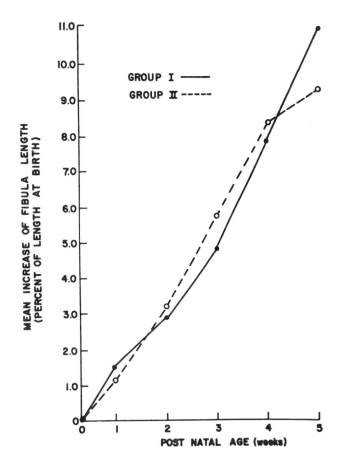

FIG. 4. Linear growth rate of the fibula in infants with fetal growth retardation (group I) and normal infants (group II).

Source: Wilson MG, Meyers HI, Peters AH. Postnatal bone growth of infants with fetal growth retardation. *Pediatrics* 1967;40:213.

TABLE 5. *Fibula length in cumulative percent increase*

Infants	Postnatal Age in Weeks				
	1	*2*	*3*	*4*	*5*
Infants with Fetal Growth Retardation (Group I)					
Cumulative percent increase in fibula length					
mean	1.5%	2.9%	4.8%	7.8%	10.9%
range	0–3.8%	.5–5.7%	1.7–9.3%	3.1–11.7%	6.7–14.6%
Number of infants	25	15	7	12	4
Normal Infants (Group II)					
Cumulative percent increase in fibula length					
mean	1.2%	3.2%	5.7%	8.3%	9.2%
range	0–2.6%	.6–4.9%	4.6–7.1%	5.3–11.2%	7.8–10.9%
Number of infants	24	21	13	15	3

Data from the graph in Fig. 4.

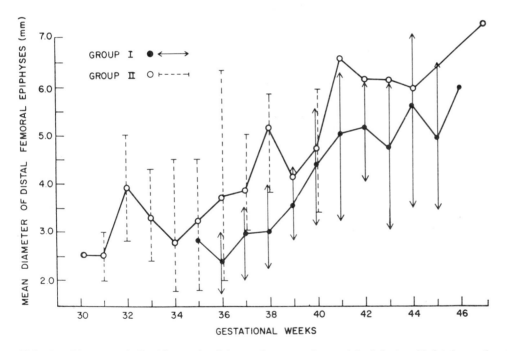

FIG. 5. Diameter of distal femoral epiphyses (mean and range) for infants with fetal growth retardation (group I) and normal infants (group II).

Source: Wilson MG, Meyers HI, Peters AH. Postnatal bone growth of infants with fetal growth retardation. *Pediatrics* 1967;40:213.

TABLE 6. *Diameter of proximal tibial epiphyses at given gestational ages*

Gestational Weeks	Number of Measurable Epiphyses	Mean Diameter of Proximal Tibial Epiphyses (mm)	Range (mm)	Number of Measurable Epiphyses	Mean Diameter of Proximal Tibial Epiphyses (mm)	Range (mm)
	91 X-rays of Infants with Fetal Growth Retardation (Group I)			*106 X-rays of Normal Infants (Group II)*		
32				1	3.0	3.0
33				—	—	—
34				1	2.0	2.0
35				1	2.4	2.4
36				2	4.15	3.0–5.
37	1	2.8	2.8	3	3.73	3.3–4.
38	2	2.40	1.8–8.0	3	4.93	3.0–7.
39	—	—	—	3	3.13	1.5–4.
40	3	4.50	4.0–5.0	3	2.20	1.8–2.
41	6	8.65	1.5–5.7	1	4.1	4.1
42	5	4.10	2.0–6.0	2	5.60	4.2–7.
43	2	8.45	3.1–3.8	1	7.0	7.0
44	4	4.30	2.3–6.1	1	4.0	4.0
45	2	4.50	2.8–6.2	1	7.0	7.0
46	1	5.1	5.1	—	—	—
Total	26			23		

Birth Measurements Only (Included above)

Gestational Weeks	Number of Measurable Epiphyses	Mean Diameter of Proximal Tibial Epiphyses (mm)	Range (mm)	Number of Measurable Epiphyses	Mean Diameter of Proximal Tibial Epiphyses (mm)	Range (mm)
	30 X-rays of Infants with Fetal Growth Retardation (Group I)			*42 X-rays of Normal Infants (Group II)*		
32				1	3.0	3.0
33				—	—	—
34				—	—	—
35				—	—	—
36				—	—	—
37	1	2.8	2.8	—	—	—
38	1	1.8	1.8	1	3.0	3.0
39	—	—	—	1	4.0	4.0
40	3	4.50	4.0–5.0	2	1.85	1.8–1.9
41	1	2.8	2.8	1	4.1	4.1
42				1	4.2	4.2
Total	6			7		

Data from the graph in Fig. 5.

Source: Wilson MG, Meyers HI, Peters AH. Postnatal bone growth of infants with fetal growth retardation. *Pediatrics* 1967;40:213.

Appearance of Ossification Centers

The numbers in Figs. 6 and 7 indicate the range from the 10th to the 90th percentile in appearance time of centers of ossification obtained from the studies on bone growth available in 1950. Statistically significant studies of the time of appearance of ossification centers had been made of relatively few portions of the skeleton after the sixth year of life. Numbers followed by an "m" indicate number of months; otherwise all numbers indicate years. Where two sets of numbers are given for one center of ossification, the upper, heavier figures refer to males and the lower, lighter figures to females. A single set of numbers applies to both sexes. "AB" indicates that the ossification center is visible at birth. Numbers in parentheses give the approximate time of fusion.

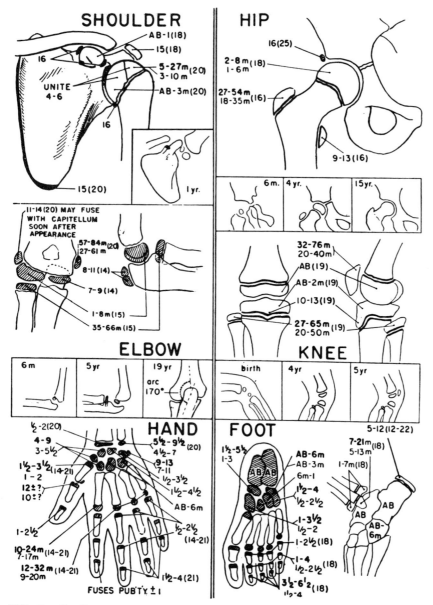

FIG. 6. Ossification centers in the shoulder, hip, elbow, knee, hand, and foot.

Source: Girdany BR, Golden R. Centers of ossification of the skeleton. *AJR* 1952;68:922–4.

References:
1. Bailey W. Persistent vertebral process epiphysis. *AJR* 1939;42:85–90.
2. Buehl CC, Pyle SI. Use of age at first appearance of three ossification centers in determining skeletal status of children. *J Pediatr* 1942;21:335–342.
3. Milamn DH, Bakwin H. Ossification of the metacarpal and metatarsal centers as a measure of maturation. *J Pediatr* 1950;36:617–620.
4. Ruckensteiner D. Die normale Entwicklung des Knochensystems im Rontgenbild. Georg Thieme, Leipzig, 1931.
5. Scammon RE, Morris H. *Morris Human Anatomy*. Edited by J.P. Schaeffer, 10th ed., Blakiston, Philadelphia, 1942.
6. Vogt EC, Vickers SV. Osseous growth and development. *Radiology* 1938;31:441–444.

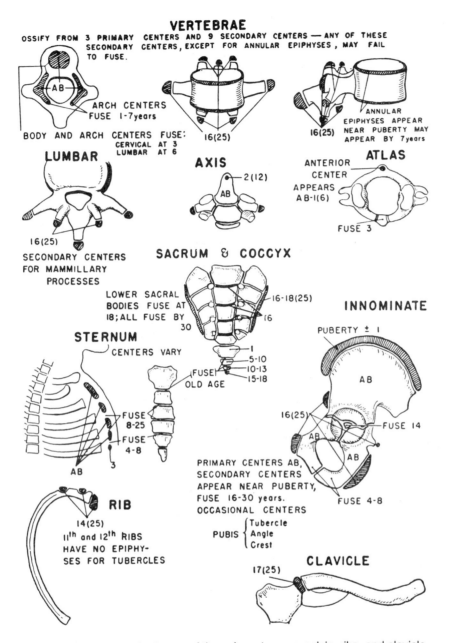

FIG. 7. Ossification centers in the bones of the spine, sternum, pelvis, ribs, and clavicle.

Source: Girdany BR, Golden R. Centers of ossification of the skeleton. *AJR* 1952;68:922–4.

Ossification Centers of Upper and Lower Extremities

This study was based on roentgenograms taken at regular intervals of all the bones and joints of the left upper and lower extremities in 149 normal children whose growth was being studied at the Samuel S. Fels Research Institute. Presented are data and curves of the time of appearance of 66 of the centers, both primary and epiphyseal, which with one or two exceptions are entirely cartilaginous at birth and in which ossification appears normally within the first 5 years of life. These 66 constitute approximately 80% of those centers of the extremities of the left side of the body which appear postnatally.

TABLE 7. Ossification centers of the upper and lower extremities

Shoulder...Coracoid	Femur.....Proximal epiphysis
Humerus...Proximal medial epiphysis	Greater trochanter
Proximal lateral epiphysis	Distal epiphysis
Capitellum	Knee......Patella
Medial epicondyle	Tibia......Proximal epiphysis
Radius.....Proximal epiphysis	Distal epiphysis
Distal epiphysis	Fibula.....Proximal epiphysis
Hand......Capitatum	Distal epiphysis
Hamatum	Foot.......Cuboid
Triquetrum	First cuneiform
Lunate	Second cuneiform
Navicula	Third cuneiform
Greater multiangular bone	Navicula
Lesser multiangular bone	Epiphysis of calcaneus
5 distal phalangeal epiphyses	5 distal phalangeal epiphyses
4 middle phalangeal epiphyses	4 middle phalangeal epiphyses
5 proximal phalangeal epiphyses	5 proximal phalangeal epiphyses
5 metacarpal epiphyses	5 metatarsal epiphyses

TABLE 8. Number of centers on left side of body ossified at a given age level

	Boys		Girls	
Age, Months	Mean Number	Standard Deviation	Mean Number	Standard Deviation
1	4.11	1.41	4.58	1.76
3	6.63	1.86	7.78	2.16
6	9.61	1.95	11.44	2.53
9	11.88	2.66	15.36	4.92
12	13.96	3.96	22.40	6.93
18	19.27	6.61	34.10	8.44
24	29.21	8.10	43.44	6.65
30	37.59	7.40	48.91	6.50
36	43.42	5.34	52.73	5.48
42	47.06	5.26	56.61	3.98
48	51.24	4.59	57.94	3.91
54	53.94	4.35	59.89	3.36
60	56.24	4.07	61.52	2.69

Source: Sontag LW, Snell D, Anderson M. Rate of appearance of ossification centers from birth to the age of five years. *Am J Dis Child* 1939;58:949–56.

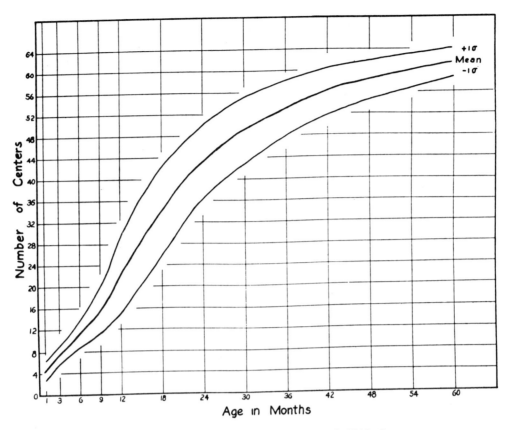

FIG. 8.   Number of ossification centers in girls, constructed from data in Table 8.

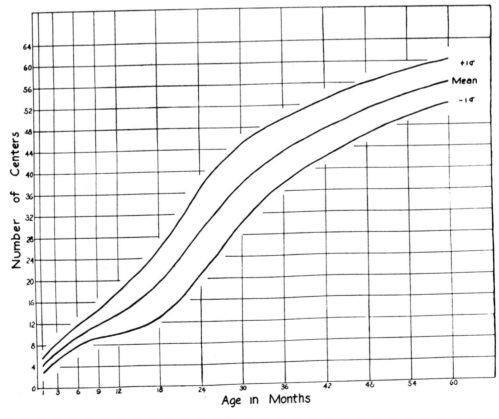

FIG. 9.   Number of ossification centers in boys, constructed from data in Table 8.

TABLE 9. *Median ages and ranges in age at which certain ossification centers appear in a group of healthy children*

Center	Median	Girls' range	No. of cases	Median	Boys' range	No. of cases
Capitate	0–2.5	0–1–0	57	0–3	0–1–0	49
Hamate	0–3	0–1–0	57	0–5	0–2–0	49
Triquetrum	2–1	0–2–5–0	62	3–1	0–4–6–0	56
Lunate	3–1	0–6–6–6	62	4–7.5	0–4–8–0	57
Greater multangular	4–2	2–0–7–6	57	6–4	3–6–10–0	54
Lesser multangular	4–6	1–6–7–0	59	6–10	4–0–10–6	62
Navicular	4–6	2–0–7–6	57	6–10	3–0–9–6	54
Pisiform	8–7.5	5–0–11–0	64	11–8	8–6–14–6	55
First metacarpal sesamoid	11–3	8–6–14–0	55	13–8	11–0–16–0	51
Tarsal cuboid	98% by 0–2	0–0–4	45	91% by 0–2	0–0–6	44
Metacarpal						
I	1–11	0–6–3–0	72	3–1	1–6–6–0	51
II	1–4	0–6–2–0	71	1–10	0–6–3–0	53
III	1–4.5	0–6–2–6	74	2–0	0–6–3–6	53
IV	1–6	0–6–2–6	74	2–1.5	1–0–4–0	54
V	1–7	0–6–3–0	73	2–5	1–0–4–0	54
Proximal phalanx						
I	2–1.5	1–0–3–0	69	3–4.5	1–0–5–6	49
II	1–2	0–4–2–0	70	1–7.5	0–6–2–6	55
III	1–1.5	0–4–2–0	72	1–7	0–6–3–0	55
IV	1–2	0–4–2–0	71	1–8	0–6–3–0	54
V	1–5.5	0–6–2–6	73	2–1.5	1–0–4–0	54
Middle phalanx						
II	1–8	0–6–3–0	64	2–6	1–0–4–0	49
III	1–7.5	0–6–2–6	69	2–4	0–6–4–0	49
IV	1–7.5	0–6–2–6	69	2–5	1–0–4–0	52
V	2–3	0–6–4–0	65	3–7	1–6–5–6	50
Distal phalanx						
I	1–5	0–4–2–6	63	1–10.5	0–6–4–0	50
II	2–5	0–6–3–0	58	3–7	1–0–6–0	45
III	1–11	0–6–3–0	65	2–7	1–0–4–0	48
IV	2–0	0–6–4–0	66	2–8	1–0–4–0	48
V	2–4	0–6–3–6	63	3–7	1–6–5–0	48
Humerus—head	81% by 0–2	0–0–4	58	78% by 0–2	0–0–6	45
Greater tuberosity	0–9	0–2–2–6	68	1–2	0–4–4–6	53
Capitellum	0–7	0–1–6	69	0–10	0–2–6	56
Lateral epicondyle	9–10	7–6–12–0	70	12–5	9–6–15–6	61
Trochlea	9–5	5–6–12–6	70	10–7	7–0–14–0	58
Medial epicondyle	3–10	2–0–6–6	64	7–1	4–6–10–0	60
Radius—head	4–10	2–0–8–0	70	6–3	2–6–9–6	57
Olecranon	8–8	6–0–11–6	69	11–3	7–6–14–0	54
Distal radius	1–1.5	0–4–3–0	69	1–4	0–4–3–6	53
Distal ulna	6–0	3–6–9–0	75	7–5	5–0–10–0	62
Femur—head	0–5	0–1–0	67	0–6	0–2–1–0	55
Greater trochanter	2–10	1–6–4–0	68	4–0	2–0–6–0	60
Distal femur	100% by 0–2	0–0–2	58	100% by 0–2	0–0–2	47
Proximal tibia	100% by 0–2	0–0–2	58	98% by 0–2	0–0–4	47
Proximal fibula	3–1.5	1–0–6–6	60	4–5	2–0–6–6	57
Distal tibia	0–5	0–1–0	68	0–5.5	0–2–1–0	56
Distal fibula	1–0.5	0–4–3–0	69	1–4	0–4–2–6	50

Source: Hansman CF. Appearance and fusion of ossification centers in the human skeleton. *AJR* 1962;88:476–482.

This material is from a longitudinal growth study of the Child Research Council, Denver, Colorado. The left upper and lower extremities were roentgenographed at 2 months, 4 months, and 6 months, and at 6-month intervals thereafter to maturity. A total of 207 children, 102 boys and 105 girls, comprised this group.

TABLE 10. *Median ages and ranges in age at which certain epiphyseal ossification centers fuse with their diaphyses in a group of healthy children*

Center		Median	Girls' Range	No. of Cases	Median	Boys' Range	No. of Cases
Metacarpal	I	14–1	11–6 to 16–0	31	16–4	14–0 to 18–6	32
	II	14–6	11–6 to 17–0	31	16–6	14–6 to 18–6	31
	III	14–6	11–6 to 17–0	31	16–6	14–6 to 18–6	31
	IV	14–5	11–6 to 17–0	31	16–5	14–6 to 19–6	31
	V	14–5	11–6 to 16–6	31	16–6	14–6 to 19–6	31
Proximal phalanx	I	14–2	11–0 to 17–0	33	16–3	14–6 to 18–6	33
	II	14–2	11–0 to 16–6	31	16–4.5	14–6 to 18–6	32
	III	14–2	11–0 to 16–6	32	16–4	14–0 to 18–6	32
	IV	14–3	11–0 to 16–6	33	16–6	14–6 to 18–6	32
	V	14–2	11–0 to 16–0	32	16–3	14–6 to 18–6	33
Middle phalanx	II	14–4.5	11–0 to 17–0	33	16–5	14–6 to 19–6	30
	III	14–4.5	11–0 to 17–0	31	16–6	14–6 to 19–6	31
	IV	14–4	11–0 to 17–0	31	16–5	14–6 to 18–6	31
	V	14–3	11–0 to 17–0	33	16–4	14–6 to 19–6	30
Distal phalanx	I	13–8	10–6 to 15–6	36	15–11	13–6 to 18–0	35
	II	13–7	10–6 to 16–0	37	15–10	13–6 to 19–6	35
	III	13–7	10–6 to 16–0	37	16–0	13–6 to 18–0	34
	IV	13–8	10–6 to 16–0	35	15–10.5	13–6 to 18–0	34
	V	13–7	10–6 to 15–6	37	15–11	13–6 to 18–0	33
Humerus—head		15–7	13–0 to 17–0	27	18–2	16–6 to 20–0	19
Greater tuberosity		4–1	2–0 to 7–6	71	5–6	3–0 to 8–6	63
Capitellum		12–5	9–6 to 14–0	62	15–2	13–6 to 17–6	58
Lateral epicondyle		12–8	9–6 to 14–0	57	15–4	13–6 to 18–0	56
Trochlea		12–4	9–6 to 14–0	58	15–1.5	13–0 to 18–0	58
Medial epicondyle		14–1	11–0 to 16–0	51	16–4	14–0 to 19–0	45
Radius—head		13–6	10–6 to 16–0	57	16–2	14–0 to 19–0	47
Olecranon		12–8	10–0 to 14–6	58	15–4.5	13–6 to 18–0	56
Distal radius		15–10.5	13–0 to 17–0	28	18–0	16–0 to 20–0	21
Distal ula		15–11	12–6 to 17–0	30	17–10.5	16–0 to 20–0	20
Femur—head		14–2	11–0 to 16–6	52	16–3	14–0 to 19–0	49
Greater trochanter		13–11	11–6 to 16–0	50	15–11	14–0 to 19–0	47
Distal femur		14–9	12–0 to 17–0	46	16–7.5	14–0 to 19–0	47
Proximal tibia		14–10	12–0 to 17–0	44	16–11	14–6 to 19–6	42
Proximal fibula		15–2	12–0 to 17–0	38	17–2	15–0 to 20–0	37
Distal tibia		14–10	12–0 to 17–0	44	16–10.5	14–0 to 20–0	46
Distal fibula		14–10.5	12–0 to 17–0	42	16–10.5	15–0 to 20–0	45

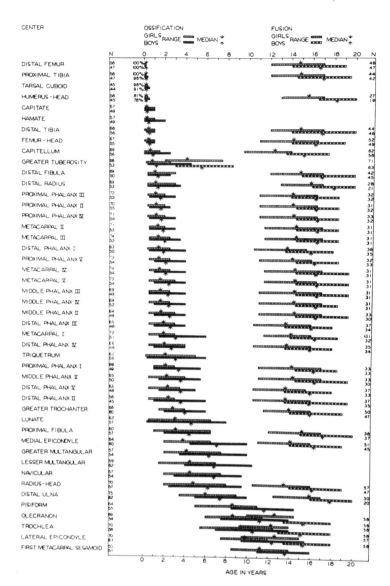

FIG. 10. Bar diagram representing the ranges in age over which certain skeletal ossification centers appeared and fused in children. The upper bar indicates the range for girls and the lower bar the range for boys. The median age of ossification or fusion of each center is indicated by an asterisk. The centers are listed in order according to the median age from earliest to latest in which they are found to ossify in girls of the group. The figure at the beginning or end of each bar is the number of children in that group.

Source: Hansman CF. Appearance and fusion of ossification centers in the human skeleton. *AJR* 1962;88:476–82.

Postnatal Ossification Centers

All values in the tables in this section were derived from a single study population, Ohio-born middle-class long-term participants in the Fels Research Institute studies of development and aging. The data are effectually free from secular trends. All values are based on the proportion of children newly showing the particular center between successive radiographs made at rigid controlled intervals with appropriate correction for the magnitude of the class interval.

TABLE 11. *Age at appearance percentiles for major postnatal ossification centers*

Ossification Center	Percentiles					
	Boys			Girls		
	5th	50th	95th	5th	50th	95th
1. Head of humerus	—	.03	.32	—	.03	.30
2. Proximal epiphysis of tibia	—	.04	.10	—	.01	.04
3. Coracoid process of scapula	—	.04	.36	—	.03	.42
4. Cuboid of tarsus	—	.07	.30	—	.05	.16
5. Capitate of carpus	—	.25	.60	—	.15	.56
6. Hamate of carpus	.03	.31	.82	—	.18	.59
7. Capitulum of humerus	.06	.33	1.07	.05	.26	.77
8. Head of femur	.06	.35	.64	.04	.33	.62
9. Third cuneiform of tarsus	.05	.46	1.58	—	.23	1.23
10. Greater tubercle of humerus	.25	.83	2.33	.20	.51	1.14
11. Primary center, middle segment of 5th toe	—	1.04	3.81	—	.74	2.08
12. Distal epiphysis of radius	.53	1.10	2.30	.38	.82	1.70
13. Epiphysis, distal segment of 1st toe	.71	1.21	2.10	.39	.78	1.68
14. Epiphysis, middle segment of 4th toe	.40	1.21	2.88	.40	.92	3.00
15. Epiphysis, proximal segment of 3d finger	.77	1.37	2.15	.41	.85	1.61
16. Epiphysis, middle segment of 3d toe	.41	1.40	4.27	.21	1.02	2.47
17. Epiphysis, proximal segment of 2d finger	.78	1.41	2.17	.40	.87	1.64
18. Epiphysis, proximal segment of 4th finger	.80	1.49	2.40	.41	.90	1.66
19. Epiphysis, distal segment of 1st finger	.75	1.51	2.70	.42	.99	1.73
20. Epiphysis, proximal segment of 3d toe	.90	1.58	2.52	.51	1.05	1.88
21. Epiphysis of 2d metacarpal	.93	1.61	2.82	.64	1.09	1.69
22. Epiphysis, proximal segment of 4th toe	.95	1.64	2.65	.61	1.24	2.06
23. Epiphysis, proximal segment of 2d toe	.97	1.74	2.65	.63	1.19	2.05
24. Epiphysis of 3d metacarpal	.95	1.79	3.01	.65	1.13	1.94
25. Epiphysis, proximal segment of 5th finger	1.00	1.85	2.82	.65	1.19	2.07
26. Epiphysis, middle segment of 3d finger	1.01	1.97	3.31	.63	1.28	2.36
27. Epiphys. 5th metacarpal	1.09	2.03	3.60	.75	1.29	2.17
28. Epiphysis, middle segment of 2d toe	.89	2.04	4.05	.49	1.18	2.24
29. Epiphysis, middle segment of 4th finger	1.00	2.05	3.24	.63	1.24	2.43
30. Epiphysis of 5th metacarpal	1.27	2.17	3.82	.86	1.37	2.35
31. First cuneiform of tarsus	.89	2.17	3.77	.50	1.43	2.82
32. Epiphysis of 1st metatarsal	1.39	2.18	3.12	.96	1.58	2.23
33. Epiphysis, middle segment of 2d finger	1.30	2.19	3.31	.67	1.36	2.54
34. Epiphysis, proximal segment of 1st toe	1.45	2.35	3.31	.89	1.55	2.47
35. Epiphysis, distal segment of 3d finger	1.31	2.41	3.72	.72	1.46	2.69
36. Triquetral of carpus	.49	2.43	5.47	.29	1.70	3.73
37. Epiphysis, distal segment of 4th finger	1.37	2.44	3.73	.73	1.52	2.82
38. Epiphysis, proximal segment of 5th toe	1.53	2.45	3.65	.97	1.73	2.67
39. Epiphysis of 1st metacarpal	1.45	2.59	4.32	.92	1.60	2.67
40. Second cuneiform of tarsus	1.19	2.65	4.21	.81	1.80	3.00
41. Epiphysis of 2d metatarsal	1.93	2.86	4.33	1.22	2.14	3.43
42. Greater trochanter of femur	1.92	2.96	4.35	.96	1.85	3.03
43. Epiphysis, proximal segment of 1st finger	1.84	3.00	4.57	.93	1.71	2.84
44. Navicular of tarsus	1.12	3.02	5.40	.77	1.94	3.58
45. Epiphysis, distal segment of 2d finger	1.80	3.17	4.97	1.06	2.50	3.29
46. Epiphysis, distal segment of 5th finger	2.06	3.29	4.98	1.01	1.96	3.45
47. Epiphysis, middle segment of 5th finger	1.94	3.40	5.84	.88	1.97	3.54

TABLE 11. *(cont'd.)*

Ossification Center	Boys			Girls		
	5th	50th	95th	5th	50th	95th
48. Proximal epiphysis of fibula	1.86	3.47	5.24	1.33	2.61	3.92
49. Epiphysis of 3d metatarsal	2.33	3.48	5.00	1.42	2.48	3.68
50. Epiphysis, distal segment of 5th toe	2.34	3.94	6.30	1.17	2.31	4.07
51. Patella of knee	2.55	4.00	5.96	1.47	2.48	4.01
52. Epiphysis of 4th metatarsal	2.92	4.02	5.74	1.77	2.84	4.05
53. Lunate of carpus	1.53	4.07	6.77	1.08	2.62	5.65
54. Epiphysis, distal segment of 3d toe	2.99	4.36	6.19	1.37	2.73	4.11
55. Epiphysis of 5th metatarsal	3.12	4.37	6.34	2.08	3.24	4.93
56. Epiphysis, distal segment of 4th toe	2.95	4.38	6.40	1.36	2.58	4.09
57. Epiphysis, distal segment of 2d toe	3.25	4.64	6.75	1.50	2.93	4.50
58. Capitulum of radius	3.00	5.21	7.97	2.26	3.87	6.28
59. Navicular of carpus	3.59	5.63	7.81	2.35	4.12	5.99
60. Greater multangular of carpus	3.53	5.87	8.97	1.94	4.08	6.36
61. Lesser multangular of carpus	3.12	6.22	8.50	2.38	4.17	6.01
62. Medial epicondyle of humerus	4.27	6.25	8.41	2.05	3.40	5.07
63. Distal epiphysis of ulna	5.25	7.10	9.07	3.29	5.37	7.63
64. Epiphysis of calcaneus	5.17	7.59	9.55	3.54	5.37	7.30
65. Olecranon of ulna	7.78	9.67	11.90	5.62	8.01	9.93
66. Lateral epicondyle of humerus	9.23	11.24	13.70	7.14	9.24	11.28
67. Tubercle of tibia	9.92	11.81	13.38	7.89	10.25	11.82
68. Adductor sesamoid of 1st finger	11.03	12.76	14.62	8.67	10.72	12.68
69. Os acetabulum of hip	11.90	13.54	15.32	9.60	11.47	13.39
70. Acromion of clavicle	12.15	13.74	15.48	10.32	11.92	13.79
71. Epiphysis, iliac crest of hip	12.03	14.03	15.91	10.81	12.79	15.31
72. Accessory epiphysis, coracoid process of scapula	12.74	14.35	16.31	10.37	12.21	14.37
73. Ischial tuberosity of hip	13.57	15.26	17.08	11.71	13.89	16.00

Source: Garn S. Radiographic standards for postnatal ossification and tooth calcification. *Med Radiogr Photogr* 1961;43:50.

When determining the correlations from which the utility rankings of the various centers were calculated, skewness was first eliminated by use of a specially written computer program. After correlating the age at appearance of every center with each of the other centers, the mean correlation coefficient for correlations involving each center in turn was used to ascertain the utility ranking.

TABLE 12. *Relative value of 73 postnatal ossification centers in skeletal assessment*

Ossification Center	Predictive Ranking		Communality	
	Boys	Girls	Boys	Girls
Epiphysis, distal segment of 5th finger	1	34	.463	.399
Epiphysis, distal segment of 4th toe	2	30	.463	.407
Epiphysis, distal segment of 4th finger	3	18	.452	.438
Epiphysis, proximal segment of 5th toe	4	23	.451	.424
Epiphysis of 3d metatarsal	5	12	.450	.459
Epiphysis, distal segment of 3d finger	6	16	.448	.440
Epiphysis of 3d metacarpal	7	3	.448	.478
Epiphysis of 5th metatarsal	8	26	.434	.419
Epiphysis, middle segment of 4th finger	9	39	.431	.388
Epiphysis, distal segment of 2d finger	10	20	.430	.433
Epiphysis of 4th metacarpal	11	5	.427	.474
Epiphysis, proximal segment of 4th toe	12	14	.424	.449
Epiphysis of 5th metacarpal	13	4	.424	.475
Epiphysis of 4th metatarsal	14	15	.424	.448
Epiphysis of 2d metacarpal	15	10	.413	.468
Epiphysis, distal segment of 3d toe	16	45	.405	.357
Epiphysis, proximal segment of 5th finger	17	7	.403	.472
Epiphysis, middle segment of 3d finger	18	33	.397	.401
Patella of knee	19	1	.397	.498
Epiphysis of 2d metatarsal	20	9	.396	.469
Epiphysis, distal segment of 1st finger	21	17	.394	.439
Epiphysis, distal segment of 2d toe	22	28	.390	.413
Epiphysis, middle segment of 2d finger	23	21	.389	.431
Epiphysis of 1st metatarsal	24	25	.387	.421
Navicular of tarsus	25	43	.378	.365
Second cuneiform of tarsus	26	22	.372	.427
Epiphysis, middle segment of 5th finger	27	40	.367	.381
Epiphysis of 1st metacarpal	28	13	.366	.455
Olecranon of ulna	29	31	.365	.406
Capitulum of radius	30	51	.365	.337
Epiphysis, distal segment of 1st toe	31	2	.359	.496
Epiphysis, proximal segment of 1st finger	32	42	.355	.378
Epiphysis of calcaneus	33	38	.345	.389
Epiphysis, proximal segment of 1st toe	34	32	.344	.403
Epiphysis, proximal segment of 4th finger	35	11	.339	.468
Lesser multangular of carpus	36	36	.338	.393
Medial epicondyle of humerus	37	50	.336	.349
Epiphysis, proximal segment of 3d finger	38	6	.335	.473
Epiphysis, proximal segment of 2d toe	39	19	.334	.435
Epiphysis, distal segment of 5th toe	40	47	.333	.351
Greater trochanter of femur	41	56	.327	.273
Greater multangular of carpus	42	24	.323	.422
Epiphysis, proximal segment of 2d finger	43	8	.321	.470
Epiphysis, proximal segment of 3d toe	44	27	.319	.415
Distal epiphysis of ulna	45	44	.316	.364
Epiphysis, iliac crest of hip	46	48	.310	.349
Tubercle of tibia	47	29	.304	.411
Os acetabulum of hip	48	53	.301	.311
Triquetral of carpus	49	55	.301	.283
Proximal epiphysis of fibula	50	41	.295	.380
Accessory epiphysis, coracoid process of scapula	51	64	.291	.203
First cuneiform of tarsus	52	46	.278	.355
Navicular of carpus	53	35	.269	.399
Primary center, middle segment of 5th toe	54	71	.269	.028
Adductor sesamoid of 1st finger	55	52	.268	.333

TABLE 12. *(cont'd.)*

Ossification Center	Predictive Ranking		Communality	
	Boys	Girls	Boys	Girls
Capitulum of humerus	56	58	.266	.270
Acromion of clavicle	57	61	.259	.228
Lateral epicondyle of humerus	58	54	.257	.295
Greater tubercle of humerus	59	59	.254	.263
Ischial tuberosity of hip	60	57	.239	.271
Distal epiphysis of radius	61	49	.235	.349
Head of humerus	62	68	.226	.150
Head of femur	63	65	.218	.179
Hamate of carpus	64	66	.199	.159
Lunate of carpus	65	60	.195	.230
Epiphysis, middle segment of 2d toe	66	37	.190	.392
Capitate of carpus	67	67	.171	.155
Epiphysis, middle segment of 3d toe	68	62	.146	.223
Epiphysis, middle segment of 4th toe	69	63	.140	.221
Cuboid of tarsus	70	69	.099	.131
Third cuneiform of tarsus	71	70	.059	.096
Coracoid process of scapula	72	73	.035	−.199
Proximal epiphysis of tibia	73	72	.030	−.106

Source: Garn S. Radiographic standards for postnatal ossification and tooth calcification. *Med Radiogr Photogr* 1961;43:50.

TABLE 13. *Sex differences in ossification timing*

Ossification Center	Sex Difference (years)	Conception-Corrected Sex Difference° (percent)	Ossification Center	Sex Difference (years)	Conception-Corrected Sex Difference° (percent)
1. Head of humerus	.00	0	35. Epiphysis, distal segment of 3d finger	.95	43
2. Proximal epiphysis of tibia	.03	4	36. Triquetral of carpus	.73	30
3. Coracoid process of scapula	.01	1	37. Epiphysis, distal segment of 4th finger	.92	40
4. Cuboid of tarsus	.02	3	38. Epiphysis, proximal segment of 5th toe	.72	29
5. Capitate of carpus	.10	11	39. Epiphysis of 1st metacarpal	.99	42
6. Hamate of carpus	.13	15	40. Second cuneiform of tarsus	.85	33
7. Capitulum of humerus	.07	7	41. Epiphysis of 2d metatarsal	.72	25
8. Head of femur	.02	2	42. Greater trochanter of femur	1.11	43
9. Third cuneiform of tarsus	.23	23	43. Epiphysis, proximal segment of 1st finger	1.29	52
10. Greater tubercle of humerus	.32	25	44. Navicular of tarsus	1.08	40
11. Primary center, middle segment of 5th toe	.30	20	45. Epiphysis, distal segment of 2d finger	.67	21
12. Distal epiphysis of radius	.28	17	46. Epiphysis, distal segment of 5th finger	1.33	49
13. Epiphysis, distal segment of 1st toe	.43	28	47. Epiphysis, middle segment of 5th finger	1.43	53
14. Epiphysis, middle segment of 4th toe	.29	17	48. Proximal epiphysis of fibula	.86	26
15. Epiphysis, proximal segment of 3d finger	.52	33	49. Epiphysis of 3d metatarsal	1.00	31
16. Epiphysis, middle segment of 3d toe	.38	21	50. Epiphysis, distal segment of 5th toe	1.63	53
17. Epiphysis, proximal segment of 2d finger	.54	33	51. Patella of knee	1.52	47
18. Epiphysis, proximal segment of 4th finger	.59	36	52. Epiphysis of 4th metatarsal	1.18	33
19. Epiphysis, distal segment of 1st finger	.52	30	53. Lunate of carpus	1.45	43
20. Epiphysis, proximal segment of 3d toe	.53	29	54. Epiphysis, distal segment of 3d toe	1.63	47
21. Epiphysis of 2d metacarpal	.52	28	55. Epiphysis of 5th metatarsal	1.13	28
22. Epiphysis, proximal segment of 4th toe	.40	20	56. Epiphysis, distal segment of 4th toe	1.80	54
23. Epiphysis, proximal segment of 2d toe	.55	28	57. Epiphysis, distal segment of 2d toe	1.71	46
24. Epiphysis of 3d metacarpal	.66	35	58. Capitulum of radius	1.34	29
25. Epiphysis, proximal segment of 5th finger	.66	34	59. Navicular of carpus	1.51	31
26. Epiphysis, middle segment of 3d finger	.69	34	60. Greater multangular of carpus	1.79	37
27. Epiphysis of 4th metacarpal	.74	36	61. Lesser multangular of carpus	2.05	42
28. Epiphysis, middle segment of 2d toe	.86	44	62. Medial epicondyle of humerus	2.85†	69†
29. Epiphysis, middle segment of 4th finger	.81	41	63. Distal epiphysis of ulna	1.73	28
30. Epiphysis of 5th metacarpal	.80	38	64. Epiphysis of calcaneus	2.22	36
31. First cuneiform of tarsus	.74	34	65. Olecranon of ulna	1.66	19
32. Epiphysis of 1st metatarsal	.60	26	66. Lateral epicondyle of humerus	2.00	20
33. Epiphysis, middle segment of 2d finger	.83	39	67. Tubercle of tibia	1.56	14
34. Epiphysis, proximal segment of 1st toe	.80	35	68. Adductor sesamoid of 1st finger	2.04	18
			69. Os acetabulum of hip	2.07	17
			70. Acromion of clavicle	1.82	14
			71. Epiphysis, iliac crest of hip	1.24	9
			72. Accessory epiphysis, coracoid process of scapula	2.14	16
			73. Ischial tuberosity of hip	1.37	9

*Percent sex difference $= \dfrac{\text{conception} - \text{corrected male median}}{\text{conception} - \text{corrected female median}} - 1.00.$

Source: Garn S. Radiographic standards for postnatal ossification and tooth calcification. *Med Radiogr Photogr* 1961;43:50.

Ossification Centers of Greatest Predictive Value

The postnatal ossification centers that have the highest statistical "communality" and hence the greatest predictive value of skeletal assessment are located in the hand, foot, and knee.

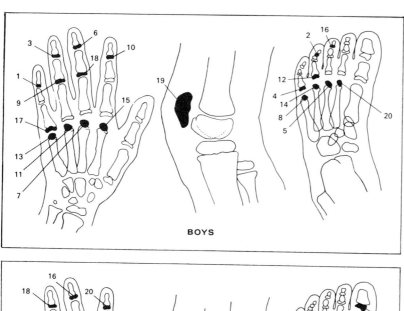

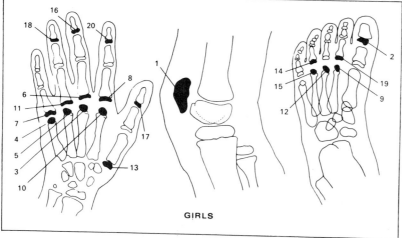

FIG. 11. The 20 ossification centers of greatest predicted value in boys and girls and their communalities.

Source: Garn S. Radiographic standards for postnatal ossification and tooth calcification. *Med Radiogr Photogr* 1961;43:58.

TABLE 14. *The 20 ossification centers and their communalities*

Boys		Girls	
Ossification Center	Internal Communality° (intra se)	Ossification Center	Internal Communality* (intra se)
Distal V, hand	0.637	Patella, knee	0.625
Distal IV, foot	0.650	Distal I, foot	0.663
Distal IV, hand	0.660	Metacarpal III, hand	0.696
Proximal V, foot	0.586	Metacarpal V, hand	0.652
Metatarsal III, foot	0.623	Metacarpal IV, hand	0.653
Distal III, hand	0.650	Proximal III, hand	0.685
Metacarpal III, hand	0.621	Proximal V, hand	0.668
Metatarsal V, foot	0.589	Proximal II, hand	0.689
Middle IV, hand	0.607	Metatarsal II, foot	0.636
Distal II, hand	0.602	Metacarpal II, hand	0.641
Metacarpal IV, hand	0.598	Proximal IV, hand	0.696
Proximal IV, foot	0.550	Metatarsal III, foot	0.616
Metacarpal V, hand	0.601	Metacarpal I, hand	0.596
Metatarsal IV, foot	0.592	Proximal IV, foot	0.623
Metacarpal II, hand	0.570	Metatarsal IV, foot	0.615
Distal III, foot	0.587	Distal III, hand	0.659
Proximal V, hand	0.551	Distal I, hand	0.619
Middle III, hand	0.583	Distal IV, hand	0.636
Patella, knee	0.477	Proximal II, foot	0.589
Metatarsal II, foot	0.542	Distal II, hand	0.620
Mean internal communality	0.595	Mean internal communality	0.645

°The term "internal communality" is defined as the mean of correlations involving a given center or a group of centers with the other centers in a given group. (Compare with Table 5, pages 56 and 57.)

Related articles:

1. Elgemmarck O. Normal development of ossific centers during infancy and childhood: clinical, roentgenographic and statistical study. *Acta Pediatr* (Suppl), 1946;133:1–79.

2. Flecker H. Time of appearance and fusion of ossification centers as observed by roentgenographic methods. *AJR* 1942;156:97–159.

3. Pyle I, Sontag LW. Variability in onset of ossification and epiphyses in short bones of the extremities. *AJR* 1943;49:759–798.

Source: Garn S. Radiographic standards for postnatal ossification and tooth calcification. *Med Radiogr Photogr* 1961;43:58.

Black/White Differences in Ossification Timing

This investigation is based on the age at which 25 postnatal ossification centers of the hand and wrist appear as seen in the radiographs of 4,988 participants in the multistate nutritional study of 1968 to 1970.

Ossification in children of largely African ancestry occurs at an earlier mean age than in boys and girls of European ancestral origin, excluding the capitate, hamate, and distal epiphysis of the radius, for which comparative data were too meager. This generalization holds for both sexes with only one exception out of 50 race-sex comparisons.

TABLE 15.

Ossification center	Male						Female					
	Black		White		Difference		Black		White		Difference	
	Num-ber	Mean age	Num-ber	Mean age	% Dif-ference	Z-score difference	Num-ber	Mean age	Num-ber	Mean age	% Dif-ference	Z-score difference
Proximal 3	62	1.15	293	1.33	+ 9	+0.52	27	0.72	91	0.94	+13	+0.69
Proximal 2	56	1.28	293	1.42	+ 6	+0.35	27	0.75	91	0.91	+10	+0.49
Proximal 4	88	1.22	293	1.51	+13	+0.71	27	0.79	91	0.96	+10	+0.55
Distal 1	202	1.26	565	1.55	+13	+0.62	27	0.72	135	1.05	+18	+1.00
Metacarpal 2	62	1.29	293	1.57	+12	+0.55	27	0.88	91	1.05	+ 9	+0.61
Metacarpal 3	94	1.37	475	1.67	+12	+0.53	27	0.86	91	1.05	+11	+0.68
Proximal 5	88	1.72	475	1.73	0	+0.02	27	0.92	91	1.17	+13	+0.84
Metacarpal 4	94	1.53	475	1.82	+11	+0.52	49	1.05	91	1.16	+ 6	+0.44
Middle 3	88	1.65	445	1.85	+ 8	+0.42	68	0.94	234	1.19	+13	+0.59
Middle 4	88	1.65	445	1.88	+ 9	+0.46	68	0.95	135	1.18	+12	+0.61
Middle 2	117	1.93	445	1.96	+ 1	+0.06	87	0.99	234	1.22	+12	+0.50
Metacarpal 5	159	1.69	565	2.08	+14	+0.55	68	1.05	234	1.19	+ 7	+0.54
Distal 3	159	1.99	445	2.11	+ 4	+0.21	68	0.99	234	1.40	+19	+0.84
Distal 4	153	2.03	445	2.12	+ 3	+0.15	68	1.14	234	1.43	+13	+0.58
Metacarpal 1	444	2.67	748	2.56	− 3	−0.12	68	1.22	392	1.33	+ 5	+0.27
Triquetral	673	2.33	1409	2.70	+11	+0.22	262	1.36	576	1.71	+14	+0.31
Proximal 1	235	2.50	646	2.74	+ 7	+0.26	68	1.18	316	1.69	+21	+0.85
Distal 2	257	2.46	748	2.97	+14	+0.59	87	1.34	384	1.86	+20	+0.83
Distal 5	187	2.49	866	3.01	+14	+0.60	87	1.35	384	1.85	+19	+0.85
Middle 5	352	2.90	866	3.01	+ 3	+0.10	87	1.22	384	1.74	+21	+0.89
Lunate	944	3.66	1379	4.01	+ 7	+0.21	934	2.46	994	2.99	+14	+0.42
Scaphoid	754	5.48	1872	6.07	+ 9	+0.42	913	3.92	942	4.38	+ 9	+0.41
Trapezoid	682	5.68	1450	6.16	+ 7	+0.41	742	4.14	911	4.40	+ 5	+0.23
Trapezium	942	5.83	1872	6.22	+ 6	+0.25	742	4.16	1174	4.24	+ 2	+0.06
Distal ulna	1008	6.72	1630	7.21	+ 6	+0.39	907	5.59	1143	5.79	+ 3	+0.17
Mean per cent difference					+ 7.8						+12.0	
Mean Z-score difference						+0.36						+0.57

Percent differences are conception-corrected using the mean + 0.75 years.

Z-score differences are expressed in standard deviation units, e.g., absolute differences divided by the standard deviation for the center in question.

Source: Garn SM, Sandusky ST, Nagy JM, McCann MB. Advanced skeletal development in low-income Negro children. *J Pediatr* 1972;80:965–9.

Status of Skeletal Maturity Based on Roentgenographic Assessment of the Pelvis and Hips

Standards presented here are the result of approximately 14,500 assessments of 8,500 serial roentgenograms of healthy American and British children. The roentgenograms were collected and the studies run by the Brush Foundation at Western Reserve University, Cleveland, Ohio, and the Institute of Social Medicine, Oxford, England. The method was also checked against roentgenograms available in the longitudinal studies of child health and development at the Harvard School of Public Health. A point is assigned for each maturity indicator, and a total maturity score is developed. The total score can be plotted on a chart (Fig. 14), thereby enabling the rate of maturation of the child to be compared with a standard.

Related Publications:
1. Buehl CC, Pyle SI. Use of age at first appearance of three ossification centers in determining the skeletal status in children. *J Pediatr* 1942;21:335–341.
2. Englemarck O. Normal development of the ossific centers during infancy and childhood. Clinical and roentgenographic and statistical study. *ACTA Pediatr Scand* 1946;33:1–79.
3. Francis CC, Werle PP. The appearance of centers of ossification from birth to 5 years. *Am J Phys Anthropol* 1939;24:273–299.
4. Garn SM, Silverman SN, Rohmann CG. A rational approach to the assessment of skeletal maturation. *Ann Radiol* 1964;7:297–307.
5. Graham CB. Assessment of bone maturation. Methods and pitfalls. *Radiol Clin North Am* 1972;10:185–202.
6. Harding CS. A method of evaluating osseous development from birth to fourteen years. *Child Devel* 1952;23:249–271.
7. Johnson GF, Dorst JP, Kuhn JP. Roche AF, Davila GH. Reliability of skeletal age assessements. *AJR* 1973;118:320–327.
8. Roche AF, Wainer H, Thissen D. *Skeletal Maturity of the Knee Joint as a Biological Indicator*. New York, Plenum, 1975.
9. Sontag LW, Reynolds EL. The Fels composite sheet. 1. A practical method for analyzing growth progress. *J Pediatr* 1945;26:327–352.
10. Sontag LW, Snell D, Anderson M. Rate of appearance of ossification centers from birth to the age of five years. *Am J Dis Child* 1939;58:949–56.
11. Tanner JM, Whitehouse RH, Marshall WA, Healy MJR, Goldstein H. *Assessment of Skeletal Maturity and Prediction of Adult Height (TW-2 Method)*. London, Academic Press, 1975.

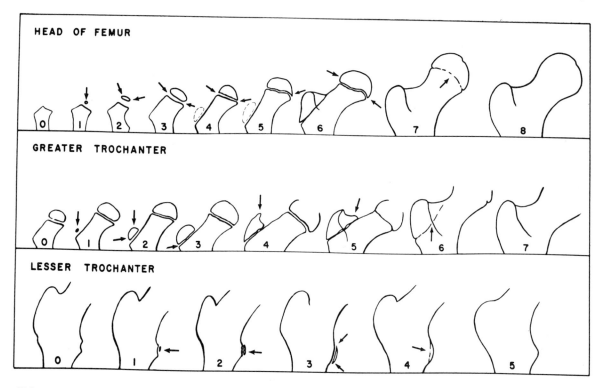

FIG. 12. Maturity indicators at the proximal end of the femur. First horizontal line is the head of the femur. Second horizontal line is the greater trochanter. Third horizontal line is the lesser trochanter. The original text should be consulted for more detailed discussion.

Source: Acheson RM. The Oxford method of assessing skeletal maturity. *Clin Orthop* 1957;10:19–39.

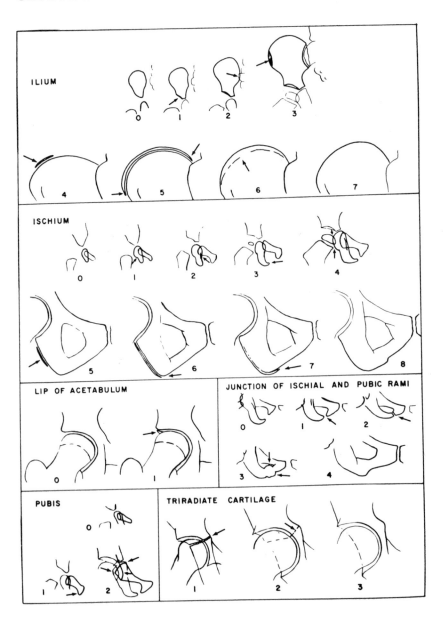

FIG. 13. Maturity indicators in the innominate bone. Original text should be consulted for more detailed explanation.

Source: Acheson RM. The Oxford method of assessing skeletal maturity. *Clin Orthop* 1957;10:19–39.

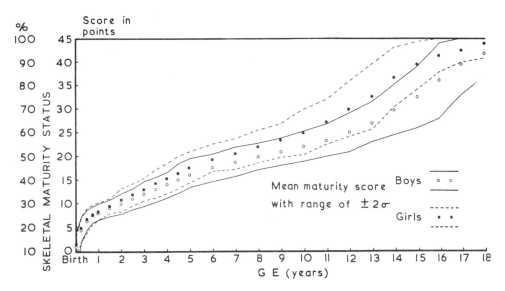

FIG. 14. Mean maturity scores of hip and pelvis of over 500 boys and girls together with the range of ±2 SD. The percentage scale has been made by taking the mature individual of 45 points as being at the 100% level and arbitrarily assuming that 0 on the point scale is at the 10% level (i.e., approximately 10% of skeletal maturation occurs in utero).

TABLE 16. *Maturity scores for hip joint and pelvis for over 500 American and British children*

AGE	BOYS Total	Maturity Score in Points Mean	S.D.	GIRLS Total	Maturity Score in Points Mean	S.D.
¼	65	4.3	1.1	40	4.6	1.3
½	134	6.5	1.0	89	6.6	1.2
¾	78	7.5	0.9	58	7.6	0.9
1	138	8.2	0.9	94	8.4	0.9
1½	128	9.2	0.9	108	9.4	0.8
2	133	10.0	1.0	108	10.7	1.2
2½	138	11.0	1.2	112	11.9	1.1
3	141	12.0	1.3	114	12.9	1.3
3½	149	12.9	1.3	115	14.1	1.5
4	161	14.0	1.4	111	15.2	1.6
4½	152	15.0	1.5	116	16.4	1.7
5	157	16.1	1.4	113	17.5	1.6
6	169	17.5	1.5	101	19.1	1.7
7	164	18.7	1.5	101	20.4	1.6
8	164	19.8	1.4	101	21.9	1.7
9	147	20.9	1.4	109	23.4	1.8
10	145	22.0	1.6	126	25.0	2.4
11	116	23.3	1.7	125	27.2	2.4
12	114	25.0	2.1	124	29.9	2.9
13	102	26.8	2.4	96	32.6	3.3
14	86	29.7	2.6	86	36.7	3.2
15	72	32.6	3.3	73	38.3	2.6
16	60	36.1	4.0	65	41.4	1.7
17	41	39.5	3.2	43	42.5	1.4
18	31	41.8	2.1	20	43.6	1.4

Data used to construct the graph in Fig. 14.

Source: Acheson RM. The Oxford method of assessing skeletal maturity. *Clin Orthop* 1957;10:19–39.

TABLE 17. *Head of femur. Children in each of eight developmental stages in various age groups*

	STAGES															
	1		2		3		4		5		6		7		8	
AGE	M	F	M	F	M	F	M	F	M	F	M	F	M	F	M	F
¼	7	38														
½	80	87	10	34												
¾	99	99	62	79												
1	100	99	84	93		4										
1½		100	99	97	7	23										
2			100	100	20	60										
2½					53	87	1	1								
3					89	96	3	11								
3½					98	100	5	28								
4					100		22	56								
4½							49	85		3						
5							76	98	1	9						
6							90	100	6	28						
7							100		28	60		1				
8									54	87		4				
9									86	97	3	19				
10									95	99	13	45				
11									98	100	33	68				
12									99		54	89		9		
13									100		78	99		37		10
14											96	100	4	74		39
15											97		34	89		74
16											100		72	96	28	86
17													88	100	50	88
18													95		66	95

TABLE 18. *Greater trochanter. Children in each of seven developmental stages at various ages*

	STAGES													
	1		2		3		4		5		6		7	
AGE	M	F	M	F	M	F	M	F	M	F	M	F	M	F
¼														
½														
¾														
1														
1½														
2		12												
2½	6	61												
3	27	88		4										
3½	48	97		15		1								
4	66	99	1	49		13								
4½	82	100	8	74		23								
5	97		23	94		60								
6	100		61	99	3	84		5						
7			85	100	7	97		16						
8			99		34	99	2	32						
9			100		70	100	12	69		7				
10					92		31	89		30				
11					100		64	98	8	58				
12							88	99	21	85		19		
13							96	100	50	100		41		12
14							100		90		9	87		34
15									98		30	98	2	72
16									99		70	100	20	91
17									100		88		36	100
18											95		76	

Source: Acheson RM. The Oxford method of assessing skeletal maturity. *Clin Orthop* 1957;10:19–39.

TABLE 19. *Lesser trochanter. Children in each of five developmental stages at various ages*

Age	1 M	1 F	2 M	2 F	3 M	3 F	4 M	4 F	5 M	5 F
¼										
½										
¾										
1										
1½										
2										
2½										
3										
3½										
4										
4½										
5										
6		3								
7		18		2						
8	1	35		15		1				
9	6	64	1	34		7				
10	22	84	7	59	1	28				
11	63	98	11	80	8	56		5		
12	78	100	61	97	20	80		16		4
13	97		75	100	63	97		44		13
14	100		98		78	100	14	78		42
15			100		97		53	94	4	67
16					100		79	99	32	90
17							92	100	51	98
18							100		71	100

TABLE 20. *Lip of acetabulum, junction of ischial and pubic rami, triradiate cartilage: developmental stages and ages indicated*

Age	Lip of Acetabulum M	Lip of Acetabulum F	Junction 1 M	Junction 1 F	Junction 2 M	Junction 2 F	Junction 3 M	Junction 3 F	Junction 4 M	Junction 4 F	Triradiate 1 M	Triradiate 1 F	Triradiate 2 M	Triradiate 2 F	Triradiate 3 M	Triradiate 3 F
¼																
½																
¾				1												
1			1	4												
1½			9	11												
2			21	23	1	2										
2½			35	36	6	4	1									
3			49	57	11	8	3	1								
3½			67	69	21	19	4	5	1							
4			78	74	31	28	7	11	2	1	1	3				
4½			89	82	51	40	15	17	2	4	6	12				
5			93	88	67	54	24	27	3	5	12	28				
6			95	90	83	71	50	47	11	11	21	40				
7			97	93	93	82	69	62	20	17	47	58				
8			98	96	95	86	84	76	34	30	69	76		1		
9			100	97	98	88	92	84	52	46	79	91		5		
10	4	7		100	99	95	95	88	65	64	92	96		20		
11	6	32			100	98	98	91	80	74	97	97	2	52		1
12	13	73				100	100	96	89	86	98	100	20	84		21
13	30	93						99	90	94	100		46	98		52
14	70	100						100	95	98			81	100	12	90
15	89								99	100			96		42	98
16	98								100				100		82	100
17	99														93	
18	100														98	

Source: Acheson RM. The Oxford method of assessing skeletal maturity. *Clin Orthop* 1957;10:19–39.

Skeletal Maturity Based on Hand-Wrist Observations

Data for skeletal maturity of the right hand-wrist in noninstitutionalized youths, aged 12 to 17 years analyzed and described by race, geographic region, size and type of community, family income, and parental education. The original data were obtained from radiographs taken during the health examination survey of 1966–1970. For this survey, a representative sample of 7,514 youths was chosen from the entire U.S. population. Ninety percent of the youths who had been chosen underwent examinations. The text of the report contains numerous charts and graphs covering this material. Only the most general charts have been reproduced here. The reader is advised to consult the original text for more detailed evaluation.

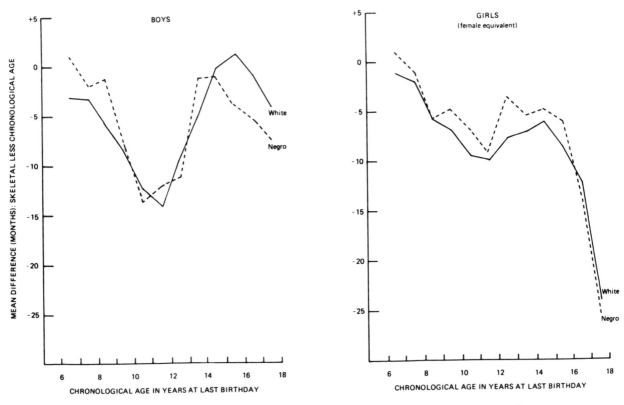

FIG. 15. Mean difference between skeletal age (hand-wrist) and chronological age for white and black boys and girls aged 6 to 17 years by chronological age in years in the United States, 1963–70.

Source: Roche AF. Skeletal maturity of youths 12–17 years, racial, geographic area, and socioeconomic differentials: U.S.—1966–70. Washington, D.C.: Government Printing Office; DHEW publ. no. (PHS)79-1654.

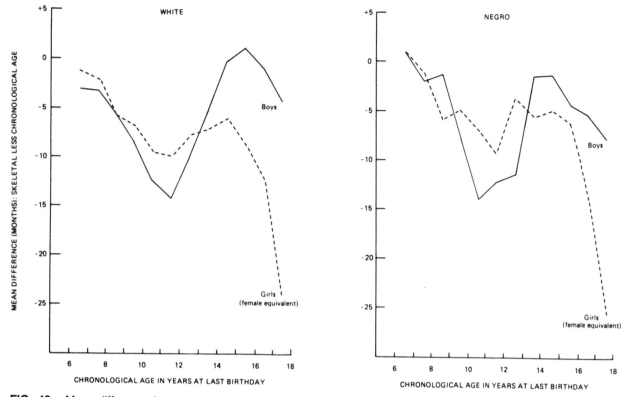

FIG. 16. Mean difference between skeletal age (hand-wrist) and chronological age for white and black boys and girls aged 6 to 17 years by chronological age in years in the United States, 1963–70.

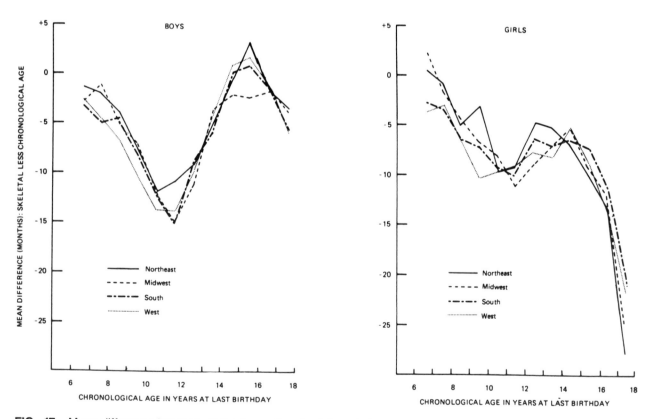

FIG. 17. Mean difference between skeletal age (hand-wrist) and chronological age for boys and girls aged 6 to 17 years by region and chronological age in years in the United States, 1963–70.

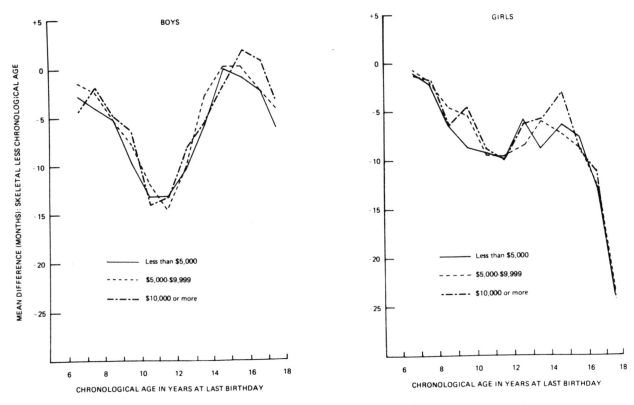

FIG. 18. Mean difference between skeletal age (hand-wrist) and chronological age for boys and girls aged 6 to 17 years by annual family income and chronological age in years in the United States, 1963–70.

TABLE 21. *Skeletal age (hand-wrist) of youths by race, chronological age at last birthday, and sex in the United States, 1966–70*

Standard of reference, sex, and chronological age at last birthday	White			Negro			Other races	
	$\bar{x}$	s_x	$s_{\bar{x}}$	$\bar{x}$	s_x	$s_{\bar{x}}$	$\bar{x}$	$s_{\bar{x}}$
Male standard				Skeletal age in months				
Boys:								
12 years	140.4	17.17	0.62	138.7	16.04	2.84	149.3	105.58
13 years	156.8	17.77	0.93	160.6	19.69	3.10	164.5	52.37
14 years	173.7	14.84	0.74	172.7	17.04	2.03	170.7	54.06
15 years	187.1	13.91	0.73	181.7	15.91	1.09	197.3	5.02
16 years	197.0	13.12	0.78	192.7	16.93	2.93	188.9	74.35
17 years	205.8	10.97	0.52	202.4	11.37	1.65	209.1	1.05
Girls:								
12 years	174.3	14.36	0.71	178.4	16.72	2.40	184.5	9.43
13 years	186.5	13.12	0.72	187.5	12.10	1.09	187.2	132.41
14 years	197.9	10.46	0.63	198.7	12.82	1.70	198.8	140.57
15 years	205.3	9.28	0.57	207.6	8.35	0.81	204.6	64.71
16 years	211.5	10.00	0.52	210.2	9.36	0.96	206.6	146.06
17 years	211.7	9.82	0.64	210.5	10.34	2.14	220.0	155.56
Actual Values:								
Boys 12-17 years	175.2	· · ·	0.40	172.6	· · ·	1.17	182.7	6.32
Girls 12-17 years	196.5	· · ·	0.38	197.1	· · ·	0.85	198.4	3.80
Expected values:								
Boys 12-17 years	175.0	· · ·	0.40	174.2	· · ·	1.18	179.2	6.29
Girls 12-17 years	196.7	· · ·	0.38	196.1	· · ·	0.84	196.0	3.78
Female equivalent								
Girls:								
12 years	142.3	11.72	0.58	146.4	13.72	1.97	152.5	7.79
13 years	154.8	10.89	0.60	156.5	10.10	0.91	156.2	110.50
14 years	167.9	8.87	0.53	169.1	10.91	1.45	168.3	119.00
15 years	177.3	8.01	0.49	179.9	7.24	0.70	175.9	55.63
16 years	185.8	8.78	0.46	184.2	8.20	0.84	178.6	126.26
17 years	186.0	8.63	0.56	184.5	9.06	1.88	197.0	139.30

NOTE: $\bar{x}$ = mean skeletal age (hand-wrist); s_x = standard deviation of skeletal age; and $s_{\bar{x}}$ = standard error of mean. Expected values remove the effect of differences in the chronological age distribution with respect to skeletal age over the 12-17-year age span by indirect adjustment.

Data used for Figs. 15 and 16.

TABLE 22. *Skeletal age (hand-wrist) of youths by geographic region, chronological age at last birthday, and sex in the United States, 1966–70.*

Standard of reference, sex, and chronological age at last birthday	Northeast			Midwest			South			West		
	$\bar{x}$	s_x	$s_{\bar{x}}$	$\bar{x}$	s_x	$s_{\bar{x}}$	$\bar{x}$	s_x	$s_{\bar{x}}$	$\bar{x}$	s_x	$s_{\bar{x}}$
Male standard	Skeletal age in months											
Boys:												
12 years	141.0	16.93	1.14	139.0	17.59	1.28	141.1	16.03	1.62	140.2	17.20	1.38
13 years	157.6	20.02	2.60	157.9	17.45	1.62	156.1	18.34	1.32	157.8	16.32	1.16
14 years	173.6	15.00	1.02	172.0	14.91	1.61	174.2	15.80	1.87	174.7	14.66	1.16
15 years	189.1	13.82	1.45	183.6	14.48	1.14	186.7	14.88	1.02	187.6	13.20	1.41
16 years	196.2	13.25	1.33	196.2	13.26	1.52	196.6	14.28	1.04	196.4	14.37	1.36
17 years	206.6	10.35	1.42	206.3	9.66	0.53	204.4	11.65	0.72	204.3	11.95	1.40
Girls:												
12 years	177.4	14.13	1.46	173.3	14.85	1.38	175.7	14.30	1.35	173.9	15.58	2.39
13 years	187.9	13.02	0.95	186.7	13.19	1.78	186.7	12.87	1.03	185.4	12.64	0.87
14 years	197.3	10.78	1.23	198.5	11.42	1.34	197.6	11.16	0.81	198.5	9.69	1.47
15 years	204.8	9.25	0.82	205.2	9.37	1.56	206.9	9.46	0.74	205.4	8.45	1.02
16 years	210.8	8.66	0.94	211.8	9.80	0.97	212.0	11.95	1.22	210.5	9.17	1.15
17 years	209.2	10.06	1.27	211.1	9.85	1.66	213.0	9.22	1.40	212.9	9.32	1.20
Actual values:												
Boys 12-17 years	174.7	- - -	0.84	174.0	- - -	0.69	175.9	- - -	0.91	175.3	- - -	0.83
Girls 12-17 years	196.4	- - -	0.72	196.0	- - -	0.66	197.5	- - -	0.96	196.6	- - -	0.86
Expected values:												
Boys 12-17 years	173.9	- - -	0.83	174.9	- - -	0.70	175.9	- - -	0.91	175.0	- - -	0.83
Girls 12-17 years	196.4	- - -	0.72	196.3	- - -	0.67	196.9	- - -	0.95	196.9	- - -	0.87
Female equivalent												
Girls:												
12 years	145.4	11.58	1.20	141.3	12.11	1.13	143.7	11.70	1.10	141.9	12.71	1.95
13 years	156.9	10.87	0.79	155.0	10.95	1.48	155.0	10.68	0.86	153.4	10.46	0.72
14 years	167.3	9.14	1.04	168.8	9.71	1.14	167.6	9.47	0.69	168.8	8.24	1.25
15 years	176.2	7.96	0.71	177.2	8.09	1.35	178.9	8.18	0.64	177.4	7.30	0.88
16 years	184.8	7.59	0.82	186.2	8.62	0.85	187.0	10.54	1.08	184.5	8.04	1.01
17 years	182.3	8.77	1.11	185.2	8.64	1.46	189.0	8.18	1.24	188.4	8.25	1.06

NOTE: $\bar{x}$ = mean skeletal age (hand-wrist); s_x = standard deviation of skeletal age; and $s_{\bar{x}}$ = standard error of mean. Expected values remove the effect of differences in the chronological age distribution with respect to skeletal age over the 12-17-year age span by indirect adjustment.

Data used for Fig. 17.

Source: Roche AF. Skeletal maturity of youths 12–17 years, racial, geographic area, and socioeconomic differentials: U.S.—1966–70. Washington, D.C.: Government Printing Office; DHEW publ. no. (PHS)79-1654.

Sexual Maturity: Genital Development in Boys

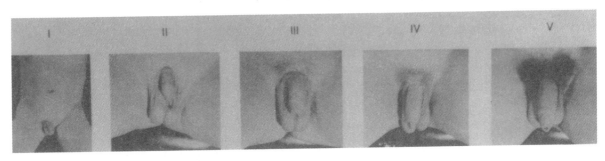

FIG. 19. Sexual maturity stages in boys shown by genital development as reported originally by Greulich et al. Somatic and Endocrine Studies of Pubertal and Adolescent Boys, 1942 (Monographs of the Society for Research in Child Development, Vol. VII, Ser. 33, No. 3). I. Penis, testes, and scrotum are essentially the same as in early childhood. II. Testes and penis have noticeably enlarged; lightly pigmented, downy hair has appeared. III. The penis has appreciably lengthened; downy hair is interspersed with straight, coarse, pigmented hair. IV. Larger testes and penis of increased diameter are apparent. Pubic hair looks adult, but its area is smaller. V. Genitalia are adult in size and shape; pubic hair is adult.

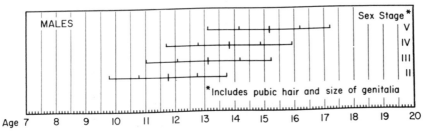

FIG. 20. Maturity indices for boys showing the normal range of occurrence of sex stages. I. Penis, testes, and scrotum are essentially the same as in early childhood. II. Testes and penis have noticeably enlarged; lightly pigmented, downy hair has appeared (mean ± SD:11.8 ± 1 year). III. The penis has appreciably lengthened; downy hair is interspersed with straight, coarse, pigmented hair (13.1 ± 1 year). IV. Larger testes and penis of increased diameter are apparent. Pubic hair looks adult, but its area is smaller (13.8 ± 1 year). V. Genitalia are adult in size and shape; pubic hair is adult.

Source: Bayer LM, Bayley N. Selected method for interpreting and predicting physical development from one year to maturity. In: *Growth diagnosis*. Chicago: University of Chicago Press, 1959.

Maturity Indices in Boys

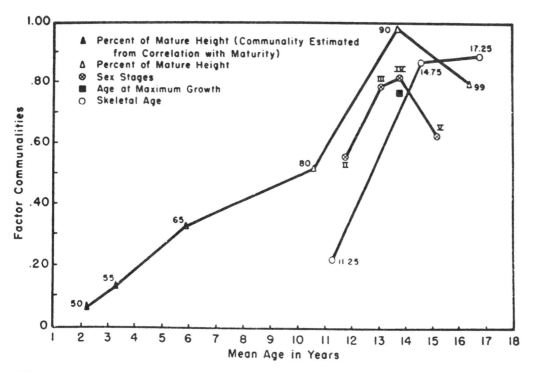

FIG. 21. Factor communalities and average chronological ages of maturity indices in boys. This chart correlates the rate of development of California children versus their age. Percent of total variance of index associated with maturity factor.

Source: Nicolson AB, Hanley C. Indices of physiologic maturity derivation and interrelationship. *Child Dev* 1953;24:3–38.

Secondary Sexual Characteristics and Skeletal Age in Boys

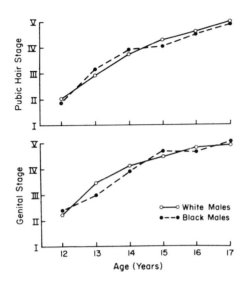

FIG. 22. Secondary sexual characteristics and their relationship to skeletal ages in a representative sample of adolescent males, aged 12 to 17 years. Data from the United States Health Examination Survey Cycle 3 were used. Concordance was found between Tanner's stages for pubic hair and genitalia. Sexual characteristics developed similarly for white and black boys; socioeconomic status did not influence their development.

TABLE 23. *Relationships among bone age, secondary sex characteristics, and serum uric acid concentration in boys 12 to 17 years of age*

Bone age (yr)	N	Percentage at each bone age with corresponding pubic hair and genital stage*					Mean uric acid (mg/dl)†
		I	II	III	IV	V	
9	7	71.4 (71.4)	28.6 (28.6)	0.0 (0.0)	0.0 (0.0)	0.0 (0.0)	3.7 *3.0-4.4*
10	92	63.0 (54.3)	35.9 (42.4)	1.1 (3.3)	0.0 (0.0)	0.0 (0.0)	4.0 *3.8-4.2*
11	217	45.2 (34.6)	48.8 (48.4)	5.5 (16.1)	0.0 (0.5)	0.5 (0.5)	4.0 *3.9-4.2*
12	216	30.6 (22.7)	53.7 (51.4)	15.3 (24.1)	0.5 (1.9)	0.0 (0.0)	4.2 *4.1-4.4*
13	318	19.2 (10.4)	47.2 (43.7)	29.2 (35.8)	4.4 (8.8)	0.0 (1.3)	4.6 *4.5-4.7*
14	455	5.7 (4.0)	23.5 (19.4)	40.0 (32.0)	28.8 (35.5)	2.0 (9.1)	5.1 *5.0-5.2*
15	644	0.2 (0.8)	3.9 (3.0)	17.1 (12.4)	54.3 (42.1)	24.5 (41.7)	5.6 *5.5-5.7*
16	410	0.0 (0.5)	0.7 (0.2)	2.0 (1.2)	42.7 (27.6)	54.6 (70.5)	5.8 *5.6-5.9*
17	577	0.0 (0.3)	0.0 (0.0)	0.5 (1.0)	15.3 (12.1)	84.2 (86.5)	6.0 *5.9-6.1*
18	408	0.0 (0.0)	0.0 (0.0)	0.0 (1.0)	7.1 (6.7)	92.9 (92.4)	6.0 *5.9-6.1*
>18	117	0.0 (0.0)	0.0 (0.0)	0.0 (0.0)	0.9 (3.4)	99.1 (96.6)	6.1 *5.8-6.3*

*Genital stage in parentheses.
†95% confidence levels in italics.

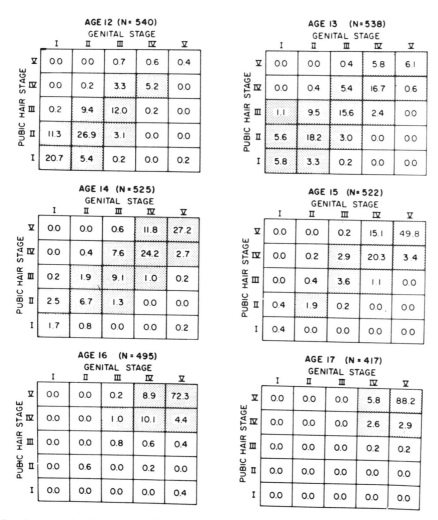

FIG. 23. Percent of white males achieving sexual maturation stage presented by age (years). These data were used to construct the graph in Fig. 22. The data are presented in a matrix format for each age with genital stage (abscissa) and pubic hair state (ordinate) being arrayed so that the concordance between these two stages can be assessed. The percentage of subjects within particular stages of development are indicated within the cells. The shaded cells represent 1% or more of the age group.

Source: Harlan WR, Girllo GP, Cornoni-Huntley G, Leaverton PE. Secondary sex characteristics of boys 12–17 years of age. *J Pediatr* 1979;95:295.

Appearance of Pubic Hair in Obese Boys

Bruch (1) used no controls, and Wolff's (4) controls were taken from a study of 664 schoolboys in Birmingham, England, by Hogben et al, 1948. Nobécourt (2) (whose data are partly longitudinal) and Quaade (3) provided controls from the records of children they examined themselves. The obese boys appear to show signs of puberty early, and there is a higher incidence of pubertal change among Burch's boys, age 11 and 12, than in any of the control groups. There is a general indication that early puberty may be associated with childhood obesity.

References:

1. Bruch H. Obesity in childhood. I. Physical growth and development of obese children. *Am J Dis Child* 1938, 58:457–84.
2. Nobécourt P. La taille des enfants et des jeunes gens obeses. *Gaz Des Hop* 1937;110:1565–73.
3. Quaade F. *Obese Children: Anthropology and Environment.* Copenhagen, Danish Science Press, 1955.
4. Wolff OH. Obesity in childhood. *Quart J Med* 1955;24:109–24.

TABLE 24. *Age incidence of appearance of pubic hair in 159 obese boys reported in the literature*

AGE	NOBÉCOURT Obese	Control	BRUCH Obese	Control	QUAADE Obese	Control	WOLFF Obese	Control	
10-	—	—	0 (10)		9.1 (11)	0 (40)	50.0 (4)	*Age (years)*	
11-	18.2 (11)	0 (10)	50 (4)		7.2 (14)	7.9 (63)	44.4 (9)		
12-	9.1 (11)	0 (12)	33 (9)		41.7 (12)	15.2 (59)	50.0 (10)	25	*11.9*
13-	15.3 (13)	41.7 (12)	} 100 (3)		46.2 (13)	53.8 (52)	} 100.0 (3)	50	*12.9*
14-	37.5 (8)	70.0 (10)			100.0 (1)	84.6 (52)		75	*14.0*
15-	66.7 (9)	80.0 (5)			100.0 (6)	100.0 (25)			
16-	{ 72.7 (11)	100 (1)							
17-									
Total No. of Cases	50	50	26	0	57	291	26	664	

Data are expressed as the percentage of boys with pubic hair at each age.

Source: Acheson RM, Dupertuis CW. The relationship between physique and rate of skeletal maturation in boys. *Hum Biol* 1957;29:167–93.

Size of Male Genitalia from Birth to Maturity

TABLE 25. *Testicular and penile size at various ages*

Age (years)	Testis Length (cm)	Testis Volume (cc)	Penis Circumference Relaxed (cm)	Penis Length Relaxed (cm)	Penis Length Stretched or Erect (cm)
Under 1	1.5	0.6	4.0		4.0
1–2	1.6	0.7	4.0		4.5
3–4	1.6	0.8	4.0	3	5.5
5–6	1.6	0.8	4.5		6.0
7–8	1.6	0.8	4.5	3–4	6.0
9–10	1.6	0.9	4.5	3–4	6.0
11	1.7	1.5	4.5		6.5
12	1.9	2	5.0	3–7	7.0
13	2.3	5	6.0		9.0
14	2.8	8	7.0		10.0
15	3.0	12	7.5		12.0
16	3.5	13	8.0		12.5
17		15	8.5		13.0
18–19		16	8.5		13.0
Over 19	4–5	16.5	8.5	6–10	13.0

Source: Schonfeld WA, Beebe GW. Normal growth and variation in the male genitalia from birth to maturity. *J Urol* 1942;48:759–77. (Originally courtesy of Dr. R. Dorfman.)

Sexual Maturity Stages in Girls

Breast stages are: I. Prepubertal breast; elevated papilla only. II. Elevated areola or minimal breast swelling. III. First swelling of the breast to a small mound formation. IV. Final stage, after which no further developmental changes in breast contour appear.
Pubic hair stages are: I. Infantile; no pigmented pubic hair. II. Hair is pigmented, straight, or only slightly curled, sparse, and primarily along the labia. III. Hair curled, slight spread on mons. IV. Hair curled; moderate amount and spread.

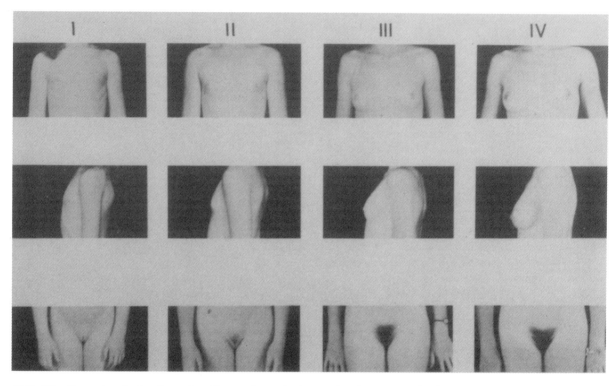

FIG. 24. Sexual maturity stages in girls, as shown by breast development and pubic hair growth. **Top:** Anterior view of the breasts at the four stages. **Center:** Corresponding side views of breast stages. **Bottom:** Stages of pubic hair development.

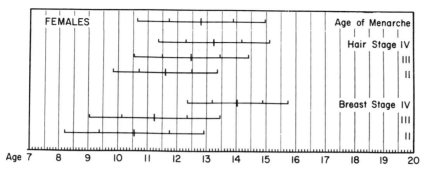

FIG. 25. Maturity indices for girls, showing normal range of occurrence of sex stages. Breast stages: I. Prepubertal breast; elevated papilla only. II. Elevated areola or minimal breast swelling (mean ± SD, 10.6 ± 1.2 years). III. First swelling of the breast to a small mound formation (11.2 ± 1.1 years). IV. Final stage, after which no further developmental changes in breast contour appear (13.9 ± 0.9 years). Pubic hair stages: I. Infantile; no pigmented pubic hair. II. Hair is pigmented, straight, or only slightly curled, sparse, and primarily along the labia (11.6 ± 0.9 years). III. Hair curled; slight spread on mons (12.5 ± 1.0 years). IV. Hair curled; moderate amount and spread (13.2 ± 0.9 years). Stages of sexual maturity (age of menarche: mean ± SD, 12.8 ± 1.1 years).

Source: Bayer LM, Bayley N. Selected methods for interpreting and predicting physical development from one year to maturity. In. *Growth Diagnosis*. Chicago; University of Chicago Press, 1959.

Maturity Indices in Girls

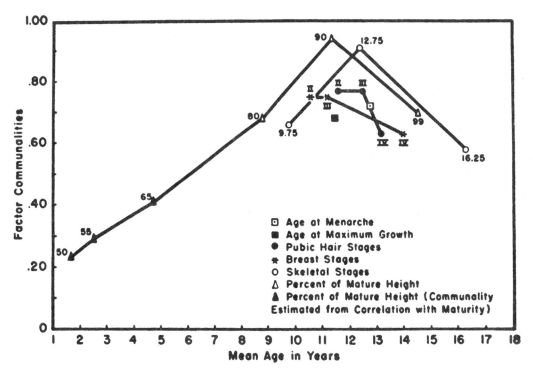

FIG. 26. Indices of physiological maturity, derivation, and interrelationships; communalities and average chronological ages of maturity indices in girls. Percentage of total variance of index associated with maturity factor.

Source: Nicolson AB, Hanley C. Indices of physiologic maturity derivation and interrelationship. *Child Dev* 1953;24:3–38.

Secondary Sexual Characteristics in Girls

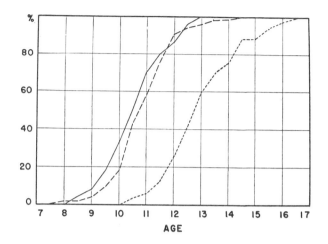

FIG. 27. Percentage distribution of age at first breast development (*solid line*) and first appearance of pubic hair (*dashed line*) of 49 girls who were regular participants in the long-term study of growth and development conducted by the Fels Research Institute. Also age at menarche (*broken line*) in 32 girls.

Source: Reynolds EL, Wines JV. Individual differences in physical changes associated with adolescence in girls. *Am J Dis Child* 1948;75:329–50.

Ossification of Iliac Crest Relative to Age at Menarche

TABLE 26. *Mean and range of onset of ossification in the iliac crest (iliac age) for 130 girls grouped according to chronologic age at menarche*

NUMBER OF CASES	MENARCHEAL AGE (YR.)	MEAN ILIAC AGE (YR.)	ILIAC AGE RANGE (YR.)
2	10.0 to 10.5	11.5	11.0 and 12.0
3	10.6 to 10.9	10.8	10.1 to 11.5
7	11.0 to 11.5	11.3	10.4 to 11.7
17	11.6 to 11.9	12.5	10.9 to 14.0
29	12.0 to 12.5	12.6	11.8 to 14.5
18	12.6 to 12.9	12.6	11.9 to 14.7
20	13.0 to 13.5	13.3	12.0 to 14.5
14	13.6 to 13.9	13.8	12.7 to 14.5
11	14.0 to 14.5	14.1	13.0 to 15.3
3	14.6 to 14.9	14.9	14.9
4	15.0 to 15.5	15.1	13.9 to 15.6
1	15.6 to 15.9	15.0	----
1	16.0 to 16.5	15.2	----

Source: Buehl CC, Pyle SI. The use of age at first appearance of 3 ossification centers in determining the skeletal status of children. *J Pediatr* 1942;21:342–55.

Breadth of Skin and Subcutaneous Tissue in the Leg of Boys and Girls

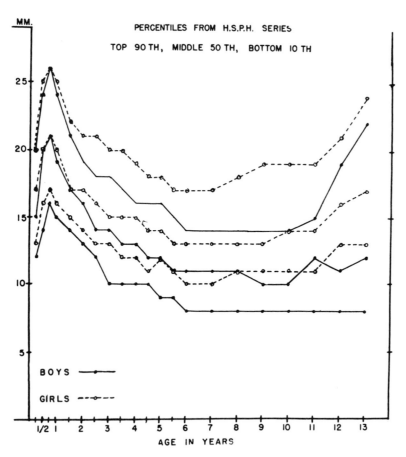

FIG. 28. Breadth of skin and subcutaneous tissue in the leg of boys and girls versus age. This was measured as the breadth of the calf less the breadth of muscle from A-P roentgenograms.

Source: Stuart HC, Sobel EH. The thickness of the skin and subcutaneous tissue by age and sex in childhood. *J Pediatr* 1946;28:637–47.

TABLE 27. *Breadth of skin and subcutaneous tissue in boys*

AGE (YR.)	PERCENTILES					NO. OF CASES	MEAN	S. D.
	10	25	50	75	90			
A. Three-Foot Tube Distance								
¼	12	13	15	18	20	66	15	3.3
½	14	17	20	22	24	64	19	3.4
¾	16	18	21	24	26	59	21	4.1
1	15	17	19	22	24	78	19	3.4
1½	14	15	17	19	21	57	17	2.7
2	13	14	16	18	19	74	16	2.8
2½	12	13	14	16	18	66	14	2.3
3	10	12	14	16	18	80	14	2.7
3½	10	12	13	15	17	60	13	2.5
4	10	11	13	14	16	71	13	2.8
4½	10	11	12	14	16	52	12	2.3
5	9	10	12	13	16	71	12	2.6
5½	9	10	11	13	15	54	12	2.6
6	8	10	11	13	16	53	11	3.0
B. Six-Foot Tube Distance								
6	8	10	11	12	14	59	10	2.0
7	8	9	11	12	14	73	10	3.0
8	8	9	11	12	14	64	11	3.0
9	8	8	10	12	14	55	11	3.6
10	8	8	10	12	14	35	10	2.4
11	8	8	12	13	15	25	11	3.1
12	8	9	11	16	19	20	12	3.8
13	8	9	12	16	22	29	14	7.0

Distributions for measurements were from anteroposterior roentgenograms.
Data used for Fig. 28.

TABLE 28. *Breadth of skin and subcutaneous tissue of girls*

AGE (YR.)	PERCENTILES					NO. OF CASES	MEAN	S. D.
	10	25	50	75	90			
A. Three-Foot Tube Distance								
¼	13	15	17	19	20	68	17	2.5
½	16	18	20	22	25	63	19	3.2
¾	17	19	21	23	26	59	21	3.2
1	16	18	20	23	25	74	19	3.2
1½	15	16	17	19	22	60	18	2.8
2	14	15	17	19	21	79	17	2.8
2½	13	15	16	19	21	62	17	2.8
3	13	14	15	18	20	79	16	2.7
3½	12	13	15	17	20	54	15	2.7
4	12	13	15	17	19	72	15	2.6
4½	11	12	14	17	18	60	14	2.7
5	12	13	14	16	18	67	14	2.5
5½	11	12	13	15	17	53	14	2.6
6	11	12	13	15	16	42	14	2.2
B. Six-Foot Tube Distance								
6	10	12	13	16	17	58	13	2.5
7	10	12	13	16	17	63	13	2.8
8	11	12	13	16	18	51	14	2.7
9	11	12	13	16	19	55	14	3.4
10	11	12	14	17	19	42	15	3.5
11	11	12	14	17	19	27	14	3.1
12	13	14	16	18	21	20	16	3.2
13	13	15	17	20	24	19	18	4.2

Distributions for measurements were from anteroposterior roentgenograms.
Data used for Fig. 28.

NEUROMUSCULAR
DEVELOPMENT

Apgar Assessment at Birth

The Apgar score is a method for evaluating a newborn infant. Each observation is scored as indicated. Total scores: 8 to 10 = good; 3 to 7 = fair; and 0 to 2 = poor. At 1-minute and 5-minute intervals after the complete birth of the neonate, Apgar scores should be obtained. If the 5-minute score is less than seven, additional scores should be obtained every 5 minutes, up to 20 minutes, unless two successive scores are 8 or greater. The longer the scoring remains low, the worse the prognosis with regard to mortality or neurologic sequela.

TABLE 1. *Apgar scoring*

Parameter	0	1	2
Heart rate	Absent	Below 100	Over 100
Respiratory effort	Absent	Slow, irregular	Good crying
Muscle tone	Limp	Some flexion of extremities	Active motion
Reflex irritability (nasal catheter)	No response	Grimace	Cough or sneeze
Color	Blue, pale	Body pink, extremities blue	Completely pink

Source: Apgar V. A proposal for a new method of evaluation of the newborn infant. *Anesth Analg* 1953;32:260.

Assessment of Gestational Age at the Time of First Examination

The scoring system in this section was originally applied to 167 newborns. The external score gave a better correlation with gestation than did the neurologic score, but the combined total score was better than either alone. The assessment is done according to the chart in Fig. 1, with the scores given, and gestational age is estimated by using the graph in Fig. 2. This was subsequently modified to simpler format by Ballard (Figs. 3 and 4) and 10 years later it was revised and expanded by Dubowitz (Fig. 5).

Posture: Observed with infant quiet and in supine position. Score 0: arms and legs extended; 1: beginning of flexion of hips and knees, arms extended; 2: stronger flexion of legs, arms extended; 3: arms slightly flexed, legs flexed and abducted; 4: full flexion of arms and legs.

Square Window: The hand is flexed on the forearm between the thumb and index finger of the examiner. Enough pressure is applied to get as full a flexion as possible, and the angle between the hypothenar eminence and the ventral aspect of the forearm is measured and graded according to diagram. (Care is taken not to rotate the infant's wrist while doing this maneuver.)

Ankle Dorsiflexion: The foot is dorsiflexed onto the anterior aspect of the leg, with the examiner's thumb on the sole of the foot and other fingers behind the leg. Enough pressure is applied to get as full flexion as possible, and the angle between the dorsum of the foot and the anterior aspect of the leg is measured.

Arm Recoil: With the infant in the supine position the forearms are first flexed for 5 seconds, then fully extended by pulling on the hands, and then released. The sign is fully positive if the arms return briskly to full flexion (score 2). If the arms return to incomplete flexion or the response is sluggish it is graded as score 1. If they remain extended or are only followed by random movements the score is 0.

Leg Recoil: With the infant supine, the hips and knees are fully flexed for 5 seconds, then extended by traction on the feet, and released. A maximal response is one of full flexion of the hips and knees (score 2). A partial flexion scores 1, and minimal or no movement scores 0.

Popliteal Angle: With the infant supine and his/her pelvis flat on the examining couch, the thigh is held in the knee-chest position by the examiner's left index finger and thumb supporting the knee. The leg is then extended by gentle pressure from the examiner's right index finger behind the ankle, and the popliteal angle is measured.

Heel to Ear Maneuver: With the baby supine, draw the baby's foot as near to the head as it will go without forcing it. Observe the distance between the foot and the head as well as the degree of extension at the knee. Grade according to diagram in Fig. 1. Note that the knee is left free and may draw down alongside the abdomen.

Scarf Sign: With the baby supine, take the infant's hand and try to put it around the neck and as far posteriorly as possible around the opposite shoulder. Assist this maneuver by lifting the elbow across the body. See how far the elbow will go across and grade according to illustrations in Fig. 1. Score 0: Elbow reaches opposite axillary line. 1: Elbow between midline and opposite axillary line. 2: Elbow reaches midline. 3: Elbow will not reach midline.

Head Lag: With the baby lying supine, grasp the hands (or the arms if a very small infant) and pull him/her slowly toward the sitting position. Observe the position of the head in relation to the trunk and grade accordingly. In a small infant the head may initially be supported by one hand. Score 0: Complete lag. 1: Partial head control. 2: Able to maintain head in line with body. 3: Brings head anterior to body.

Ventral Suspension: The infant is suspended in the prone position, with examiner's hand under the infant's chest (one hand in a small infant, two in a large infant). Observe the degree of extension of the back and the amount of flexion of the arms and legs. Also note the relation of the head to the trunk. Grade according to diagram in Fig. 1. If score differs on the two sides, take the mean.

Source: Dubowitz LMS. *The neurological assessment of the preterm and full-term newborn infant.* London: Spastics International Medical Publications, 1981. Reproduced in Dubowitz LMS, Dubowitz V, and Goldberg C. Clinical assessment of gestational age. *J Pediatr* 1970;77:1–10.

GESTATIONAL AGE CHART

(Dubowitz Score)

Name

Hospital No.

Sex _____ Race

Date/time of birth

Date/time of examination

Age

Weight

Length

Head circumference

Score
    Neurological _____
    Superficial _____
             Total _____

FDD (certain/uncertain)

Gest by dates

Gest by Assessment

Comments

Neurological Criteria

NEURO-LOGICAL SIGN	SCORE					
	0	1	2	3	4	5
POSTURE						
SQUARE WINDOW	90°	60°	45°	30°	0°	
ANKLE DORSI-FLEXION	90°	75°	45°	20°	0°	
ARM RECOIL	180°	90–180°	<90°			
LEG RECOIL	180°	90–180°	<90°			
POPLITEAL ANGLE	180°	160°	130°	110°	90°	<90°
HEEL TO EAR						
SCARF SIGN						
HEAD LAG						
VENTRAL SUSPEN-SION						

External (superficial) Criteria

EXTERNAL SIGN	SCORE				
	0	1	2	3	4
OEDEMA	Obvious oedema hands and feet, pitting over tibia	No obvious oedema hands and feet, pitting over tibia	No oedema		
SKIN TEXTURE	Very thin, gelatinous	Thin and smooth	Smooth, medium thickness. Rash or superficial peeling	Slight thickening. Superficial cracking and peeling esp. hands and feet	Thick and parchment-like, superficial or deep cracking
SKIN COLOUR (infant not crying)	Dark red	Uniformly pink	Pale pink, variable over body	Pale. Only pink over ears, lips, palms or soles	
SKIN OPACITY (trunk)	Numerous veins and venules clearly seen esp. over abdomen	Veins and tributaries seen	A few large vessels clearly seen over abdomen	A few large vessels seen indistinctly over abdomen	No blood vessels seen
LANUGO (over back)	No lanugo	Abundant, long and thick over whole back	Hair thinning especially over lower back	Small amount of lanugo and bald areas	At least half of back devoid of lanugo
PLANTAR CREASES	No skin creases	Faint red marks over anterior half of sole	Definite red marks over more than anterior half, indentations over less than anterior third	Indentations over more than anterior third	Definite deep indentations over more than anterior third
NIPPLE FORMA-TION	Nipple barely visible, no areola	Nipple well defined, areola smooth and flat, diameter <0.75 cm	Areola stippled, edge not raised, diameter <0.75 cm	Areola stippled, edge raised, diameter >0.75cm	
BREAST SIZE	No breast tissue palpable	Breast tissue on one or both sides 0.5 cm diameter	Breast tissue both sides, one or both 0.5–1.0 cm	Breast tissue both sides, one or both >1 cm	
EAR FORM	Pinna flat and shapeless, little or no incurving of edge	Incurving of part of edge of pinna	Partial incurving whole of upper pinna	Well-defined incurving whole of upper pinna	
EAR FIRMNESS	Pinna soft, easily folded, no recoil	Pinna soft, easily folded, slow recoil	Cartilage to edge of pinna, but soft in places, ready recoil	Pinna firm, cartilage to edge, instant recoil	
GENITALIA MALE	Neither testis in scrotum	At least one testis high in scrotum	At least one testis right down		
FEMALES (with hips half abducted)	Labia majora widely separated, labia minora protruding	Labia majora almost cover labia minora	Labia majora completely cover labia minora		

(Adapted from Farr et al. Develop Med Child Neurol 1966, 8, 507)

FIG. 1. Scoring system for gestational age, based on 10 neurologic and 11 external criteria.

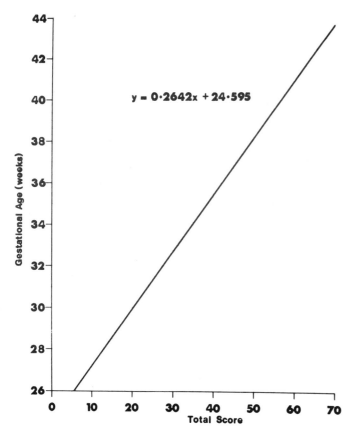

FIG. 2. Graph of Dubowitz score versus gestational age.

Source: Dubowitz LMS. *The neurological assessment of the preterm and full-term newborn infant*. London: Spastics International Medical Publications, 1981. Reproduced in Dubowitz LMS, Dubowitz V, and Goldberg C. Clinical assessment of gestational age. *J Pediatr* 1970;77:1–10.

Simplified Assessment of Gestational Age

This score was developed by condensing the methods of Dubowitz and others. It consists of six neurologic and six physical criteria. The physical criteria were combined into single observations; the neurologic signs which required active muscle tone were eliminated, as they are misleading in sick infants. To test the accuracy of the simplified system, the Dubowitz method was used as a standard, and 284 babies were examined by both methods by unbiased observers. Ages ranged from 12 to 96 with weights ranging from 760 to 5,460 g. Correlation *(r)* between the two examinations was 0.975, p = 0.001. Individual criteria of the simplified score on a second group of 85 infants were then weighed for predictive value according to their correlation with known dates. The gestational age tended to be more closely related to the individual components of the physical assessment *(r* = 0.614 to 0.784) than to the neurologic criteria *(r* = 0.437 to 0.756). The correlation for the score obtained for the total assessment *(r* = 0.952) was greater than that for any examination of the individual components. The average time required for the Dubowitz examination was 10 to 15 min and for the simplified method 3 to 4 min.

PHYSICAL MATURITY

Physical sign	SCORE					
	0	1	2	3	4	5
Skin	gelatinous red, transparent	smooth pink, visible veins	superficial peeling &/or rash few veins	cracking pale area rare veins	parchment deep cracking no vessels	leathery cracked wrinkled
Lanugo	none	abundant	thinning	bald areas	mostly bald	
Plantar Creases	no crease	faint red marks	anterior transverse crease only	creases ant. 2/3	creases cover entire sole	
Breast	barely percept.	flat areola no bud	stippled areola 1–2 mm bud	raised areola 3–4 mm bud	full areola 5–10 mm bud	
Ear	pinna flat, stays folded	sl. curved pinna; soft with slow recoil	well-curv. pinna; soft but ready recoil	formed & firm with instant recoil	thick cartilage ear stiff	
Genitals ♂	scrotum empty no rugae		testes descending, few rugae	testes down good rugae	testes pendulous deep rugae	
Genitals ♀	prominent clitoris & labia minora		majora & minora equally prominent	majora large minora small	clitoris & minora completely covered	

MATURITY RATING

Score	Wks
5	26
10	28
15	30
20	32
25	34
30	36
35	38
40	40
45	42
50	44

FIG. 3. Classification of the low-birth-weight infant; an abbreviated version in which certain neurologic criteria are retained which do not require the infant to be alert and vigorous.

NEUROMUSCULAR MATURITY

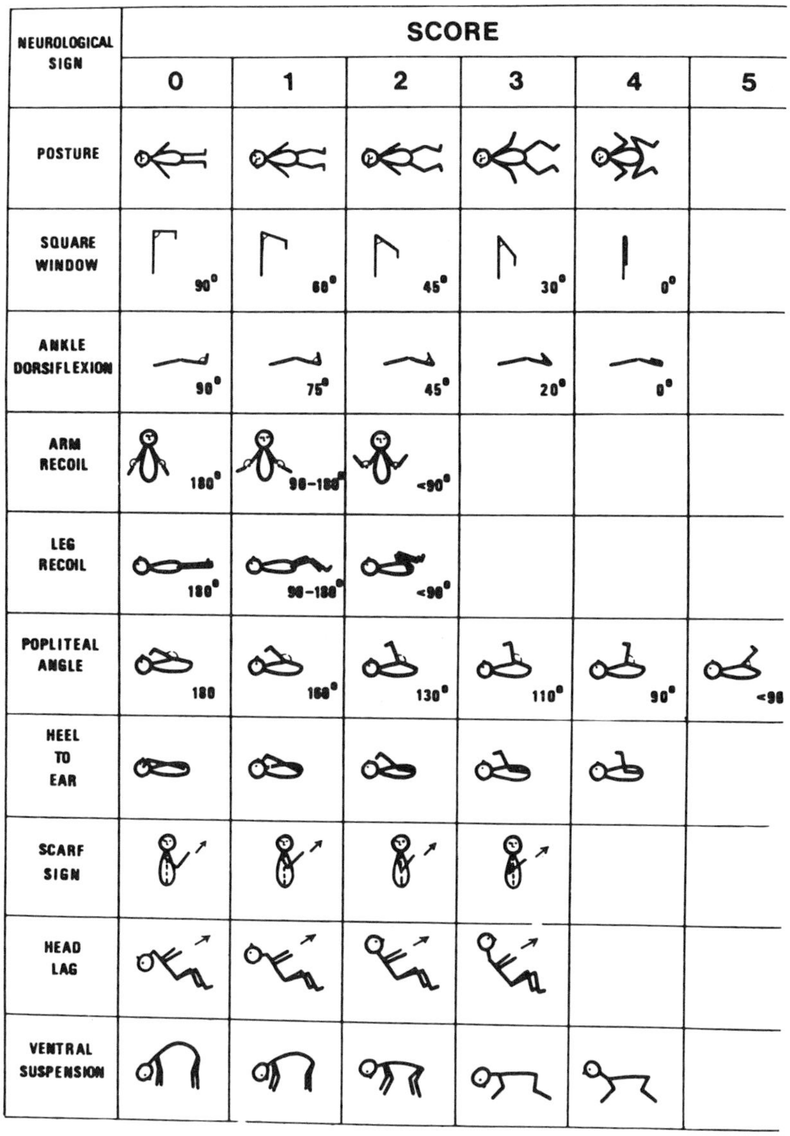

NEUROLOGICAL SIGN	SCORE					
	0	1	2	3	4	5
POSTURE						
SQUARE WINDOW	90°	60°	45°	30°	0°	
ANKLE DORSIFLEXION	90°	75°	45°	20°	0°	
ARM RECOIL	180°	90-180°	<90°			
LEG RECOIL	180°	90-180°	<90°			
POPLITEAL ANGLE	180	160°	130°	110°	90°	<90
HEEL TO EAR						
SCARF SIGN						
HEAD LAG						
VENTRAL SUSPENSION						

FIG. 4. Continuation of scoring system of the low-birth-weight infant.

Sources: Ballard JL, Kazmaier K, Driver M, Light IJ. A simplified assessment of gestational age. *Pediatr Res* 1977;11:374.

Sweet AY. Classification of low-birth-weight infant. In: Klaus MH, Faranoff WB (eds). *Care of the high risk infant*. Philadelphia: W. B. Saunders, 1977;79.

Neurological Assessment of the Newborn

NAME		D.O.B./TIME	WEIGHT	E.D.D. L.N.M.P.	E.D.D. U/snd.				
HOSP.	NO.	DATE OF EXAM	HEIGHT						
RACE	SEX	AGE	HEAD CIRC.	GESTATIONAL SCORE WEEKS ASSESSMENT					

STATES
1. Deep sleep, no movement, regular breathing.
2. Light sleep, eyes shut, some movement.
3. Dozing, eyes opening and closing.
4. Awake, eyes open, minimal movement.
5. Wide awake, vigorous movement.
6. Crying.

						STATE	COMMENT	ASYMMETRY

HABITUATION (≤state 3)

LIGHT Repetitive flashlight stimuli (10) with 5 sec. gap. Shutdown 2 consecutive negative responses	No response	A. Blink response to first stimulus only. B. Tonic blink response C. Variable response.	A. Shutdown of movement but blink persists 2-5 stimuli. B. Complete shutdown 2-5 stimuli.	A. Shutdown of movement but blink persists 6-10 stimuli. B. Complete shutdown 6-10 stimuli.	A. Equal response to 10 stimuli. B. Infant comes to fully alert state. C. Startles + major responses throughout.			
RATTLE Repetitive stimuli (10) with 5 sec. gap.	No response	A. Slight movement to first stimulus. B. Variable response.	Startle or movement 2-5 stimuli, then shutdown	Startle or movement 6-10 stimuli, then shutdown	A. B. C. Grading as above			

MOVEMENT & TONE   Undress infant

POSTURE (At rest predominant) ✱				(hips abducted)	(hips adducted)	Abnormal postures. A. Opisthotonus. B. Unusual leg extension. C. Asymm. tonic neck reflex		
ARM RECOIL Infant supine. Take both hands, extend parallel to the body, hold approx. 2 secs and release	No flexion within 5 sec.	Partial flexion at elbow >100° within 4-5 sec.	Arms flex at elbow to <100° within 2-3 sec.	Sudden jerky flexion at elbow immediately after release to <60°	Difficult to extend; arm snaps back forcefully			
ARM TRACTION Infant supine, head midline, grasp wrist, slowly pull arm to vertical. Angle of arm scored and resistance noted at moment infant is initially lifted off and watched until shoulder off mattress. Do other arm	Arm remains fully extended	Weak flexion maintained only momentarily	Arm flexed at elbow to 140° and maintained 5 sec.	Arm flexed at approx. 100° and maintained	Strong flexion of arm <100° and maintained			
LEG RECOIL First flex hips for 5 secs, then extend both legs of infant by traction on ankles, hold down on the bed for 2 secs and release	No flexion within 5 sec	Incomplete flexion of hips within 5 sec.	Complete flexion within 5 sec.	Instantaneous complete flexion	Legs cannot be extended; snap back forcefully			
LEG TRACTION Infant supine. Grasp leg near ankle and slowly pull toward vertical until buttocks 1-2" off. Note resistance at knee and score angle. Do other leg.	No flexion	Partial flexion, rapidly lost	Knee flexion 140-160° and maintained	Knee flexion 100-140° and maintained	Strong resistance; flexion <100°			

POPLITEAL ANGLE Infant supine. Approximate knee and thigh to abdomen; extend leg by gentle pressure with index finger behind ankle.	180-160°	150-140°	130-120°	110-90°	<90°			
HEAD CONTROL (post. neck m.) Grasp infant by shoulders and raise to sitting position; allow head to fall forward; wait 30 sec.	No attempt to raise head	Unsuccessful attempt to raise head upright	Head raised smoothly to upright in 30 sec. but not maintained.	Head raised smoothly to upright in 30 sec. and maintained	Head cannot be flexed forward			
HEAD CONTROL (ant. neck m.) Allow head to fall backward as you hold shoulders; wait 30 secs.	Grading as above	Grading as above	Grading as above	Grading as above				
HEAD LAG ✱ Pull infant toward sitting posture by traction on both wrists. Also note arm flexion.								
VENTRAL SUSPENSION ✱ Hold infant in ventral suspension; observe curvature of back, flexion of limbs and relation of head to trunk.								
HEAD RAISING IN PRONE POSITION Infant in prone position with head in midline.	No response	Rolls head to one side	Weak effort to raise head and turns raised head to one side	Infant lifts head, nose and chin off	Strong prolonged head lifting			
ARM RELEASE IN PRONE POSITION Head in midline. Infant in prone position; arms extended alongside body with palms up.	No effort	Some effort and wriggling	Flexion effort but neither wrist brought to nipple level	One or both wrists brought at least to nipple level without excessive body movement	Strong body movement with both wrists brought to face, or 'press-ups'			
SPONTANEOUS BODY MOVEMENT during examination (supine). If no spont. movement try to induce by cutaneous stimulation.	None or minimal Induced	A. Sluggish. B. Random, incoordinated. C. Mainly stretching.	Smooth movements alternating with random, stretching, athetoid or jerky	Smooth alternating movements of arms and legs with medium speed and intensity	Mainly: A. Jerky movement. B. Athetoid movement. C. Other abnormal movement.	1 2		
TREMORS Mark: Fast (>6/sec.) or Slow (<6/sec.)	No tremor	Tremors only in state 5-6	Tremors only in sleep or after Moro and startles	Some tremors in state 4	Tremulousness in all states			
STARTLES	No startles	Startles to sudden noise, Moro, bang on table only	Occasional spontaneous startle	2-5 spontaneous startles	6+ spontaneous startles			
ABNORMAL MOVEMENT OR POSTURE	No abnormal movement	A. Hands clenched but open intermittently. B. Hands do not open with Moro.	A. Some mouthing movement. B. Intermittent adducted thumb	A. Persistently adducted thumb. B. Hands clenched all the time.	A. Continuous mouthing movement. B. Convulsive movements.			

	STATE	COMMENT	ASYMMETRY

REFLEXES

TENDON REFLEXES Biceps jerk Knee jerk Ankle jerk	Absent			Present		Exaggerated		Clonus				
PALMAR GRASP Head in midline. Put index finger from ulnar side into hand and gently press palmar surface. Never touch dorsal side of hand.	Absent		Short, weak flexion		Medium strength and sustained flexion for several secs.		Strong flexion; contraction spreads to forearm		Very strong grasp. Infant easily lifts off couch				
ROOTING Infant supine, head midline. Touch each corner of the mouth in turn (stroke laterally).	No response		A. Partial weak head turn but no mouth opening. B. Mouth opening, no head turn.		Mouth opening on stimulated side with partial head turning		Full head turning, with or without mouth opening		Mouth opening with very jerky head turning				
SUCKING Infant supine; place index finger (pad towards palate) in infant's mouth; judge power of sucking movement after 5 sec.	No attempt		Weak sucking movement: A. Regular. B. Irregular.		Strong sucking movement, poor stripping: A. Regular. B. Irregular.		Strong regular sucking movement with continuing sequence of 5 movements. Good stripping.		Clenching but no regular sucking.				
WALKING (state 4, 5) Hold infant upright, feet touching bed, neck held straight with fingers.	Absent				Some effort but not continuous with both legs		At least 2 steps with both legs		A. Stork posture; no movement. B. Automatic walking.				
MORO One hand supports infant's head in midline, the other the back. Raise infant to 45° and when infant is relaxed let his head fall through 10°. Note if jerky. Repeat 3 times.	No response, or opening of hands only		Full abduction at the shoulder and extension of the arm		Full abduction but only delayed or partial adduction		Partial abduction at shoulder and extension of arms followed by smooth adduction	A. Abd>Add B. Abd=Add C. Abd<Add	A. No abduction or adduction; extension only. B. Marked adduction only.		J S		

NEUROBEHAVIOURAL ITEMS

EYE APPEARANCES	Sunset sign Nerve palsy		Transient nystagmus. Strabismus. Some roving eye movement.		Does not open eyes		Normal conjugate eye movement		A. Persistent nystagmus. B. Frequent roving movement C. Frequent rapid blinks.				
AUDITORY ORIENTATION (state 3, 4) To rattle. (Note presence of startle.)	A. No reaction. B. Auditory startle but no true orientation		Brightens and stills; may turn toward stimuli with eyes closed		Alerting and shifting of eyes; head may or may not turn to source		Alerting; prolonged head turns to stimulus; search with eyes		Turning and alerting to stimulus each time on both sides		S		
VISUAL ORIENTATION (state 4) To red woollen ball	Does not focus or follow stimulus		Stills; focuses on stimulus; may follow 30° jerkily; does not find stimulus again spontaneously		Follows 30-60° horizontally; may lose stimulus but finds it again. Brief vertical glance		Follows with eyes and head horizontally and to some extent vertically, with frowning		Sustained fixation; follows vertically, horizonally, and in circle				

ALERTNESS (state 4)	Inattentive; rarely or never responds to direct stimulation	When alert, periods rather brief; rather variable response to orientation	When alert, alertness moderately sustained; may use stimulus to come to alert state	Sustained alertness; orientation frequent, reliable to visual but not auditory stimuli	Continuous alertness, which does not seem to tire, to both auditory and visual stimuli			
DEFENSIVE REACTION A cloth or hand is placed over the infant's face to partially occlude the nasal airway.	No response	A. General quietening. B. Non-specific activity with long latency.	Rooting; lateral neck turning; possibly neck stretching.	Swipes with arm	Swipes with arm with rather violent body movement			
PEAK OF EXCITEMENT	Low level arousal to all stimuli; never > state 3	Infant reaches state 4-5 briefly but predominantly in lower states	Infant predominantly state 4 or 5; may reach state 6 after stimulation but returns spontaneously to lower state	Infant reaches state 6 but can be consoled relatively easily	A. Mainly state 6. Difficult to console, if at all. B. Mainly state 4-5 but if reaches state 6 cannot be consoled.			
IRRITABILITY (states 3, 4, 5) Aversive stimuli: Uncover Ventral susp. Undress Moro Pull to sit Walking reflex Prone	No irritable crying to any of the stimuli	Cries to 1-2 stimuli	Cries to 3-4 stimuli	Cries to 5-6 stimuli	Cries to all stimuli			
CONSOLABILITY (state 6)	Never above state 5 during examination, therefore not needed	Consoling not needed. Consoles spontaneously	Consoled by talking, hand on belly or wrapping up	Consoled by picking up and holding; may need finger in mouth	Not consolable			
CRY	No cry at all	Only whimpering cry	Cries to stimuli but normal pitch	Lusty cry to offensive stimuli; normal pitch	High-pitched cry, often continuous			

FIG. 5. Neurological assessment of the preterm and fullterm newborn infant.

Source: Dubowitz L, Dubowitz V. Neurological assessment of the preterm and fullterm newborn infant. *Clin Develop Med* 79. Spastics International Medical Publications, London; 1981.

Related Reference:

Brazelton TB. Neonatal behavioral assessment scale. *Clin Develop Med* 50. Spastics International Medical Publications, London; 1973.

Bayley Scales of Infant Development

There are 163 items on the mental scale and 81 items on the motor scale of Bayley's chart. As this section is directed to the muscle and skeletal system, only the motor scale has been reproduced here. This scale has been developed from a standardized sample of 1,262 children distributed in approximately equal numbers among 14 age groups ranging from 2 to 30 months. The sample was selected to be representative of the United States population within this age range and was accomplished with the collaboration of well-trained, highly qualified psychologists located in each of the major geographic regions of the country. The mental scale is designed to assess sensory perception acuities, discriminations, and the abilities to respond to these, the early acquisition of "object consistancy" and memory, learning, and problem solving ability; vocalizations and the beginnings of verbal communication, and early evidence of the ability to form generalizations and classifications, which is the basis of abstract thinking.

The motor scale is designed to provide a measure of the degree of control of the body, coordination for the large muscles, and finer manipulatory skills for the hands and fingers. As the motor skill is specifically directed toward behaviors reflecting motor coordination and skills, it is not concerned with functions that are commonly thought of as mental or intelligent in nature. The results of the administration of the motor scale are expressed as a standard score, the Psychomotor Developmental Index (PDI). The chart consists of the item number, the activity to be assessed, the age placement value (mean or the age at which 50% of the children attained the skill), and the age range values (Table 2). The latter provide estimates of the ages at which each item was passed by 5 and 95%, respectively, of the children in the standardization sample. The first few items have age placement values below 2 months, the lowest age for children in the sample.

TABLE 2. *Bayley scales of infant development*

Item	Activity	Percentiles (months)		
		Mean (50%)	5%	95%
1	Lifts when held at shoulder	0.1	—	—
2	Postural adjustment when held at shoulder	0.1	—	—
3	Lateral head movements	0.1	—	—
4	Crawling movements	0.4	0.1	3
5	Retains red ring	0.8	0.3	3
6	Arm thrusts in play	0.8	0.3	2
7	Leg thrusts in play	0.8	0.3	2
8	Head erect: vertical	0.8	0.3	3
9	Head erect and steady	1.6	0.7	4
10	Lifts head: dorsal suspension	1.7	0.7	4
11	Turns from side to back	1.8	0.7	5
12	Elevates self by arms: prone	2.1	0.7	5
13	Sits with support	2.3	1.0	5
14	Holds head steady	2.5	1.0	5
15	Hands predominantly open	2.7	0.7	6
16	Cube: ulnar-palmar prehension	3.7	2.0	7
17	Sits with slight support	3.8	2.0	6
18	Head balanced	4.2	2.0	6
19	Turns from back to side	4.4	2.0	7
20	Effort to sit	4.8	3.0	8
21	Cube: partial thumb opposition (radial-palmar)	4.9	4.0	8
22	Pulls to sitting position	5.3	4.0	8
23	Sits alone momentarily	5.3	4.0	8
24	Unilateral reaching[a]	5.4	4.0	8
25	Attempts to secure pellet[b]	5.6	4.0	8

TABLE 2. *(Cont'd)*

26	Rotates wrist	5.7	4.0	8
27	Sits alone 30 seconds or more	6.0	5.0	8
28	Rolls from back to stomach	6.4	4.0	10
29	Sits alone, steadily	6.6	5.0	9
30	Scoops pellet*b*	6.8	5.0	9
31	Sits alone, good coordination	6.9	5.0	10
32	Cube: complete thumb opposition (radial-digital)	6.9	5.0	9
33	Prewalking progression	7.1	5.0	11
34	Early stepping movements	7.4	5.0	11
35	Pellet: partial finger*b* prehension (inferior pincer)	7.4	6.0	10
36	Pulls to standing position	8.1	5.0	12
37	Raises self to sitting position	8.3	6.0	11
38	Stands up by furniture	8.6	6.0	12
39	Combines spoons or cubes:*b* midline	8.6	6.0	12
40	Stepping movements	8.8	6.0	12
41	Pellet: fine prehension*b* (neat pincer)	8.9	7.0	12
42	Walks with help	9.6	7.0	12
43	Sits down	9.6	7.0	14
44	Pak-a-Cake: midline skill*b*	9.7	7.0	15
45	Stands alone	11.0	9.0	16
46	Walks alone	11.7	9.0	17
47	Stands up: I	12.6	9.0	18
48	Throws ball*b*	13.3	9.0	18
49	Walks sideways	14.1	10	20
50	Walks backward	14.6	11	20
51	Stands on right foot with help	15.9	12	21
52	Stands on left foot with help	16.1	12	23
53	Walks up stairs with help	16.1	12	23
54	Walks down stairs with help	16.4	13	23
55	Tries to stand on walking board	17.8	13	26
56	Walks with one foot on walking board	20.6	15	29
57	Stands up: II	21.9	11	30+
58	Stands on left foot alone	22.7	15	30+
59	Jumps off floor, both feet	23.4	17	30+
60	Stands on right foot alone	23.5	16	30+
61	Walks on line, general direction	23.9	18	30+
62	Walking board: stands with both feet	24.5	17	30+
63	Jumps from bottom step	24.8	19	30+
64	Walks up stairs alone: both feet on each step	25.1	18	30+
65	Walks on tiptoe, few steps	25.7	16	30+
66	Walks down stairs alone: both feet on each step	25.8	19	30+
67	Walking board: attempts step	27.6	19	30+
68	Walks backward, 10 feet	27.8	20	30+
69	Jumps from second step	28.1	21	30+
70	Distance jump: 4 to 14 inches	29.1	22	30+
71	Stands up: III	30+	22	30+
72	Walks up stairs: alternating forward foot	30+	23	30+
73	Walks on tiptoe, 10 feet	30+	20	30+
74	Walking board: alternates steps part way	30+	24	30+
75	Keeps feet on line, 10 feet	30+	23	30+
76	Distance jump: 14 to 24 inches	30+	25	30+
77	Jumps over string 2 inches high	30+	24	30+
78	Distance jump: 24 to 34 inches	30+	24	30+
79	Hops on one foot, 2 or more hops	30+	30+	—
80	Walks down stairs: alternating one forward foot	30+	30+	—
81	Jumps over string 8 inches high	30+	28	30+

*a*May be observed incidentally.
*b*May be presented during administration of Mental Scale.

Source: Bayley N. Manual for the Bayley scales of infant development. New York: The Psychological Corporation, 1969.

Comparisons of Mental and Motor Test Scores for Ages 1 to 15 Months

The Bayley scale of mental and motor development was administered in 12 metropolitan areas to 1,409 infants, aged 1 to 15 months. Babies tested were drawn primarily from hospital well-baby clinics. Comparisons of means and standard deviations and total scores were made for a series of subsamples. No differences in scores were found for either scale between boys and girls, firstborn and laterborn, education of either father or mother, or geographic residence. No differences were found between blacks and whites on a mental scale, but the black babies tend to consistently score above the whites on the motor scale.

TABLE 3. *Bayley Infant Scales of mental and motor development by age*

AGE (MONTHS)	NUMBER	MENTAL TOTAL BABIES			MOTOR TOTAL BABIES			INTERNAL CONSISTENCY RELIABILITIES	
		M	σ	Range	M	σ	Range	Mental	Motor
1......	87	13.83	4.57	3–29	6.40	2.03	3–10	.79	.57
2......	91	22.78	6.21	6–40	9.69	2.28	4–15	.86	.65
3......	88	33.56	8.55	10–58	12.75	2.72	6–19	.92	.74
4......	89	43.10	8.03	18–64	15.16	3.07	7–22	.90	.77
5......	85	56.13	8.32	39–74	20.08	3.52	13–31	.92	.81
6......	93	69.61	9.00	49–86	25.71	4.64	14–36	.94	.89
7......	97	74.87	7.06	59–90	29.58	4.93	20–39	.90	.89
8......	123	80.74	6.35	59–93	35.04	5.41	21–43	.89	.90
9......	103	84.30	5.94	61–98	37.69	4.35	25–45	.88	.90
10......	99	90.66	6.02	75–104	41.31	3.73	25–46	.86	.88
11......	81	94.46	5.68	76–105	43.70	2.92	35–49	.84	.83
12......	100	99.65	6.86	67–116	45.41	3.77	35–52	.90	.90
13......	90	103.68	6.13	91–115	46.21	5.15	38–53	.87	.97
14......	90	107.39	6.93	83–120	48.42	3.23	34–60	.90	.86
15......	87	110.68	7.47	92–132	49.18	3.18	39–55	.90	.90

The totals in Table 3 and other tables in this section are less than 1,409 because complete scores were not obtained for all cases.

TABLE 4. *Bayley scales of mental development: comparison of mean point scores by sex of child*

Age (Months)	Boys			Girls			C.R.
	No.	M	σ	No.	M	σ	
1.......	42	6.07	1.87	44	6.86	2.74	1.58
2.......	44	10.05	2.30	46	9.41	2.20	1.36
3.......	41	12.76	3.03	48	12.81	2.41	.09
4.......	43	15.60	3.22	46	14.72	2.86	1.35
5.......	42	19.67	3.34	44	20.59	3.58	1.23
6.......	52	26.27	4.52	43	24.88	4.75	1.45
7.......	32	29.34	4.75	65	29.69	5.01	.34
8.......	46	36.57	4.61	77	34.14	5.63	2.61
9.......	50	38.14	3.96	53	37.64	4.65	.59
10.......	53	40.25	3.98	46	41.28	3.63	1.34
11.......	41	43.02	3.05	39	43.79	2.72	1.18
12.......	52	45.65	3.16	48	44.63	4.29	1.34
13.......	51	46.67	2.99	39	46.38	3.35	.43
14.......	46	48.37	3.60	44	48.36	2.78	.01
15.......	44	48.59	3.23	43	49.37	3.09	1.15

Data used to construct the graph in Fig. 6.

TABLE 5. *Bayley scale of motor development: comparison of means of point scores, by sex of child*

Age (Months)	Boys			Girls			C.R.
	No.	M	σ	No.	M	σ	
1.......	42	13.29	5.15	45	14.33	6.08	.86
2.......	45	22.84	4.67	46	22.72	7.42	.09
3.......	41	32.56	9.49	47	34.60	7.72	1.10
4.......	43	45.23	7.45	46	41.30	8.26	2.35
5.......	40	56.03	9.35	45	56.51	7.29	.26
6.......	51	70.88	8.25	44	68.43	9.56	1.32
7.......	32	75.81	7.00	65	74.62	6.93	.79
8.......	46	80.76	5.69	77	80.77	6.70	.01
9.......	50	85.22	4.82	53	84.40	6.76	.71
10.......	53	87.89	5.86	46	91.43	5.57	3.08
11.......	41	93.49	6.36	40	95.43	4.68	1.56
12.......	52	100.48	6.14	48	98.88	7.51	1.16
13.......	51	103.53	6.41	39	103.87	5.74	.27
14.......	46	107.59	6.95	44	107.25	6.90	.23
15.......	44	110.05	6.85	43	112.70	7.85	1.68

Data used to construct the graph in Fig. 6.

Source: Bayley N. Manual for the bayley scales of infant development. New York: The Psychological Corporation, 1969.

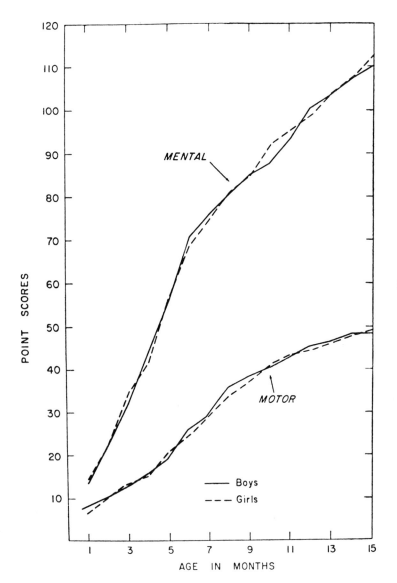

FIG. 6. Mean mental and motor point scores in boys compared with girls.

Source: Bayley N. Manual for the bayley scales of infant development. New York: The Psychological Corporation, 1969.

Related References:

1. Illingworth RS. The development of the infant and young child. 7th ed. London: Churchill Livingstone, 1980.

2. Knoblock H, Stevens F, Malone AF. Manual of developmental diagnosis. The administration and interpretation of the revised Gesell and Amatruda developmental and neurological examination. Hagerstown, MD: Harper & Row, 1980.

Reflex Maturation Chart

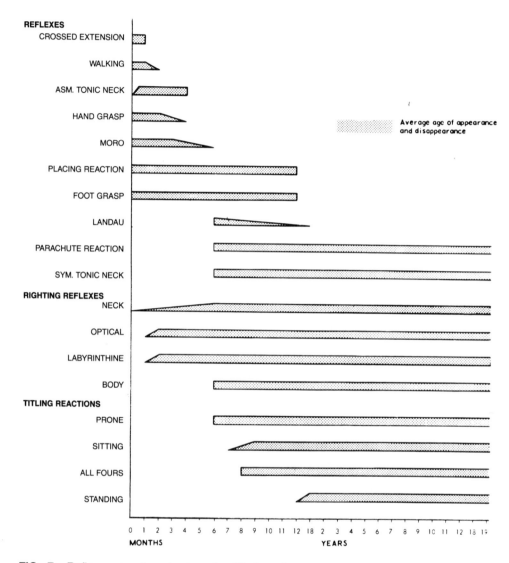

FIG. 7. Reflex maturation chart, a simplified version noting the average age of appearance and disappearance of the individual reflex.

Source: Tachdjian MO. *Pediatric Orthopaedics*. Philadelphia: W. B. Saunders, 1972.

Developmental Chart for Routine Examination of Children

Divided into two sections, the upper section is a behavioristic scale modified from Koupernik (1954), and the lower section contains the primitive reactions and specific reactions. Entries in the chart are made by writing the chronological age in months below the functional finding indicated at the head of the columns. The chart was developed over a 5-year experience in regular weekly sessions in a children's clinic. (Koupernik C. *Developpement Psychomoteur du Premier Age*. Paris: Presses Universitaires, 1954.)

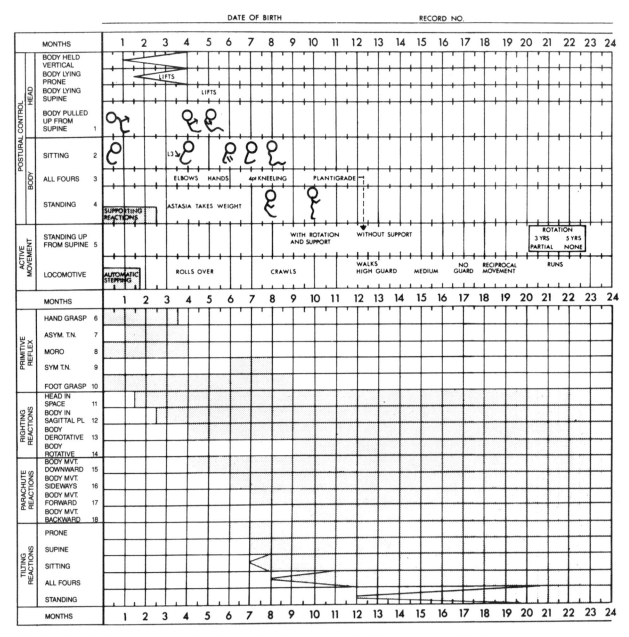

FIG. 8. The first letter of any word in the chart is aligned vertically with the age at which the phenomenon usually appears.

(1) The figurines indicate that from birth until 4 months the head lags when gentle traction is applied to the arms of the supine child; at 4 months the head is maintained in alignment with the trunk as it is raised; at 5 months the child 'collaborates' with the examiner by flexing the head and exerting traction through the shoulders, and elbows.

(2) L3 against the second figurine indicates that the progressive craniocaudal uncurving of the vertebral column has normally extended downwards to the level of the third lumbar segment at the age of four months.

(3) The words "elbows" and "hands" imply that at 3½ months the normal infant extends the trunk by thrust through the elbows; at 5 months through the hands with extended elbows. These are considered to be the earliest phases of the adoption of the quadrupedal position. (4)

The *hatched area* (supporting reaction) is in fact a primitive reflex. These are assessed separately (*see* below), but it is convenient to record the supporting reactions in the examination of standing.

(5) Standing up without support is achieved in two different ways. The supine child rotates into the prone position, gets into four-foot kneeling, and then either climbs up using the hands as a support, or straightens the knees so that the plantigrade position is assumed, and from this position the trunk is lifted without support. This second alternative is recorded by putting the figure for the month on the arrow connecting "plantigrade" to "standing without support." The box is a convenience to extend the time covered by the chart. *N.B.* The conditions for performing tests in the bottom half of the chart are critical, because we are not so much interested in whether a particular reaction can be elicited, but rather in whether its presence under certain conditions and at a particular stage of development is interfering with the "funczione statica."

(6) Hand grasp is assessed by placing the child in the prone position and stimulating the palms by contact with the couch. The grasp-reflex normally ceases to interfere with the supporting function of the arm at 3½ months *(shading)*.

(7) The Asymmetric Tonic Neck Reflex is assessed by placing the child supine and by rotating the head (without flexion). It is marked as positive if the elbow on the "occipital" side is more flexed than the elbow on the "chin" side.

(8) The Moro reflex is elicited by holding the child in a sitting position and tilting the trunk backwards. The effective stimulus is the falling back of the head when the examiner arrests the tilting movement at the shoulder level. The minimum positive reaction is a slight extention of the fingers. No parachute or tilting reactions usually exist until this minimal sign in the fingers has disappeared. The leg and foot response to this maneuver persists longer.

(9) The Symmetric Tonic Neck Reflex is assessed in the "all-fours" position. The presence of the S.T.N. at 6 months is indicated by flexion of the hips when the head is passively extended. The disappearance of the S.T.N. is seen when the child can lift the buttocks from the heels without flexing the head and upper limbs.

(10) Foot Grasp is assessed with the child standing and by stimulating the sole of the foot by contact with the couch.

(11) We consider head-righting in space to be present when we see lifting of the head with the child in the prone position, or righting of the head when the vertically held child is tilted.

(12) The child is suspended prone with the upper abdomen on the examiner's hand. A positive reaction is indicated by extension of the head, trunk, and legs (first phase of the Landau Reflex).

(13) The child is supine, and the examiner rotates the pelvis by using one flexed leg as a crank, alternatively he may rotate the flexed head. A positive reaction is indicated by "derotation" of the applied rotation, starting with flexion of the shoulder on the raised side. When this reaction appears the mother must be warned that the child should not be left alone lying on a bed because spontaneous rolling over is on the point of appearing.

(14) The child is placed supine and the normal 9 month infant tries to get out of this position and stand up by a sequence of movements ("chain reaction") starting with a flexion of the head and shoulder girdle. In cases where it is difficult to see this reaction on a couch in the clinic the mother may ask if, when waking up, the child immediately stands.

(15) The child is held vertically under the armpits and rapidly lowered; the normal reaction as seen in the lower limbs is extension, abduction, and external rotation. (*N.B.* Reaction in the upper limbs is impeded with this type of suspension.)

(16) The child is placed sitting and is pushed sideways on one shoulder with sufficient force to make it lose balance. The positive reaction is abduction of the opposite arm, with extension of the elbow, wrist, and fingers.

(17) The child is held with the trunk vertical and not inclined head-down as more usually described for testing the "sprungbereitschaft." In the vertical position the child is tilted forwards towards the couch. The arms project forwards with extended elbows, wrist, and fingers.

(18) The child is sitting and is pushed backwards. The full reaction is backward extension of both arms, but more frequently an element of trunk rotation comes in, and the reaction is seen in one arm only.

(19) The stimulus for all the tilting reactions is a slow tilt of the couch, either done smoothly, or in a series of small jerks. The examiner's attention is focused only on the reactive curving of the spine. Reactions in the limbs are ignored as it is difficult to separate the reaction to tilting from parachute reactions. With the "all-fours tilting reaction" the arrows should taper to 12 months and for the "standing tilting reaction" they should taper to 21 months.

Source: Milani-Comparetti A, Gidoni EA. Routine developmental examination in normal and retarded children. *Dev Med Child Neurol* 1967;9:631–8.

Denver Developmental Screening Test

A total of 105 test items were drawn from 12 developmental and preschool intelligence tests in order to select simple, economical, and typical activities and materials for inclusion in this screening test. The items were administered to a sample of 1,036 infants and preschool children between the ages of 2 weeks and 6 years who were matched to approximate percentages of both parental occupation and social culture characteristics of the Denver, Colorado population. The ages at which 25, 50, 75 and 90% passed each item were calculated for the entire sample. Norms were developed for the children whose fathers were laborers, service workers, or unemployed and for children whose fathers were in professional, managerial, or sales occupations.

The results in 237 children were validated by testing with the revised Bayley Infant Scale or the Stanford Binet Intelligence Scale. 186 children, varying in ages from 1.5 to 76 months, were also tested on two occasions 7 days apart. Use of the revised method of interpretation yielded 97% agreement.

The number of children involved in the standardization, the matching of community characteristics, the spread of age range, and careful item selection make this one of the better standardized survey instruments available. If there is a weakness, it is in the substantial difference in characteristics between the Denver population and other major urban areas in the United States.

Source: Frankenburg WK, Dodds JB. The Denver developmental screening test. *J Pediatr* 1967;71:181–91.

Related References:
1. Frankenburg WK, Camp BW, VanNatte PA. Validity of the Denver developmental screening test. *Child Develop* 1971;42:475.
2. Frankenburg WK, Goldstein AD, Camp BW. The revised Denver developmental screening test: its accuracy as a screening instrument. *J Pediatr* 1971;79:995–8.
3. Frankenburg WK, Dodds JB, Fandal A. The revised Denver developmental screening test manual. Denver: University of Colorado Press, 1970.
4. Frankenburg WK, Camp BW. Pediatric screening tests. Springfield, IL: Charles C Thomas, 1975.

TABLE 6 *Items in Denver developmental screening test: fine motor-adaptive and personal–social skills*

Item	25 per cent	50 per cent	75 per cent	90 per cent
Fine motor-adaptive				
Follows to midline			0.7 mo.	1.3 mo.
Symmetrical movements*				
Follows past midline		1.3 mo.	1.9 mo.	2.5 mo.
Follows 180 degrees	1.8 mo.	2.4 mo.	3.2 mo.	4.0 mo.
Hands together	1.3 mo.	2.2 mo.	3.0 mo.	3.7 mo.
Grasps rattle	2.5 mo.	3.3 mo.	3.9 mo.	4.2 mo.
Regards raisin	2.5 mo.	3.3 mo.	4.2 mo.	5.0 mo.
Reaches for object	2.9 mo.	3.6 mo.	4.5 mo.	5.0 mo.
Sits, looks for yarn	4.8 mo.	5.6 mo.	6.9 mo.	7.5 mo.
Sits, takes 2 cubes	5.1 mo.	6.1 mo.	7.0 mo.	7.5 mo.
Rakes raisin, attains	5.0 mo.	5.6 mo.	6.2 mo.	7.8 mo.
Transfers cube hand to hand	4.7 mo.	5.6 mo.	6.6 mo.	7.5 mo.
Bangs 2 cubes held in hands	7.0 mo.	8.4 mo.	9.8 mo.	12.3 mo.
Thumb-finger grasp	7.1 mo.	8.3 mo.	9.1 mo.	10.6 mo.
Neat pincer grasp of raisin	9.4 mo.	10.7 mo.	12.3 mo.	14.7 mo.
Scribbles spontaneously	11.9 mo.	13.3 mo.	15.8 mo.	2.1 yr.
Tower of 2 cubes	12.1 mo.	14.1 mo.	17.0 mo.	20.0 mo.
Dumps raisin from bottle—spontaneous	12.7 mo.	13.4 mo.	16.4 mo.	2.0 yr.
Dumps raisin from bottle—demonstrative	13.7 mo.	14.8 mo.	2.1 yr.	3.0 yr.
Tower of 4 cubes	15.5 mo.	17.9 mo.	20.5 mo.	2.2 yr.
Imitates vertical line within 30 degrees	18.4 mo.	21.7 mo.	2.2 yr.	3.0 yr.
Tower of 8 cubes	21.0 mo.	23.8 mo.	2.4 yr.	3.4 yr.
Copies circle	2.2 yr.	2.6 yr.	2.9 yr.	3.3 yr.
Imitates bridge	2.3 yr.	2.7 yr.	3.1 yr.	3.4 yr.
Copies +	2.9 yr.	3.4 yr.	3.8 yr.	4.4 yr.
Copies square	4.1 yr.	4.7 yr.	5.5 yr.	6.0 yr.
Imitates square, demonstrative	3.5 yr.	4.1 yr.	4.7 yr.	5.7 yr.
Draws man, 3 parts	3.3 yr.	4.0 yr.	4.7 yr.	5.2 yr.
Draws man, 6 parts	4.6 yr.	4.8 yr.	5.4 yr.	6.0 yr.
Picks longer line, 3 of 3	2.6 yr.	2.9 yr.	3.4 yr.	4.4 yr.
Personal-social				
Regards face				1.0 mo.
Smiles responsively			1.5 mo.	1.9 mo.
Smiles spontaneously	1.4 mo.	1.9 mo.	3.0 mo.	5.0 mo.
Initially shy with strangers	5.5 mo.	9.5 mo.	9.8 mo.	10.0 mo.
Feeds self cracker	4.7 mo.	5.3 mo.	6.2 mo.	8.0 mo.
Resists toy pull	4.1 mo.	5.4 mo.	6.5 mo.	10.0 mo.
Plays peek-a-boo		5.7 mo.	7.3 mo.	9.7 mo.
Works for toy out of reach	4.9 mo.	5.8 mo.	7.0 mo.	9.0 mo.
Plays pat-a-cake	7.0 mo.	9.1 mo.	9.8 mo.	13.0 mo.
Plays ball with examiner	9.7 mo.	11.6 mo.	13.5 mo.	16.0 mo.
Indicates wants (not crying)	10.4 mo.	12.2 mo.	13.4 mo.	14.3 mo.
Drinks from cup	10.0 mo.	11.7 mo.	14.4 mo.	16.5 mo.
Imitates housework	12.5 mo.	13.8 mo.	16.3 mo.	19.5 mo.
Uses spoon, spilling little	13.3 mo.	14.4 mo.	18.0 mo.	23.5 mo.
Helps in house—simple tasks	14.8 mo.	19.3 mo.	21.8 mo.	23.5 mo.
Removes garment	13.7 mo.	15.8 mo.	19.2 mo.	21.9 mo.
Dons shoes, not tied	20.1 mo.	22.3 mo.	2.6 yr.	3.0 yr.
Washes and dries hands	19.0 mo.	23.0 mo.	2.5 yr.	3.2 yr.
Plays interactive games, e.g., tag	20.0 mo.	2.0 yr.	3.0 yr.	3.5 yr.
Buttons up	2.6 yr.	3.0 yr.	3.7 yr.	4.2 yr.
Dresses with supervision	2.2 yr.	2.7 yr.	3.1 yr.	3.5 yr.
Separates from mother easily	23.0 mo.	3.0 yr.	3.5 yr.	4.7 yr.
Dresses without supervision	2.6 yr.	3.6 yr.	4.1 yr.	5.0 yr.

*All 100 per cent.

TABLE 7 *Items in Denver developmental screening test: gross motor and language skills*

Item	25 per cent	50 per cent	75 per cent	90 per cent
Gross motor				
Prone, lifts head				0.7 mo.
Prone, head up 45 degrees			1.9 mo.	2.6 mo.
Prone, head up 90 degrees	1.3 mo.	2.2 mo.	2.6 mo.	3.2 mo.
Prone, chest up, arm support	2.0 mo.	3.0 mo.	3.5 mo.	4.3 mo.
Sits—head steady	1.5 mo.	2.9 mo.	3.6 mo.	4.2 mo.
Rolls over	2.3 mo.	2.8 mo.	3.8 mo.	4.7 mo.
Bears some weight on legs	3.4 mo.	4.2 mo.	5.0 mo.	6.3 mo.
Pulls to sit, no head lag	3.0 mo.	4.2 mo.	5.2 mo.	7.7 mo.
Sits without support	4.8 mo.	5.5 mo.	6.5 mo.	7.8 mo.
Stands holding on	5.0 mo.	5.8 mo.	8.5 mo.	10.0 mo.
Pulls self to stand	6.0 mo.	7.6 mo.	9.5 mo.	10.0 mo.
Gets to sitting	6.1 mo.	7.6 mo.	9.3 mo.	11.0 mo.
Stands momentarily	9.1 mo.	9.8 mo.	12.1 mo.	13.0 mo.
Walks holding on furniture	7.3 mo.	9.2 mo.	10.2 mo.	12.7 mo.
Stands alone well	9.8 mo.	11.5 mo.	13.2 mo.	13.9 mo.
Stoops and recovers	10.4 mo.	11.6 mo.	13.2 mo.	14.3 mo.
Walks well	11.3 mo.	12.1 mo.	13.5 mo.	14.3 mo.
Walks backwards	12.4 mo.	14.3 mo.	18.2 mo.	21.5 mo.
Walks up steps	14.0 mo.	17.0 mo.	21.0 mo.	22.0 mo.
Kicks ball forward	15.0 mo.	20.0 mo.	22.3 mo.	2.0 yr.
Throws ball overhand	14.9 mo.	19.8 mo.	22.8 mo.	2.6 yr.
Balances on 1 foot 1 second	21.7 mo.	2.5 yr.	3.0 mo.	3.2 yr.
Jumps in place	20.5 mo.	22.3 mo.	2.5 yr.	3.0 yr.
Pedals trike	21.0 mo.	23.9 mo.	2.8 yr.	3.0 yr.
Broad jump	2.0 yr.	2.8 yr.	3.0 yr.	3.2 yr.
Balances on 1 foot 5 seconds	2.6 yr.	3.2 yr.	3.9 yr.	4.3 yr.
Balances on 1 foot 10 seconds	3.0 yr.	4.5 yr.	5.0 yr.	5.9 yr.
Hops on 1 foot	3.0 yr.	3.4 yr.	4.0 yr.	4.9 yr.
Catches bounced ball	3.5 yr.	3.9 yr.	4.9 yr.	5.5 yr.
Heel-to-toe walk	3.3 yr.	3.6 yr.	4.2 yr.	5.0 yr.
Backward heel-toe	3.9 yr.	4.7 yr.	5.6 yr.	6.3 yr.
Language				
Responds to bell				1.6 mo.
Vocalizes—not crying			1.3 mo.	1.8 mo.
Laughs	1.4 mo.	2.0 mo.	2.6 mo.	3.3 mo.
Squeals	1.5 mo.	2.2 mo.	3.0 mo.	4.5 mo.
"Dada" or "mama," nonspecific	5.6 mo.	6.9 mo.	8.7 mo.	10.0 mo.
Turns to voice	3.8 mo.	5.6 mo.	7.3 mo.	8.3 mo.
Imitates speech sounds	5.7 mo.	7.0 mo.	9.2 mo.	11.2 mo.
"Dada" or "mama," specific	9.2 mo.	10.1 mo.	11.9 mo.	13.3 mo.
3 words other than "mama," "dada"	11.8 mo.	12.8 mo.	15.0 mo.	20.5 mo.
Combines 2 different words	14.0 mo.	19.6 mo.	22.0 mo.	2.3 yr.
Points to 1 named body part	14.0 mo.	17.0 mo.	21.0 mo.	23.0 mo.
Names 1 picture	15.9 mo.	20.3 mo.	2.1 yr.	2.5 yr.
Follows 2 of 3 directions	14.8 mo.	19.8 mo.	22.0 mo.	2.7 yr.
Uses plurals	20.0 mo.	2.3 yr.	2.8 yr.	3.2 yr.
Gives first and last name	2.0 yr.	2.7 yr.	3.2 yr.	3.8 yr.
Comprehends "cold," "tired," "hungry"	2.6 yr.	2.9 yr.	3.5 yr.	4.1 yr.
Comprehends 3 prepositions	2.7 yr.	3.1 yr.	3.4 yr.	4.5 yr.
Recognizes 3 colors	2.7 yr.	3.0 yr.	3.7 yr.	4.9 yr.
Opposite analogies, 2 of 3	2.9 yr.	3.2 yr.	4.8 yr.	5.3 yr.
Defines 6 words	3.4 yr.	4.8 yr.	6.1 yr.	6.3 yr. (87%)
Composition of materials	3.9 yr.	4.9 yr.	5.7 yr.	6.3 yr. (87%)

Source: Frankenburg WK, Dodds JB. The Denver developmental screening test. *J Pediatr* 1967;71:181–91.

1. Try to get child to smile by smiling, talking or waving to him. Do not touch him.
2. When child is playing with toy, pull it away from him. Pass if he resists.
3. Child does not have to be able to tie shoes or button in the back.
4. Move yarn slowly in an arc from one side to the other, about 6" above child's face.
   Pass if eyes follow 90° to midline. (Past midline; 180°)
5. Pass if child grasps rattle when it is touched to the backs or tips of fingers.
6. Pass if child continues to look where yarn disappeared or tries to see where it went. Yarn
   should be dropped quickly from sight from tester's hand without arm movement.
7. Pass if child picks up raisin with any part of thumb and a finger.
8. Pass if child picks up raisin with the ends of thumb and index finger using an over hand
   approach.

 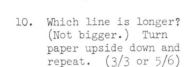 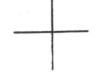

9. Pass any en-
   closed form.
   Fail continuous
   round motions.

10. Which line is longer?
    (Not bigger.) Turn
    paper upside down and
    repeat. (3/3 or 5/6)

11. Pass any
    crossing
    lines.

12. Have child copy
    first. If failed,
    demonstrate

When giving items 9, 11 and 12, do not name the forms. Do not demonstrate 9 and 11.

13. When scoring, each pair (2 arms, 2 legs, etc.) counts as one part.
14. Point to picture and have child name it. (No credit is given for sounds only.)

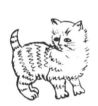 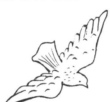 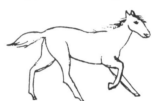 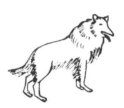 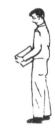

15. Tell child to: Give block to Mommie; put block on table; put block on floor. Pass 2 of 3.
    (Do not help child by pointing, moving head or eyes.)
16. Ask child: What do you do when you are cold? ..hungry? ..tired? Pass 2 of 3.
17. Tell child to: Put block <u>on</u> table; <u>under</u> table; <u>in front</u> of chair, <u>behind</u> chair.
    Pass 3 of 4. (Do not help child by pointing, moving head or eyes.)
18. Ask child: If fire is hot, ice is ?; Mother is a woman, Dad is a ?; a horse is big, a
    mouse is ?. Pass 2 of 3.
19. Ask child: What is a ball? ..lake? ..desk? ..house? ..banana? ..curtain? ..ceiling?
    ..hedge? ..pavement? Pass if defined in terms of use, shape, what it is made of or general
    category (such as banana is fruit, not just yellow). Pass 6 of 9.
20. Ask child: What is a spoon made of? ..a shoe made of? ..a door made of? (No other objects
    may be substituted.) Pass 3 of 3.
21. When placed on stomach, child lifts chest off table with support of forearms and/or hands.
22. When child is on back, grasp his hands and pull him to sitting. Pass if head does not
    hang back.
23. Child may use wall or rail only, not person. May not crawl.
24. Child must throw ball overhand 3 feet to within arm's reach of tester.
25. Child must perform standing broad jump over width of test sheet. (8-1/2 inches)
26. Tell child to walk forward, ⟨⟩⟨⟩⟨⟩⟨⟩→ heel within 1 inch of toe.
    Tester may demonstrate. Child must walk 4 consecutive steps, 2 out of 3 trials.
27. Bounce ball to child who should stand 3 feet away from tester. Child must catch ball with
    hands, not arms, 2 out of 3 trials.
28. Tell child to walk backward, ←⟨⟩⟨⟩⟨⟩ toe within 1 inch of heel.
    Tester may demonstrate. Child must walk 4 consecutive steps, 2 out of 3 trials.

<u>DATE AND BEHAVIORAL OBSERVATIONS</u> (how child feels at time of test, relation to tester, attention
span, verbal behavior, self-confidence, etc,):

FIG. 9A. Ways of testing for items in the Denver developmental screening test.

Source: Frankenberg WK, Fandel AW, Sciarillo W, Burgess D. The newly abbreviated
and revised Denver Developmental Screening Test. *J Pediatr* 1981;99:995–9.

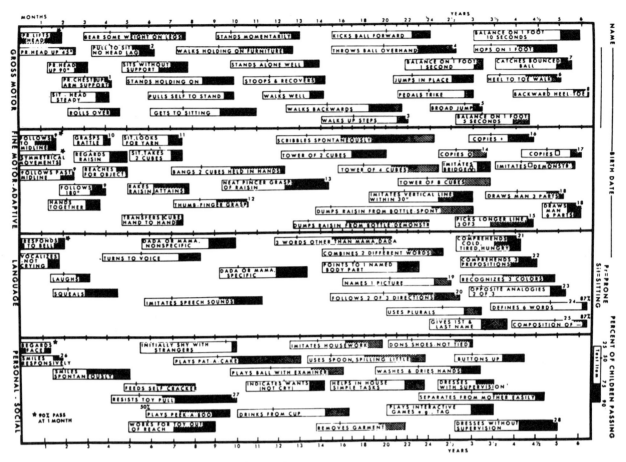

FIG. 9B.   Items in the Denver developmental screening test.

Revised Denver Developmental Screening Test (DDST)

This was devised to make it easier for the clinician to administer the test as part of a routine medical evaluation. A computer simulation using previous results showed that a prescreen test consisting of the administration of 12 items would identify 100% of children having "suspect" DDST results. The 12 items consist of three items from each four sectors that are immediately to the left of but not touching the age line. If this abbreviated version is employed, only 25% of the children screened would receive a "suspect" result and thus need the full DDST. In a test of 200 children, the agreement between the two tests in classifying the abbreviated test as negative (nonsuspect) and positive (suspect) was 98%.

Source: Frankenburg WK, Dodds JB. The Denver developmental screening test. *J Pediatr* 1967;71:181–91.

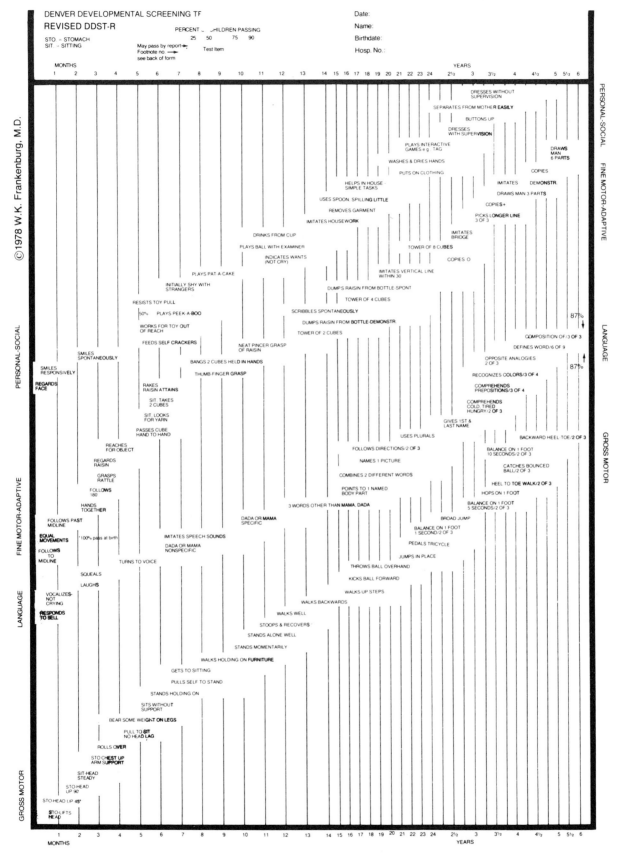

FIG. 10. Revised DDST.

Motor Maturity Tests

TABLE 8. *Basic motor maturity tests performed supine, prone, and pull-to-sit at 3 to 10 months*

Age (mo.)	Supine	Prone	Pull-to-sit
3	Limb posture is flexion Limb and trunk postures becoming symmetrical	Holds chin and shoulders off table, weight on forearms Pelvis is flat when plane of face is 45° to 90° to table	Head lag in beginning of movement, then keeps head in line with trunk Head will bob forward when sit is completed Lower limbs are flexed
4	Bilateral activities at mid-line (Resting) legs are in flexion, abduction, and outward rotation (Active) able to flex hips and extend legs, lifting them an inch	Head in mid-line Prone swimming, jerky movements	Slight head lag in beginning of movement, then keeps head in line with trunk (lower limbs flexed)
5	Back arches and child raises hips (bridges, no progression)	Arms forward, fully extended for support Arms retracted and flexed (hands off support) Support on one forearm and reaches for toys Free kicking of legs	Assists and brings head forward, no head lag (lower limbs flexed)
6	Rolls supine to prone Reaches forward with extended arms to be picked up Lifts legs and plays with feet	Rolls prone to supine (purposeful)	Spontaneous lifting of head Pulls him/herself to sitting Raises extended leg (hips are flexed, knees are extended)
7	Lifts head off table	Commando-crawls Assumes quadruped position	
8	Does not like supine position	Pivots	
9		Goes from prone to sitting	
10		Creeps on hands and knees	

TABLE 9. *Basic motor tests performed sitting and standing, 3 to 15 months*

Age (mo.)	Sitting	Standing
3	Back somewhat rounded Head mostly held up	Does not accept weight
4	Holds head steady, but set forward Head wobbles when child is swayed Back shows only a lumbar curvature (slight rounding)	Accepts some weight

5	No arm support, arms retracted at
	   shoulders with elbows flexed
	Child tends to fall backwards (does not
	   push back)
	Head stable when body is mildly rocked
	   by examiner
		Takes almost full weight

6	May sit alone unsupported briefly when placed Arm support forward Sits well when propped	Bounces

8	Sits unsupported, without hand support
	   for 1 minute
	Sits erect
	Has arm support sideways
		Readily bears whole weight when
		   supported (not rigid)

9	Adjusts posture to reach Good sitting balance, sits 10 min	Pulls self to standing
10	Pivots to pick up objects Arm support backwards Leans forward and recovers Can lean over sideways and recover Goes forward from sitting to prone	Stands holding on and lifts one foot Lowers self to floor by holding on Collapses if not holding on
11		Walks holding on to furniture
12		Walks with one hand held; attempts to stand alone
13		Stands alone well; walks alone
14		Gets to standing unsupported
15		Stoops and recovers

Source: Bleck EE. *Orthopaedic management of cerebral palsy.* Philadelphia: W. B. Saunders, 1979.

Order of Developmental Sequence

TABLE 10. *Order of developmental sequence or approximate age when a child accomplishes specific activities*

Activity	Order of dev. seq. (~age: yr, mo)
Feeding	
Swallow (liquids)	Birth
Drooling under control	1.0
Suck and use straw	2.0
Chew (semisolids, solids)	1.6
Finger foods	0.10
Utensils	
Bottle	0.10
Spoon	3.0
Cup	1.6
Glass	2.0
Fork	3.0
Knife	6.0–7.0
Hygiene	
Turn faucets on/off	3.0
Wash/dry hands/face	4.9
Wash ears	8.0
Bathing	8.0
Deodorant	12.0
Care for teeth	4.9
Care for nose	6.0
Care for hair	7.6
Care for nails	8.0
Feminine hygiene	Puberty
Dressing	
Lower body	
Put on socks	4.0
Put on pulldown garment	4.0
Put on shoe	4.0
Lace shoe	4.0–5.0
Tie bow	6.0
Upper body	
Put on pullover garment	5.0
Fasten	
Button	
Large front	2.6
Series	3.6
Back	6.3
Zipper	
Front, lock tab	4.0
Separating front	4.6
Separating back	5.6
Buckle	
Belt	4.0
Shoe	4.0
Insert belt in loops	4.6

TABLE 10. *(Contd.)*

Tie	
Front	6.0
Back	8.0
Neck tie	10.0
Snaps	
Front	3.0
Back	6.0
Undressing	
Remove socks	1.6
Remove pulldown garment	2.6
Upper body	
Remove pullover garment	4.0
Lower body	
Untie shoe bow	2.0–3.0
Remove shoes	2.0–3.0
Toileting	
Bowel control	1.6
Bladder control	2.0
Sit on toilet	2.9
Arrange clothing	4.0
Cleanse self	5.0
Flush toilet	3.3–5.0

Source: Bleck EE, *Orthopeadic management of cerebral palsy.* Philadelphia: W. B. Saunders, 1979.

Behavioral Patterns During Years 1 Through 5

TABLE 11. *Emerging patterns of behavior during the first year of life*

NEONATAL PERIOD (FIRST 4 WEEKS)

Prone:	Lies in flexed attitude; turns head from side to side; head sags on ventral suspension
Supine:	Generally flexed and a little stiff
Visual:	May fixate face or light in line of vision; "doll's-eye" movement of eyes on turning of the body
Reflex:	Moro response active; stepping and placing reflexes; grasp reflex active

---

AT 4 WEEKS

Prone:	Legs more extended; holds chin up; turns head; head lifted momentarily to plane of body on ventral suspension
Supine:	Tonic neck posture predominates; supple and relaxed; head lags on pull to sitting position
Visual:	Watches person; follows moving object a few degrees

AT 8 WEEKS

Prone:	Raises head slightly farther; head sustained in plane of body on ventral suspension
Supine:	Tonic neck posture predominates; head lags on pull to sitting position
Visual:	Follows moving object 180 degrees
Social:	Smiles on social contact; listens to voice and coos

AT 12 WEEKS

Prone:	Lifts head and chest, arms extended; head above plane of body on ventral suspension
Supine:	*Tonic neck posture predominates*; reaches toward and misses objects; waves at toy
Sitting:	Head lag partially compensated on pull to sitting position; early head control with bobbing motion; back rounded
Reflex:	Typical Moro response has not persisted; makes defense movements or selective withdrawal reactions
Social:	Sustained social contact; listens to music; says "aah, ngah"

AT 16 WEEKS

Prone:	Lifts head and chest, head in approximately vertical axis; legs extended
Supine:	*Symmetrical posture predominates*, hands in midline; reaches and grasps objects and brings them to mouth
Sitting:	No head lag on pull to sitting position; head steady, held forward; enjoys sitting with full truncal support
Standing:	When held erect, pushes with feet
Adaptive:	Sees pellet, but makes no move to it
Social:	Laughs out loud; may show displeasure if social contact is broken; excited at sight of food

---

AT 28 WEEKS

Prone:	Rolls over; may pivot
Supine:	Lifts head; rolls over; squirming movements
Sitting:	Sits briefly, with support of pelvis; leans forward on hands; back rounded
Standing:	May support most of weight; bounces actively
Adaptive:	Reaches out for and grasps large object; *transfers* objects from hand to hand; grasp uses radial palm; rakes at pellet
Language:	Polysyllabic vowel sounds formed
Social:	Prefers mother; babbles; enjoys mirror; responds to changes in emotional content of social contact

---

AT 40 WEEKS

Sitting:	Sits up alone and indefinitely without support, back straight
Standing:	Pulls to standing position
Motor:	Creeps or crawls
Adaptive:	Grasps objects with *thumb and forefinger*; pokes at things with forefinger; picks up pellet with assisted pincer movement; uncovers hidden toy; attempts to retrieve dropped object; releases object grasped by other person
Language:	Repetitive consonant sounds (mama, dada)
Social:	Responds to sound of name; plays peek-a-boo or pat-a-cake; waves bye-bye

---

AT 52 WEEKS (1 YEAR)

Motor:	Walks with one hand held; "cruises" or walks holding on to furniture
Adaptive:	Picks up pellet with unassisted pincer movement of forefinger and thumb; releases object to other person on request or gesture
Language:	2 "words" besides mama, dada
Social:	Plays simple ball game; makes postural adjustment to dressing

---

TABLE 12. *Emerging patterns of behavior from 1 to 5 years of age*

15 MONTHS

Motor: Walks alone; crawls up stairs
Adaptive: Makes tower of 2 cubes; makes a line with crayon; inserts pellet in bottle
Language: Jargon; follows simple commands; may name a familiar object (ball)
Social: Indicates some desires or needs by pointing

18 MONTHS

Motor: Runs stiffly; sits on small chair; walks up stairs with one hand held; explores drawers and waste baskets
Adaptive: Piles 3 cubes; imitates scribbling; imitates vertical stroke; dumps pellet from bottle
Language: 10 words (average); names pictures
Social: Feeds self; seeks help when in trouble; may complain when wet or soiled

24 MONTHS

Motor: Runs well; walks up and down stairs, one step at a time; opens doors; climbs on furniture
Adaptive: Tower of 6 cubes; circular scribbling; imitates horizontal stroke; folds paper once imitatively
Language: Puts 3 words together (pronoun, verb, object)
Social: Handles spoon well; often tells immediate experiences; helps to undress; listens to stories with pictures

30 MONTHS

Motor: Jumps
Adaptive: Tower of 8 cubes; makes vertical and horizontal strokes, but generally will not join them to make a cross; imitates circular stroke, forming closed figure
Language: Refers to self by pronoun "I"; knows full name
Social: Helps put things away

36 MONTHS

Motor: Goes up stairs alternating feet; rides tricycle; stands momentarily on one foot
Adaptive: Tower of 9 cubes; imitates construction of "bridge" of 3 cubes; copies a circle; imitates a cross
Language: Knows age and sex; counts 3 objects correctly; repeats 3 numbers or a sentence of 6 syllables
Social: Plays simple games (in "parallel" with other children); helps in dressing (unbuttons clothing and puts on shoes); washes hands

48 MONTHS

Motor: Hops on one foot; throws ball overhand; uses scissors to cut out pictures; climbs well
Adaptive: Copies bridge from model; imitates construction of "gate" of 5 cubes; copies cross and square; draws a man with 2 to 4 parts besides head; names longer of 2 lines
Language: Counts 4 pennies accurately; tells a story
Social: Plays with several children with beginning of social interaction and role-playing; goes to toilet alone

60 MONTHS

Motor: Skips
Adaptive: Draws triangle from copy; names heavier of 2 weights
Language: Names 4 colors, repeats sentence of 10 syllables; counts 10 pennies correctly
Social: Dresses and undresses; asks questions about meaning of words; domestic role-playing

After 5 years the Stanford-Binet, Wechsler-Bellevue and other scales offer the most precise estimates of developmental level. In order to have their greatest value, they should be administered only by an experienced and qualified person.

Source: Vaughn VC III, Nelson WE. *Textbook of pediatrics.* Philadelphia: W. B. Saunders, 19xx.

Related Reference:

Rosenbaum MS, Chau-Lim C, Wilhit J, Mankad BN. Applicability of the Denver pre-screening developmental questionnaire in low income population. *Pediatrics* 1983;71:359–363.

Breadths of Muscle, Skin, Subcutaneous Tissue, and Bone During Childhood

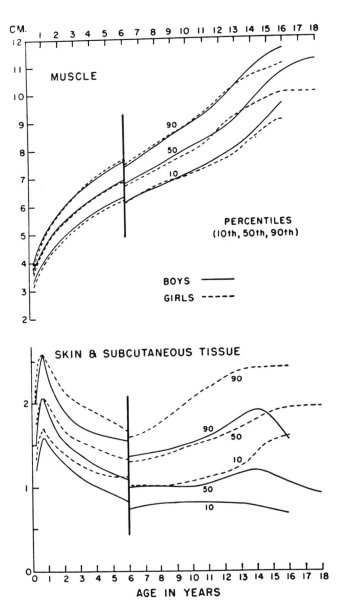

FIG. 11. Breadths of muscle and of double layers of skin and subcutaneous tissue at the greatest width of calf by age and sex from 3 months to 18 years of age. The graphs reveal the close similarity in curves for muscle and general growth, but a unique pattern of increase and decrease and a sex difference in those for skin and subcutaneous tissue. Data were derived from A-P roentgenograms of the leg.

Source: Nelson WE. *Textbook of pediatrics,* 1975. Adapted from Stuart HC and Sobel EHJ *J Pediatr* 1946;28:637–647; Lombar OM. Child Develop 1950;21:229–239; and Reynolds EL. *Monogr Soc Res Child Dev* 1951:15.

The growth of muscle and skin and subcutaneous tissue is analyzed by breadth measurements. Measurements are taken on a plane through the center of the leg. X-rays were taken at the 3-foot distance for children up to 6 years; in older children, the 6-foot distance is used. The norms are given for breadth of bone and muscle for boys and girls throughout the period of growth, demonstrating the mean, standard deviation, and 10th, 25th, 75th, and 90th percentiles.

TABLE 13. *Norms for breadth of bone and muscle (in cm) by age and sex during childhood*

Age	BOYS Percentiles 10th	25th	M	75th	90th	m	S.D.	n	GIRLS Percentiles 10th	25th	M	75th	90th	m	S.D.	n
	THREE-FOOT TUBE								DISTANCE							
3 months	3.3	3.4	3.6	3.8	3.9	3.59	0.24	84	3.1	3.2	3.4	3.6	3.7	3.40	0.26	92
6	3.6	3.6	3.9	4.2	4.3	3.91	0.28	78	3.4	3.6	3.8	4.0	4.2	3.79	0.31	87
9	3.9	4.0	4.2	4.4	4.6	4.24	0.29	73	3.7	3.8	4.1	4.3	4.6	4.11	0.41	76
1 year	4.2	4.4	4.6	4.8	5.1	4.61	0.39	96	4.0	4.2	4.5	4.8	5.0	4.46	0.44	96
1½	4.5	4.8	5.0	5.2	5.5	5.03	0.35	74	4.4	4.6	5.0	5.2	5.4	4.90	0.40	75
2	4.8	5.0	5.2	5.5	5.7	5.27	0.36	96	4.6	5.0	5.2	5.4	5.6	5.18	0.37	99
2½	4.9	5.4	5.6	5.9	6.1	5.60	0.45	86	4.9	5.4	5.6	5.8	6.0	5.54	0.42	82
3	5.3	5.6	5.8	6.1	6.4	5.83	0.46	96	5.2	5.5	5.8	6.2	6.4	5.80	0.45	97
3½	5.6	5.6	6.2	6.4	6.6	6.10	0.47	71	5.5	5.8	6.2	6.4	6.8	6.13	0.49	73
4	5.7	5.8	6.2	6.6	6.8	6.25	0.49	88	5.6	6.0	6.3	6.6	7.0	6.30	0.52	89
4½	5.7	6.1	6.5	6.8	7.1	6.49	0.52	68	5.8	6.1	6.5	6.8	7.2	6.49	0.54	77
5	5.8	6.2	6.5	6.9	7.2	6.54	0.53	86	5.9	6.2	6.5	7.0	7.2	6.57	0.55	84
5½	6.1	6.4	6.8	7.2	7.4	6.81	0.54	66	6.0	6.4	6.8	7.3	7.5	6.79	0.58	74
6	6.3	6.6	7.0	7.3	7.6	6.98	0.48	70	6.2	6.4	6.8	7.2	7.6	6.84	0.51	64
	SIX-FOOT TUBE								DISTANCE							
6	6.2	6.4	6.8	7.2	7.4	6.81	0.55	62	6.0	6.4	6.9	7.2	7.5	6.84	0.55	62
7	6.4	6.6	7.0	7.5	7.7	7.04	0.54	81	6.4	6.8	7.1	7.5	7.9	7.13	0.57	76
8	6.6	7.1	7.4	7.8	8.2	7.41	0.61	77	6.4	6.8	7.4	7.8	8.3	7.35	0.65	69
9	7.0	7.2	7.7	8.0	8.5	7.68	0.63	61	6.8	7.1	7.4	8.0	8.5	7.56	0.67	66
10	7.0	7.6	8.0	8.6	8.9	8.06	0.72	46	6.8	7.1	7.6	8.2	8.8	7.68	0.75	57
11	7.5	7.8	8.3	8.8	9.4	8.32	0.68	39	7.2	7.4	7.9	8.9	9.2	8.11	0.84	46
12	7.7	8.3	8.6	9.0	9.5	8.57	0.70	38	7.3	7.8	8.7	9.2	10.1	8.64	0.95	36
13	7.9	8.4	8.9	9.4	10.3	9.07	0.90	48	7.6	8.1	9.1	9.9	10.6	9.06	1.09	37
14	8.4	8.9	9.5	10.3	10.9	9.59	0.95	35	8.4	8.6	9.2	10.1	10.8	9.40	0.82	27
15	8.3	9.6	10.2	10.8	11.3	10.19	1.02	30	8.7	9.1	9.6	10.1	11.3	9.72	0.84	25
16	9.0	9.8	10.3	11.2	11.4	10.40	1.07	25	8.3	9.0	9.3	10.1	10.8	9.57	0.89	14

TABLE 14. *Breadths of skin and subcutaneous tissue (in cm) during childhood*

Age	SIX-FOOT TUBE 10th	25th	M	75th	90th	m	S.D.	n	DISTANCE 10th	25th	M	75th	90th	m	S.D.	n
6	0.8	0.9	1.0	1.1	1.3	1.03	0.22	62	1.0	1.1	1.3	1.5	1.6	1.29	0.26	62
7	0.7	0.9	1.0	1.2	1.4	1.04	0.30	81	1.0	1.2	1.3	1.5	1.6	1.33	0.28	76
8	0.8	0.9	1.0	1.2	1.5	1.08	0.30	77	1.0	1.2	1.4	1.5	1.8	1.37	0.31	69
9	0.8	0.8	1.0	1.2	1.4	1.09	0.36	61	1.0	1.2	1.4	1.6	1.9	1.43	0.35	66
10	0.8	0.9	1.0	1.2	1.4	1.04	0.24	46	1.1	1.2	1.5	1.7	2.2	1.55	0.41	57
11	0.8	0.8	1.1	1.2	1.5	1.09	0.27	39	1.1	1.3	1.5	1.7	2.0	1.50	0.33	46
12	0.8	0.9	1.1	1.5	1.7	1.20	0.35	38	1.1	1.3	1.6	1.8	2.2	1.63	0.39	36
13	0.7	0.9	1.2	1.6	1.9	1.32	0.59	48	1.3	1.5	1.8	1.8	2.4	1.74	0.42	37
14	0.7	1.0	1.2	1.6	1.9	1.37	0.65	35	1.4	1.6	1.8	2.0	2.6	1.89	0.47	27
15	0.7	0.9	1.0	1.5	1.8	1.22	0.50	30	1.5	1.7	1.9	2.1	2.4	1.94	0.45	25
16	0.6	0.8	1.0	1.2	1.5	1.05	0.44	25	1.7	1.7	1.9	2.1	2.3	1.94	0.24	14

Source: Stuart HC, Sobel EH. The thickness of the skin and subcutaneous tissue by age and sex in childhood. *J Pediatr* 1946;28:637–47.

Related Reference:

Reynolds EL. The distribution of subcutaneous fat in childhood and adolescence. *Monogr Soc Res Child Dev* 1951;15:1–189.

Growth of Bone, Muscle and Overlying Tissues in Children 6 to 10 Years of Age

A method is described for evaluating relative amounts of three principal tissues of the body (subcutaneous, muscle, and bone) from the study of the X-ray film of the leg. The method involves taking an anterior-posterior roentgenogram of the leg, including the knee and the ankle, with the tube set at a 3-foot distance. The tibial shaft area of the film is then bound by prescribed lines, and the tissue shadows within these lines are outlined. Tibial length and breadth measurements are first taken, and then areas of tissue shadows are cut out and weighed on a chemical balance. This is the technique used in children 3 months to 7 years of age; in those over 6 to 7 years of age, a technique with a 6-foot tube distance is used.

TABLE 15. *Tissue areas as percent of total area in children 6 to 10 years of age*

| | | BOYS | | | | | GIRLS | | |
No.	10th	Percentiles 50th	90th	Age in Years	10th	Percentiles 50th	90th	No.
				BONE AREA				
59	41.3	43.4	47.2	6	37.6	40.6	44.4	58
73	40.2	44.3	48.0	7	37.7	41.3	45.2	63
64	40.1	44.4	48.1	8	37.8	41.6	45.7	52
45	40.9	45.1	48.7	9	38.6	41.8	46.3	37
25	40.7	45.5	48.8	10	37.4	42.3	47.0	24
				MUSCLE AREA				
59	36.2	39.6	43.1	6	33.9	38.6	41.9	58
73	35.1	40.6	42.6	7	33.7	38.6	42.4	63
64	35.3	39.2	43.3	8	34.0	37.9	41.9	52
45	34.6	38.2	43.3	9	34.3	37.5	41.6	37
25	34.8	38.4	43.5	10	31.0	36.6	42.0	24
				SKIN + SUBCUTANEOUS AREA				
59	13.6	17.2	21.3	6	16.6	20.8	24.7	58
73	12.7	16.6	20.9	7	16.2	20.4	24.9	63
64	12.4	16.6	20.9	8	16.5	20.5	24.7	52
45	11.9	16.1	21.1	9	16.5	19.9	26.3	37
25	12.2	16.2	20.5	10	16.2	20.8	24.8	24

Source: Stuart HC, Dwinell PH. The growth of bone, muscle and overlying tissues in children six to ten years of age as revealed by studies of roentgenograms of the leg area. *Child Dev* 1942;13:195–213.

TABLE 16. *Areas for earlier ages by young child technique*

TOTAL AREA

	BOYS				GIRLS			
No.	**10th**	**Percentiles 50th**	**90th**	**Age in Months**	**10th**	**Percentiles 50th**	**90th**	**No.**
66	32.0	38.8	44.7	3	32.0	38.2	43.8	68
63	43.1	51.9	57.8	6	42.6	50.0	56.5	64
57	51.9	60.2	66.5	9	49.7	58.6	66.5	59
77	58.1	67.4	74.9	12	56.6	65.6	74.2	74
58	66.5	77.0	86.3	18	65.2	75.6	88.0	60
74	73.6	85.6	96.0	24	75.8	85.4	101.1	79
66	82.3	92.2	103.0	30	77.6	92.5	111.8	62
79	88.2	100.9	115.8	36	89.4	101.8	119.8	79
60	95.3	106.3	121.0	42	96.0	111.1	129.2	55
72	99.9	114.9	132.1	48	102.8	119.1	143.2	75
52	105.8	124.8	142.8	54	108.0	126.7	149.0	60
72	111.8	130.0	147.0	60	115.3	132.2	153.5	67
54	116.4	138.0	159.1	66	120.1	140.6	163.3	54
53	126.3	141.5	164.1	72	125.8	147.3	169.1	45

BONE AREA

No.	**10th**	**50th**	**90th**	**Age in Months**	**10th**	**50th**	**90th**	**No.**
66	10.9	12.4	13.9	3	10.2	11.8	13.0	68
63	13.7	15.2	17.4	6	12.7	14.6	16.8	65
57	15.8	18.3	20.1	9	14.3	17.4	20.2	59
77	17.4	21.1	23.9	12	17.4	20.5	23.9	73
58	23.3	27.0	30.8	18	21.8	26.1	30.4	60
74	27.1	31.7	35.7	24	26.7	31.4	36.1	79
66	30.8	36.0	40.7	30	30.4	34.8	41.6	62
79	34.5	39.8	45.6	36	34.2	38.8	45.0	79
60	37.6	42.6	49.1	42	37.9	41.9	48.5	55
72	41.0	46.9	55.3	48	39.8	46.6	54.4	75
52	43.2	51.2	58.7	54	43.5	50.3	57.5	60
72	46.6	53.5	62.7	60	46.0	54.4	62.4	67
54	48.7	56.3	65.2	66	50.0	57.6	67.0	54
52	52.6	60.3	68.3	72	52.1	60.9	69.3	45

MUSCLE AREA

No.	**10th**	**50th**	**90th**	**Age in Months**	**10th**	**50th**	**90th**	**No.**
66	11.5	13.7	14.9	3	10.9	12.4	14.9	68
63	13.7	16.8	18.6	6	13.7	15.5	18.3	64
58	16.1	19.6	22.1	9	15.2	18.9	22.3	59
77	19.6	23.0	27.0	12	18.3	21.7	26.4	74
58	22.6	27.1	30.5	18	21.4	25.5	29.5	60
74	24.9	29.5	35.4	24	23.9	28.3	33.6	79
66	28.3	33.2	39.5	30	26.1	32.3	38.9	62
79	31.1	36.3	42.8	36	30.7	35.7	43.5	79
59	33.2	40.1	46.9	42	33.6	40.1	49.1	55
73	37.3	44.1	50.6	48	36.4	44.4	52.5	75
52	40.4	46.6	55.6	54	39.8	48.2	56.6	60
72	42.6	48.7	58.4	60	42.6	50.4	60.3	67
54	45.6	54.4	65.8	66	43.8	54.1	63.0	54
53	49.1	56.5	66.5	72	46.3	55.9	64.6	45

SKIN + SUBCUTANEOUS AREA

No.	**10th**	**50th**	**90th**	**Age in Months**	**10th**	**50th**	**90th**	**No.**
66	9.9	12.7	17.4	3	10.9	14.0	16.8	68
63	14.6	19.6	23.6	6	15.8	19.9	23.6	64
57	16.5	22.4	27.6	9	17.1	22.7	27.6	59
77	17.4	23.3	28.0	12	18.0	23.0	28.6	74
58	17.7	24.2	28.0	18	19.3	24.2	29.5	60
74	19.2	24.5	29.2	24	20.8	26.1	33.6	79
66	19.6	23.9	29.8	30	21.8	27.0	34.2	62
79	18.9	24.8	30.7	36	22.0	28.0	34.2	79
59	18.9	24.2	32.6	42	22.3	28.3	37.6	55
72	19.2	24.2	32.3	48	22.3	29.5	38.5	75
52	20.5	25.5	33.2	54	23.9	29.5	38.8	60
72	19.2	24.2	33.2	60	24.5	29.8	39.8	67
54	19.2	24.5	33.2	66	22.3	30.7	41.0	54
53	18.6	24.5	34.8	72	24.2	31.1	40.1	45

Development of Strength

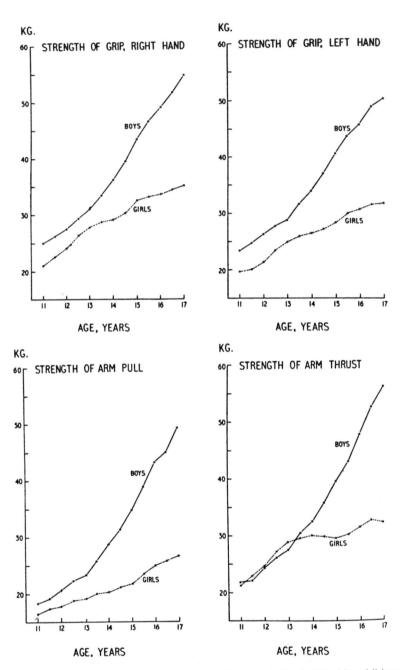

FIG. 12. Strength in relation to age and maturity in a study of 183 white children, studied serially, aged 11 to 18.

TABLE 17. *Manual strength (thrust) by age in boys*

Age	N	I			II	III	IV
		Mean	S.D.	Coeff. of variation	Mean	Relative gain	Percentage of terminal score
		kg.			*S.D. scale units*	*per cent*	
11.0	65	21.86	4.78	21.87	0	...	37.6
11.5	86	22.14	5.00	22.58	.1	1.3	38.0
12.0	92	24.30	5.26	21.65	.5	9.8	41.8
12.5	87	26.14	5.56	21.27	.9	7.6	44.9
13.0	93	27.46	6.22	22.65	1.2	5.0	47.2
13.5	90	30.49	7.08	23.22	1.8	9.9	52.4
14.0	86	32.51	9.34	28.73	2.2	6.2	55.9
14.5	84	35.75	8.65	24.30	2.9	10.0	61.4
15.0	84	39.61	10.61	26.79	3.7	10.8	68.1
15.5	77	42.97	10.58	24.62	4.4	8.5	73.8
16.0	75	47.70	10.87	22.79	5.4	11.0	82.0
16.5	77	52.45	10.00	19.07	6.4	10.0	90.1
17.0	78	56.04	10.40	18.56	7.1	6.8	96.3
17.5	61	58.20	10.49	18.02	7.6	3.9	100.0

Data used to construct graphs in Fig. 12.

TABLE 18. *Manual strength (pull) by age in boys*

Age	N	I			II	III	IV
		Mean	S.D.	Coeff. of variation	Mean	Relative gain	Percentage of terminal score
		kg.			*S.D. scale units*	*per cent*	
11.0	65	18.41	3.71	20.15	0	...	36.5
11.5	86	19.16	4.31	22.49	.2	4.1	38.0
12.0	93	20.72	4.42	21.33	.6	8.1	41.1
12.5	87	22.24	5.42	24.37	1.0	7.3	44.1
13.0	93	23.26	6.26	26.91	1.3	4.6	46.1
13.5	90	25.69	6.63	25.81	2.0	10.4	50.9
14.0	86	28.79	7.33	25.46	2.8	12.1	57.1
14.5	83	31.28	7.53	24.07	3.5	8.6	62.0
15.0	84	34.71	7.98	22.99	4.4	11.0	68.8
15.5	77	38.82	8.63	22.23	5.5	11.8	77.0
16.0	75	43.10	9.53	22.11	6.6	11.0	85.5
16.5	76	45.02	8.74	19.41	7.2	4.4	89.3
17.0	76	49.25	9.17	18.62	8.3	9.4	97.7
17.5	62	50.42	9.30	18.44	8.6	2.4	100.0

Data used to construct graphs in Fig. 12.

Source: Jones HE. Motor performance and growth. A developmental study of static dynamometric strength. Berkeley: University of California, Publications in Child Development, 1949.

TABLE 19. *Gripping strength (right grip) by age in boys*

Age[a]	N	I			II	III	IV
		Mean	S.D.	Coeff. of variation	Mean	Relative gain	Percentage of terminal score
		kg.			*S.D. scale units*	*per cent*	
11.0	65	25.14	4.09	16.27	0	...	44.7
11.5	87	26.28	3.89	14.80	.3	4.5	46.7
12.0	93	27.62	3.71	13.43	.6	5.1	49.1
12.5	90	29.37	4.42	15.05	1.0	6.3	52.2
13.0	92	30.96	4.60	14.86	1.4	5.4	55.0
13.5	92	33.39	5.68	17.01	2.0	7.8	59.3
14.0	89	36.33	6.96	19.16	2.7	8.8	64.6
14.5	84	39.55	7.24	18.31	3.5	8.9	70.3
15.0	84	43.40	7.15	16.47	4.5	9.7	77.1
15.5	77	46.62	7.35	15.77	5.2	7.4	82.9
16.0	76	49.10	7.09	14.44	5.8	5.3	87.3
16.5	77	51.74	6.82	13.18	6.5	5.4	92.0
17.0	77	54.50	7.06	12.95	7.2	5.3	97.0
17.5	62	56.26	7.25	12.89	7.6	3.2	100.0

[a] The class interval is 10.75 to 11.24, etc.

Data used to construct graphs in Fig. 12.

TABLE 20. *Gripping strength (left grip) by age in boys*

Age	N	I			II	III	IV
		Mean	S.D.	Coeff. of variation	Mean	Relative gain	Percentage of terminal score
		kg.			*S.D. scale units*	*per cent*	
11.0	65	23.46	3.93	16.75	0	...	44.9
11.5	88	24.91	3.63	14.57	.4	6.2	47.7
12.0	93	26.29	3.69	14.04	.7	5.5	50.3
12.5	90	27.69	4.06	14.66	1.1	5.3	53.0
13.0	94	28.77	4.58	15.91	1.4	3.9	55.0
13.5	92	31.50	5.15	16.35	2.1	9.5	60.3
14.0	88	33.82	6.11	18.07	2.6	7.4	64.7
14.5	85	37.06	6.06	16.35	3.5	9.6	70.9
15.0	84	40.48	7.03	17.37	4.3	9.2	77.4
15.5	78	43.61	7.25	16.62	5.1	7.7	83.4
16.0	74	45.65	6.77	14.83	5.7	4.7	87.3
16.5	75	48.73	6.48	13.30	6.4	6.7	93.2
17.0	78	50.08	7.03	14.04	6.8	2.8	95.8
17.5	61	52.28	6.94	13.27	7.3	4.4	100.0

Data used to construct graphs in Fig. 12.

TABLE 21. *Manual strength (pull) by age in girls*

Age	N	I			II	III	IV
		Mean	S.D.	Coeff. of variation	Mean	Relative gain	Percentage of terminal score
		kg.			*S.D. scale units*	*per cent*	
11.0	66	16.51	3.86	23.38	0	...	65.0
11.5	89	17.40	4.74	27.24	.2	5.4	68.5
12.0	93	17.60	4.87	27.67	.3	1.1	69.3
12.5	89	18.84	5.04	26.75	.6	7.0	74.1
13.0	93	19.20	5.61	29.22	.7	1.9	75.6
13.5	80	20.05	5.36	26.73	.9	4.4	78.9
14.0	81	20.25	5.40	26.66	1.0	1.0	79.7
14.5	79	21.15	5.99	28.32	1.2	4.4	83.2
15.0	76	21.68	6.29	29.01	1.3	2.5	85.3
15.5	78	23.42	6.39	27.28	1.8	8.0	92.2
16.0	73	24.90	6.37	25.58	2.2	6.3	98.0
16.5	76	25.74	5.59	21.72	2.4	3.4	101.3
17.0	72	26.53	6.31	23.78	2.6	3.1	104.4
17.5	59	25.41	5.99	23.57	2.3	−4.2	100.0

Data used to construct graphs in Fig. 12.

TABLE 22. *Manual strength (thrust) by age in girls*

Age	N	I			II	III	IV
		Mean	S.D.	Coeff. of variation	Mean	Relative gain	Percentage of terminal score
		kg.			*S.D. scale units*	*per cent*	
11.0	66	21.30	5.78	27.14	0	...	67.9
11.5	89	22.86	6.34	27.73	.3	7.3	72.9
12.0	93	24.39	6.36	26.08	.5	6.7	77.8
12.5	88	27.11	6.10	22.50	1.0	11.2	86.4
13.0	93	28.82	6.76	23.46	1.3	6.3	91.9
13.5	80	29.62	6.28	21.20	1.4	2.8	94.4
14.0	81	30.02	6.52	21.72	1.5	1.4	95.7
14.5	79	29.78	6.06	20.34	1.5	−0.8	94.9
15.0	76	29.39	6.62	22.52	1.4	−1.3	93.7
15.5	78	30.10	6.75	22.43	1.5	2.4	96.0
16.0	73	31.44	6.27	19.94	1.7	4.5	100.2
16.5	76	32.53	6.33	19.46	1.9	3.5	103.7
17.0	72	32.19	6.16	19.14	1.9	−1.0	102.6
17.5	59	31.37	6.07	19.35	1.7	−2.5	100.0

Data used to construct graphs in Fig. 12.

Source: Jones HE. Motor performance and growth. A developmental study of static dynamometric strength. Berkeley: University of California, Publications in Child Development, 1949.

TABLE 23. *Gripping strength (right grip) by age in girls*

Age	N	I			II	III	IV
		Mean	S.D.	Coeff. of variation	Mean	Relative gain	Percentage of terminal score
		kg.			*S.D. scale units*	*per cent*	
11.0	66	21.04	3.86	18.35	0	...	58.8
11.5	89	22.62	4.82	21.30	.4	7.5	63.2
12.0	92	24.15	4.89	20.25	.8	6.8	67.5
12.5	88	26.36	5.03	19.08	1.4	9.2	73.7
13.0	92	27.72	5.20	18.76	1.7	5.2	77.5
13.5	80	28.72	4.97	17.31	2.0	3.6	80.2
14.0	79	29.19	5.21	17.85	2.1	1.6	81.6
14.5	79	30.34	5.60	18.46	2.4	3.9	84.8
15.0	76	32.50	5.32	16.37	3.0	7.1	90.8
15.5	77	33.08	5.62	16.99	3.1	1.8	92.4
16.0	72	33.69	5.59	16.59	3.3	1.8	94.1
16.5	75	34.61	5.19	15.00	3.5	2.7	96.7
17.0	71	35.15	5.47	15.56	3.7	1.6	98.2
17.5	58	35.79	5.05	14.11	3.8	1.8	100.0

Data used to construct graphs in Fig. 12.

TABLE 24. *Gripping strength (left grip) by age in girls*

Age	N	I			II	III	IV
		Mean	S.D.	Coeff. of variation	Mean	Relative gain	Percentage of terminal score
		kg.			*S.D. scale units*	*per cent*	
11.0	66	19.73	3.52	17.84	0	...	62.0
11.5	89	20.16	4.78	23.71	.1	2.2	63.4
12.0	93	21.41	4.61	21.53	.5	6.2	67.3
12.5	89	23.48	4.43	18.87	1.1	9.7	73.8
13.0	93	24.92	5.69	22.83	1.5	6.1	78.4
13.5	80	25.90	5.05	19.50	1.8	3.9	81.4
14.0	81	26.41	5.21	19.72	1.9	2.0	83.0
14.5	79	27.11	5.90	21.76	2.1	2.6	85.2
15.0	76	28.26	5.65	19.99	2.4	4.2	88.9
15.5	78	29.82	4.74	15.90	2.9	5.5	93.8
16.0	73	30.78	5.19	16.86	3.1	3.2	96.8
16.5	76	31.42	5.75	18.30	3.3	2.1	98.9
17.0	72	31.78	4.93	15.51	3.4	1.1	99.9
17.5	59	31.81	5.51	17.32	3.4	.1	100.0

Data used to construct graphs in Fig. 12.

Source: Jones HE. Motor performance and growth. A developmental study of static dynamometric strength. Berkeley: University of California, Publications in Child Development, 1949.

Working Capacity of Toronto Schoolchildren: Strength of Selected Muscle Groups (Mean ± SD)

TABLE 25. *Strength of selected muscle groups (kg) (mean ± SD)*

	Boys				Girls			
	9-10 yrs. (n = 8)	11 yrs. (n = 12)	12-13 yrs. (n = 10)	All boys (n = 30)	9-10 yrs. (n = 15)	11 yrs. (n = 9)	12-13 yrs. (n = 9)	All girls
R. hand grip	19.0 ± 2.6	21.0 ± 4.7	23.3 ± 3.3	21.2 ± 4.1	15.5 ± 3.0	18.7 ± 4.0	23.1 ± 6.0	18.4 ± 5.5
R. arm flexion	15.5 ± 2.9	20.0 ± 4.7	18.7 ± 5.9	18.5 ± 4.9	11.6 ± 2.1	15.0 ± 3.4	18.9 ± 5.6	14.5 ± 4.9
R. arm extension	14.0 ± 3.6	15.9 ± 4.7	16.3 ± 4.1	15.5 ± 4.2	10.8 ± 4.1	13.4 ± 4.4	14.4 ± 3.6	12.5 ± 4.2
Trunk flexion	14.2 ± 5.1	20.0 ± 7.7	17.6 ± 4.4	17.7 ± 6.3	16.0 ± 6.5	19.4 ± 5.8	23.3 ± 5.9	18.9 ± 6.7
Trunk extension	17.2 ± 5.5	21.1 ± 6.7	19.7 ± 3.6	19.6 ± 5.6	15.6 ± 3.1	16.3 ± 5.2	22.5 ± 7.2	17.7 ± 5.7
R. leg extension	33.4 ± 13.5	41.2 ± 10.9	36.9 ± 10.1	37.7 ± 11.4	28.2 ± 6.8	34.8 ± 5.2	46.2 ± 16.5	34.9 ± 12.4
Other authors	Howell *et al.*, Edmonton	Montpetit *et al.*, Saginaw, U.S.A.	Jones, Calif., U.S.A.	Asmussen *et al.*, Denmark	Clarke & Wickens, Oregon, U.S.A.		Bookwalter, U.S.A.	Hasegawa *et al.*, Japan
Handgrip	*kg.*	*kg.*	*kg.*	*kg.*	*kg.*		*kg.*	*kg.*
Boys 9-10	18.3	16.5	—	24.5	21.1		21.4	15.0
11	19.7	19.8	25.0	25.5	23.5		24.2	18.0
12-13	24.3	24.0	29.5	27.0	25.7		26.4	21.28
Girls 9-10	15.5	14.8	—	21.5	—		—	—
11	19.6	18.9	20.5	25.5	—		—	—
12-13	22.9	20.6	26.0	28.5	—		—	24.5

Data from 57 boys and 72 girls in Toronto, aged 11 to 13 years.

Asmussen E, Heeboll-Nielsen K, Molbech S. Muscle strength in children. In: *International Research in Sport and Physical Education*, edited by E Jokl, E Simon. Springfield, Charles C Thomas, 1964, p. 384.

Hasegawa J et al. Physical fitness status of Japanese youth through sport test. In: *Proceedings of the International Congress of Sports Sciences, Tokyo, Japan*, edited by K. Kato. Hirata Institute of Health, Mino-City 2234, Gifu Prefecture, Japan, 1964, p. 326.

Howell ML, Loisselle DS, Lucas WG. Strength of Edmonton schoolchildren. University of Alberta Fitness Research Unit, Edmonton, 1964.

Jones HE. Motor performance and growth: a developmental study of static dynamometric strength. University of California Press, Berkeley 1949.

Montepetit RR, Montoye HJ, Laeding L. *Res Q Amer Assoc Health Phys Ed* 1967;38:231.

Source: Shephard RJ, Allen C, Barror O, et al. Working capacity of Toronto schoolchildren. *Can Med Assoc J* 1969;100:705–14.

Grip and Arm Strength in Males and Females

This study represents a survey of over 6,000 males and females aged 10 to 69 in the total community of Tecumseh, Michigan. The values over age 20 have been omitted for this publication.

Grip strength was measured using an adjustable Stoelting grip dynamometer. Two trials with each hand were made with suitable rest periods between. The score for each hand is the force in kilograms exerted in the better of two trials. The two grip strengths (right and left) were then summed for the chart in Table 26.

TABLE 26. *Percentile scores for sum of grip strengths (kg)*

Percentile										Age
	10	11	12	13	14	15	16	17	18	19
Males										
90	34	42	52	69	89	96	106	111	117	118
80	30	37	47	60	80	90	99	105	106	113
70	26	34	41	53	72	84	95	99	101	109
60	24	32	38	48	66	80	91	93	98	104
50	22	29	34	44	61	76	87	89	96	101
40	20	26	31	42	58	73	84	85	93	98
30	18	23	30	39	54	69	78	81	90	94
20	15	21	27	34	49	64	74	76	86	90
10	11	16	23	28	39	55	68	70	81	84
Mean	23.6	30.2	37.4	47.5	64.3	76.6	87.6	91.5	97.1	102.0
SD	8.8	9.9	11.9	14.4	18.1	15.1	15.5	18.2	15.5	13.7
N	104	116	120	97	97	92	106	85	55	54
Females										
90	30	37	44	49	65	60	58	61	59	63
80	25	33	40	44	50	54	53	54	55	59
70	22	30	36	41	48	49	49	50	52	54
60	20	27	33	38	44	45	48	47	49	50
50	18	25	31	36	41	43	43	44	46	48
40	17	23	28	34	39	41	41	42	43	46
30	15	20	26	32	36	38	39	39	39	42
20	14	17	22	30	32	36	36	36	36	39
10	10	12	18	26	27	31	33	31	31	36
Mean	19.9	26.2	32.5	37.8	43.6	45.7	45.8	46.8	47.1	49.9
SD	7.5	9.7	10.9	9.5	13.4	10.8	10.1	12.1	9.7	10.3
N	73	102	114	83	85	89	89	64	48	47

The arm strength test was designed to measure the strength of flexors of the upper arm but involved other muscle groups as well. A cable connected to a dynamometer passed directly overhead and was adjusted so that the angle of the elbow was 90° and the upper arm was parallel to the floor while the child was standing. The subject exerted a maximum pull gradually without jerking, and the force in kilograms was recorded. Trials were allowed, and the larger reading constituted the subject's score. Also reported in this publication is the sum of the grip strengths and arm strengths recorded as strength index. The relative strength index reflects the sum of the grip and arm strengths adjusted for size and body fatness.

TABLE 27. *Percentile scores for arm strength (kg)*

Percentile									Age	
	10	11	12	13	14	15	16	17	18	19
Males										
90	48	52	58	66	86	90	98	100	106	115
80	42	47	52	60	77	84	91	93	98	104
70	38	44	48	56	71	80	86	88	94	98
60	36	42	46	53	67	77	83	86	90	93
50	35	40	44	50	64	74	80	83	87	90
40	34	38	43	49	61	71	77	81	84	87
30	32	36	41	47	58	67	74	78	80	84
20	29	33	38	44	53	63	72	72	74	81
10	25	29	34	41	46	58	67	62	65	77
Mean	36.1	40.9	46.1	52.8	65.3	74.5	81.5	83.4	88.0	94.1
SD	7.0	8.0	8.8	10.6	14.7	13.4	12.6	14.3	15.2	15.4
N	104	116	120	97	97	92	106	85	55	54
Females										
90	40	43	49	50	56	54	53	57	55	56
80	36	41	45	48	52	51	48	52	53	54
70	33	38	43	45	48	48	47	49	51	52
60	31	36	41	43	46	45	45	47	49	49
50	30	34	38	41	44	43	43	46	47	47
40	29	32	36	39	42	41	42	44	45	45
30	27	30	34	37	40	39	40	43	44	43
20	25	27	32	34	36	36	37	39	40	40
10	23	25	29	30	33	33	33	33	36	36
Mean	31.3	34.9	39.3	42.0	45.2	44.8	44.0	47.0	47.3	47.7
SD	6.2	6.8	7.9	8.9	9.8	8.2	7.4	8.8	7.6	7.7
N	73	102	114	83	85	89	89	64	48	47

Source: Montoye HJ, Lamphear DE. Grip and arm strength in males and females aged 10 to 69. *Res Q* 1977;48:109.

National Norms for Youth Fitness and Performance: Physical Fitness and Performance for Boys and Girls, Grades 5 Through 12 (Ages 9 Through 17)

The original test battery of seven tests was developed in 1957 by a special committee of the American Alliance for Health, Physical Education, Recreation and Dance (AAHPERD) Research Council. Originally seven test items were chosen, and subsequently these have been modified to the present six: pullups (with flexed-arm hang for girls) for judging arm and shoulder girdle strength; flexed-leg situp for judging efficiency of abdominal and hip flexor muscles; shuttle turn for judging speed and change of direction; standing long jump for judging explosive muscle power of leg extensors; 50 yard dash for judging speed; and 600 yard run (with optional runs of 1 mile or 9 min for ages 10 to 12, or 1½ mile or 12 min for ages 13 and older) for judging endurance. The first national survey was finished in 1957–1958 on a representative sample of 8,500 boys and girls in grades 5 through 12. It was subsequently repeated in 1965 and most recently in 1975. For the purposes of this supplement, only the 1975 norms are reproduced. Mean scores are given in all cases. The complete text includes comparisons between the decades.

Related References:
1. Canadian Association for Health, Physical Education and Recreation: Fitness-Performance Test Manual. CAHPER, Ottawa, Canada, 1966.
2. Clarke, HH, Deguitis, EW. Comparison of skeletal age and various physical and motor factors with the pubescent development of ten 13 and 16 year old boys. *Res Q*, 1962, 33:356–8.
3. Curetun TK, Barry AK. Improving the physical fitness of youth. A reprint of research in the sports school of the University of Illinois. *Monogr Soc Res Child Dev*, 1964, 29:1–221.

An overhand grasp is used and the child hangs on a bar equal to her standing height. The child raises her body off the floor to a position where the chin is above the bar, the elbows are flexed, and the chest is close to the bar. The time the child maintains this position is recorded in seconds.

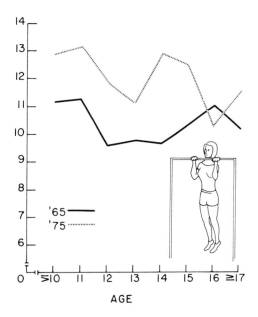

FIG. 13. Flexed-arm hang in girls.

An overhand grasp of the bar is used. The bar should be high enough so that the child can hang with his arms and legs fully extended and his feet free from the floor. He raises his body by his arms until the chin can be placed over the bar; he then lowers his body to the starting position. The number completed in 1 min is recorded.

FIG. 14. Pullups in boys.

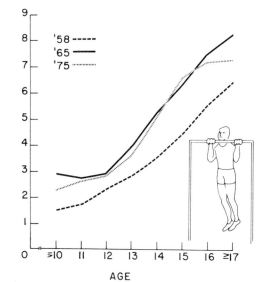

Source: Hunsicker P, Reiff GG. AAHPERD Young Fitness Test Manual. AAHPERD 1900 Association, Reston, Virginia, 1976.

The child lies on the floor, with heels no more than 12 inches from the buttocks. The child curls up, touching elbows to the knees (constituting one situp), and returns to the starting position. The number of correctly executed situps performed in 60 sec is recorded.

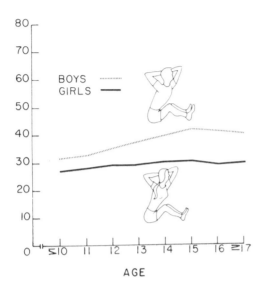

FIG. 15. Situps in boys and girls (flexed knee), 1975.

Two parallel lines, 30 feet apart (width of a regulation volleyball court), are used. The child starts from behind the first line, runs to the second line, picks up a block, runs back to the starting line, and places the block behind the line. This is repeated, with the child going back to pick up the second block and carrying it back across the starting line. Time is measured in seconds. The best of two trials is recorded.

FIG. 16. Shuttle run, 1975.

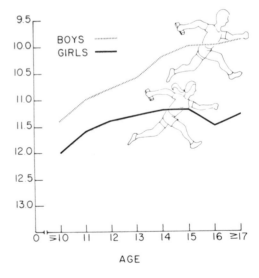

The child stands behind a line and swings the arms backward and bends the knees. The jump is accomplished by simultaneously extending the knees and swinging forward with the arms. The best of three trials, measured in feet and inches, is recorded.

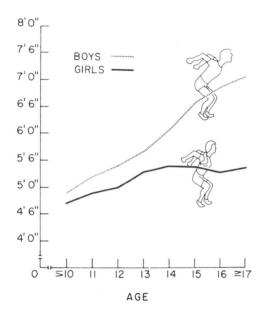

FIG. 17. Standing long jump, 1975.

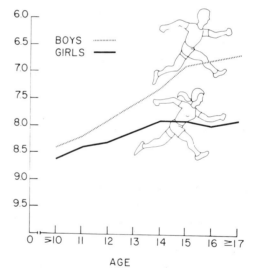

FIG. 18. Fifty-yard dash, 1975, recorded in seconds.

MEAN SCORES

Source: Hunsicker P, Reiff GG. AAHPERD Youth Fitness Test Manual. AAHPERD 1900 Association, Reston, Virginia, 1976.

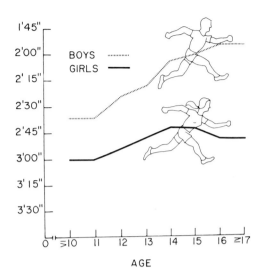

FIG. 19. Six-hundred-yard run, 1975, recorded in minutes and seconds.

TABLE 28. *Boys: data used to construct the graphs in Figs. 14–19*

	Pullups (no/60 sec)			Situps (no/60 sec)			Shuttle run (sec)			Long jump (ft/in)			50 yd dash (sec)			600 yd run (min/sec)		
Age	Mean	5%	95%	Mean	5%	95%	Mean	5%	95%	Mean	5%	95%	Mean	5%	95%	Mean	5%	95%
9–10	1	0	9	31	13	47	11.2	13.1	10.0	4'11"	3'10"	6'0"	9.9	8.2	7.3	2:33	3:22	2:50
11	2	0	8	34	15	48	10.9	12.9	9.7	5'2"	4'0"	6'2"	9.5	8.0	7.1	2:27	3:29	2:20
12	2	0	9	35	18	50	10.7	12.4	9.6	5'5"	4'2"	6'6"	9.5	7.8	6.8	2:19	3:06	1:52
13	3	0	10	38	20	53	10.4	12.4	9.3	5'9"	4'4"	7'1"	9.0	7.5	6.5	2:10	3:00	1:52
14	4	0	12	41	24	55	10.1	11.9	8.9	6'2"	4'8"	7'6"	8.8	7.2	6.2	2:03	3:51	1:39
15	6	0	15	42	28	57	9.9	11.7	8.9	6'8"	5'2"	8'0"	8.0	6.9	6.0	1:56	2:30	1:36
16	7	1	14	41	28	55	9.9	11.9	8.6	7'0"	5'5"	8'2"	7.7	6.7	6.0	1:52	2:31	1:34
17	7	0	15	41	26	54	9.8	11.7	8.6	7'2"	5'5"	8'5"	7.9	6.6	5.9	1:52	2:38	1:32

TABLE 29. *Girls: data used to construct the graphs in Figs. 13–19*

	Flexed-arm hang (sec)			Situps (no/60 sec)			Shuttle run (sec)			Long jump (ft/in)			50 yd dash (sec)			600 yd run (min/sec)		
Age	Mean	5%	95%	Mean	5%	95%	Mean	5%	95%	Mean	5%	95%	Mean	5%	95%	Mean	5%	95%
9–10	9	0	42	27	10	45	11.8	14.3	10.2	4'8"	3'5"	5'10"	8.6	10.3	7.4	2:56	4:00	2:20
11	10	0	39	29	9	43	11.5	14.0	10.0	4'11"	3'8"	6'0"	8.3	10.0	7.3	2:53	4:15	2:14
12	9	0	33	29	13	44	11.4	13.3	9.9	5'0"	3'10"	6'2"	8.1	10.0	7.0	2:47	3:59	2:06
13	8	0	34	30	15	45	11.2	13.2	9.9	5'3"	4'0"	6'5"	8.0	10.0	6.9	2:41	3:49	2:04
14	9	0	35	30	16	45	11.0	13.1	9.7	5'4"	4'0"	6'8"	7.8	9.6	6.8	2:40	3:49	2:02
15	9	0	36	31	15	45	11.0	13.3	9.9	5'5"	4'2"	6'7"	7.8	9.2	6.9	2:37	3:28	2:00
16	7	0	31	30	15	43	11.2	13.7	10.0	5'3"	4'0"	6'6"	7.9	9.3	7.0	2:43	3:49	2:08
17	8	0	34	30	14	45	11.1	14.0	9.6	5'5"	4'1"	6'9"	7.9	9.5	6.8	2:41	3:45	2:02

TABLE 30. *Nine-minute, one-mile run by boys and girls aged 10–12 years*

Age	9-Minute run (yd)			1-Mile run (min/sec)		
	Mean	5%	95%	Mean	5%	95%
Boys						
10	1,717	1,140	2,294	9:07	12:19	5:55
11	1,779	1,202	2,356	8:44	11:56	5:32
12	1,841	1,264	2,418	8:21	11:33	5:09
Girls						
10	1,514	1,059	1,969	10:29	13:30	7:28
11	1,537	1,082	1,992	9:58	12:59	6:57
12	1,560	1,105	2,015	9:24	12:24	6:23

TABLE 31. *Twelve-minute, 1.5-mile run by boys and girls 13 years and older*

Age	12-Minute run (yd)			1.5-Mile run (min/sec)		
	Mean	5%	95%	Mean	5%	95%
Boys	2,592	1,888	3,297	11:29	14:20	8:37
Girls	1,861	1,274	2,448	16:57	21:36	12:17

Source: Hunsicker P, Reiff GG. AAHPERD Youth Fitness Test Manual. AAHPERD 1900 Association, Reston, Virginia, 1976.

Physical Performance of 106 Boys Tested Annually From 10 Through 16 Years

Three performance tests were utilized: (1) Standing broad jump: Two trials were given and the best trial recorded. Measurements were made in inches from the take-off line to the heel of the foot landing nearest the take-off line. (2) Flexed arm hang test: The subject was required to take a reverse grip on the bar. He was then assisted to a fixed position where his eyes were level with the bar and his arms fully bent. The total time the subject maintained this starting position was recorded to the nearest second. The trial was terminated as soon as the subject's eyes fell below the bar level. (3) One minute speed situps: The subject's knees were bent and the feet placed flat on a tumbling mat and held by the experimenter. A situp consisted of a movement upward, touching both elbows to the knees, and return with both shoulders touching the mat. The score recorded was the number of complete excutions completed in 60 sec.

TABLE 32. *Standing broad jumps, flexed-arm hang, and bent-knee situps of 106 boys tested, 10–16 years of age, in this Saskachewan child growth and development study*

Age	Standing Broad Jump Mean ± S.D. (cm)	Increase	Percent Increase	Flexed Arm Hang Mean ± S.D. (sec)	Increase	Percent Increase	Bent Knee Sit Ups Mean ± S.D. no./min.	Increase	Percent Increase
10	164.08 ± 14.22			30.6 ± 19.9			37.8 ± 10.2		
		5.34	3.3		5.5	17.9		1.6	4.2
11	169.42 ± 14.99			36.1 ± 22.9			39.4 ± 10.5		
		8.64	5.1		10.3	28.5		2.5	6.3
12	178.05 ± 15.49			46.4 ± 22.8			41.9 ± 8.4		
		9.14	5.1		4.5	9.7		1.4	3.3
13	187.20 ± 17.27			50.9 ± 23.5			43.3 ± 8.1		
		7.62	4.1		5.2	10.2		1.8	4.2
14	194.82 ± 19.56			56.1 ± 23.1			45.1 ± 8.3		
		14.22	7.3		9.6	17.1		2.7	6.0
15	209.04 ± 19.56			65.7 ± 25.1			47.8 ± 8.7		
		9.14	4.4		− 1.2	− 1.8		1.1	2.3
16	218.19 ± 28.19			64.5 ± 22.3			48.9 ± 8.9		

Source: Ellis JD, Carron AV, Bailey DA. Physical performance in boys from 10 to 16 years *Hum Biol* 1975;47:263–81.

ged 7 to 15 Years

...n the source text were the standing broad
...jh jump, chins, and dips.

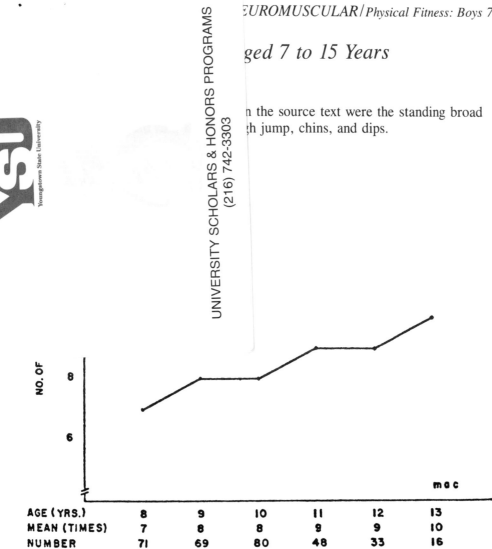

AGE (YRS.)	8	9	10	11	12	13
MEAN (TIMES)	7	8	8	9	9	10
NUMBER	71	69	80	48	33	16
σ	4.3	5.7	5.6	5.1	6.1	6.6

FIG. 20. Floor pushups completed in 1 min versus age.

Source: Curetun TK, Barry AK. Improving the physical fitness of youths: a report of research in the sports fitness school of the University of Illinois. *Monogr Soc Res Child Dev* 1964;29:1–221.

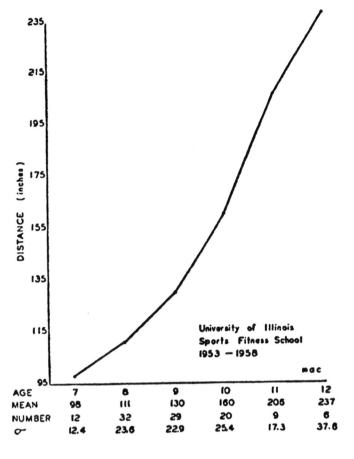

FIG. 21.   Shotput (8 lb) in inches versus age.

University of Illinois
Sports Fitness School
1953 — 1958

AGE	7	8	9	10	11	12
MEAN	98	111	130	160	206	237
NUMBER	12	32	29	20	9	6
σ	12.4	23.6	22.9	25.4	17.3	37.8

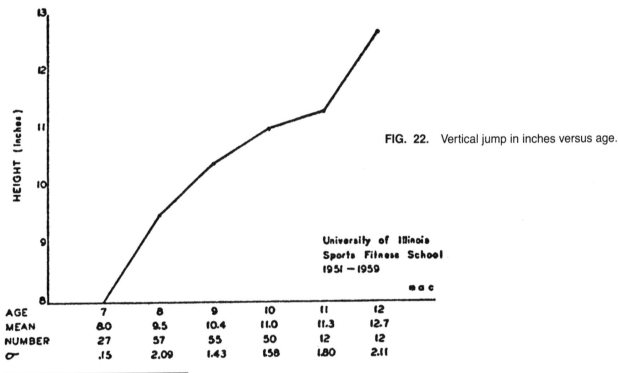

FIG. 22.   Vertical jump in inches versus age.

University of Illinois
Sports Fitness School
1951 — 1959

AGE	7	8	9	10	11	12
MEAN	8.0	9.5	10.4	11.0	11.3	12.7
NUMBER	27	57	55	50	12	12
σ	.15	2.09	1.43	1.58	1.80	2.11

Source: Curetun TK, Barry AK. Improving the physical fitness of youths: a report of research in the sports fitness school of the University of Illinois. *Monogr Soc Res Child Dev* 1964;29:1–221.

Summary of Basic Data for the 35-Yard Dash

Fourth, fifth, and sixth grade boys and girls (792) from five public elementary schools in Kansas City, Missouri, were tested. Of these, 390 were white and 402 were black. They were all tested in a 35-yard dash.

TABLE 33. *Differences in speed between American black and white children in the 35-yard dash*

	N	Grade 4				Grade 5				Grade 6			
		Boys	N	Girls	N	Boys	N	Girls	N	Boys	N	Girls	N
Black	402	5.76	84	6.28	84	5.72	72	5.98	66	5.62	46	5.68	50
White	390	6.37	78	6.58	68	6.11	62	6.40	71	5.82	57	6.12	54
Differences between mean scores													
		0.61		0.30		0.39		0.42		0.20		0.44	

N, number tested.

Source: Huntinger PW. Differences in speed between American Negro and white children in performance of thirty-five yard dash. *Res Q*, 1959;30:366–8.

Motor Performance in Girls

The subjects were limited to approximately 125 for whom there were performance scores for at least three consecutive years. (1) Running ability: The score for each girl was the average of the times of two trials in a 30-yard run. The watch was started as the runner reached a line 5 yards from the starting line and stopped when she reached a line 35 yards from the starting line. The procedure was followed to eliminate reaction time and the time required to develop speed. (2) Jumping ability: The jump was measured in inches. The individual score is the average distance of the two best jumps in four trials. (3) Throwing ability: Throwing was measured in feet per second. The score was the average of the velocities of the two best-of-four trials. A regulation hard baseball was used, and velocity rather than distance of throw was scored because it is a more valid measure of the force developed by the throwing pattern.

TABLE 34. *Performance scores of girls in grades 1 to 8*

Grade	Run (in seconds)			Jump (in inches)			Throw (in feet per second)			
	No.	Mean	SD	No.	Mean	SD	No.	Mean	SD	Distance[a]
1	52	6.18	.652	59	41.67	5.90	22	28.3	5.2	28.1
2	42	5.63	.472	64	46.31	5.85	48	33.7	5.1	38.5
3	58	5.32	.372	82	50.7	5.21	72	34.5	5.4	40.2
4	72	5.07	.409	72	56.55	7.13	69	38.7	5.9	49.9
5	71	4.89	.417	74	59.91	6.51	61	41.9	6.4	58.0
6	67	4.74	.472	64	63.40	6.40	50	47.2	8.1	73.0
7	46	4.47	.443	47	65.00	6.87	47	50.1	7.5	81.9
8	45	4.28	.396	46	68.3	6.63	31	54.3	10.6	95.6

[a] Estimated if projected at 40 degrees above horizontal.

TABLE 35. *Performance scores at ages 6 to 14 years*

Age	Run—30 yd. (in seconds)			Jump (in inches)			Throw (in feet per second)		
	No.	Mean	S.D.	No.	Mean	S.D.	No.	Mean	S.D.
6	26	6.37	.70	26	40.5	7.1	22	29.1	7.3
7	49	5.85	.58	59	43.5	6.6	41	30.5	6.2
8	54	5.56	.50	67	47.7	5.8	63	34.7	6.5
9	64	5.24	.41	81	52.9	7.6	68	36.4	6.9
10	80	5.02	.44	77	57.6	7.4	65	40.7	7.1
11	73	4.79	.61	73	61.5	7.4	63	44.0	8.3
12	42	4.60	.42	47	63.9	6.0	36	48.6	7.6
13	24	4.42	.48	22	68.0	6.2	25	51.9	10.3
14	12	4.25	.5	12	69.7	6.2	13	58.7	11.9

[a] Each age represents a 12-month span beginning with 67-78 months.

Source: Glassow RB, Kruse P. Motor performance of girls aged 6 to 14 years. *Res Q*, 1960;31:426–33.

Mean Score of Test Items for All Age/Grade Groups

Three hundred girls in Georgia, ranging from 12 to 18 years of age and enrolled in physical education from seventh grade through freshman year in college (CF), were given 8 motor performance test items to measure running, jumping, throwing, speed, and agility. Test items included: (1) Ball bounce: the subject bounces a ball from the starting line to one side of an obstacle 9 feet away, to the opposite side of a second obstacle 9 feet away, to the opposite side and around a third obstacle 9 feet away, and returns in the same manner. Score is the best of three trials in seconds and tenths of seconds. (2) Jump rope: the subject complete as many jumps as possible in a 30 sec period. The best score of three trials is used. (3) Jump for height: the subject stands against wall, reaches as high as possible and marks wall, then jumps as high as possible and again marks wall. The best jump in three trials is used. (4) Wall ball: the subject stands behind a restraining line 5 feet from wall, throws the ball against wall, and catches it as many times as possible in 30 sec. (5) Throw for accuracy: subject stands behind restraining line 30 ft from wall and attempts to hit a target, using any type throw, 4 ft square with its center 3 ft from the floor. The best of three trials is the recorded score, with six throws constituting one trial. (6) Side Step: three parallel lines 4 ft apart are drawn on the floor. Subject starts astride the center line and moves sideward until foot has touched the side line, then moves to the other side in the same manner, facing in the same direction throughout a 30 sec trial. Counting one for each trip over the center line, the score is the best of three trials. (7) Throw for distance: subject starts within a 10 ft area behind a restraining line, uses an overarm throw, and throws a 2.5 lb bag (5.5 inch square) as far as possible. Score is the greatest distance in feet for three trials. (8) Base run: four bases are placed in a diamond shape, 35 ft apart. Subject starts at home and runs outside the bases to return to home. Score is time in seconds and tenths for the best of three trials.

TABLE 36. *Mean score of test items for all age/grade groups*

Grade	Age	Number	Ball bounce	Jump rope	Jump-height	Wall ball	Accuracy throw	Side step	Distance throw	Base run
7	12.3	69	8.88	46.98	12.24	28.07	2.33	21.72	33.93	9.60
8	13.5	43	8.41	46.53	11.21	28.12	2.44	21.81	34.23	9.83
9	14.4	51	8.02	46.43	12.61	31.04	2.69	21.71	38.16	9.55
10	15.3	37	7.48	52.84	12.15	33.65	2.89	24.54	43.85	10.46
11	16.4	30	7.62	49.07	11.58	32.67	2.77	26.17	42.82	10.38
12	17.2	30	7.63	52.07	11.95	32.20	2.63	27.27	43.73	10.37
CF	18.4	40	7.66	58.92	11.75	33.35	2.85	33.67	33.77	10.02

Source: Vincent MF. Motor performance of girls from 12 to 18 years of age. *Res Q* 1968;39:1094–100.

Development of Audio and Visual Reactions

Reaction times versus age were determined from data obtained in 707 boys, aged 7 to 15 years, at the University of Illinois Sport Fitness Summer Day School during 1951–1958.

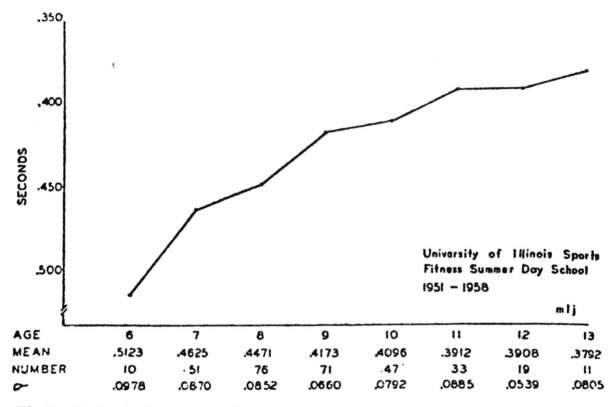

AGE	6	7	8	9	10	11	12	13
MEAN	.5123	.4625	.4471	.4173	.4096	.3912	.3908	.3792
NUMBER	10	· 51	76	71	.47	33	19	11
σ	.0978	.0870	.0852	.0660	.0792	.0885	.0539	.0805

FIG. 23. Visual rection time versus age (boys).

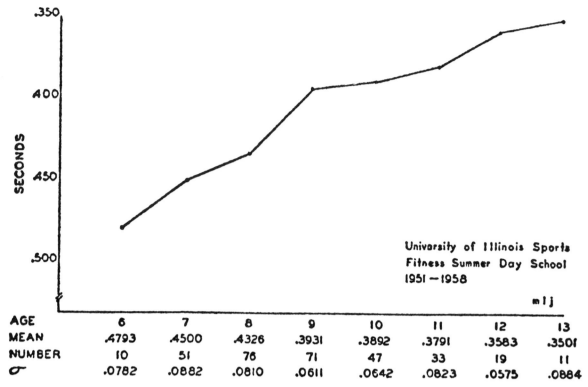

AGE	6	7	8	9	10	11	12	13
MEAN	.4793	.4500	.4326	.3931	.3892	.3791	.3583	.3501
NUMBER	10	51	76	71	47	33	19	11
σ	.0782	.0882	.0810	.0611	.0642	.0823	.0575	.0884

FIG. 24. Auditory reaction time versus age (boys).

Source: Curetun TK, Barry AJ. Improving the physical fitness of youths: a report of research in the sports fitness school of the University of Illinois. *Monogr Soc Res Child Dev* 1964;29:Serial #95.

Related Reference:

Johnson, RD. Measurement of achievement in fundamental skills in elementary school children. *Res Q*, 1962,33:94–103.

Longitudinal Examination of Reaction and Speed of Movement

Hand reaction time (RT) and movement time (MT) measures were secured annually in a sample of 146 boys ages 7 to 13 as part of the Saskatchewan child growth and development study. Total body reaction time (BRT) increases were secured on the same subjects for ages 10 through 13 years of age. Reaction time: The subject responded by lifting his hand from the response pad and continuing upward through a narrow beam of light that activated a photoelectric cell. One chronoscope recorded the time taken to remove the hand from the pad (RT), and a second chronoscope recorded the time taken to move upward from the response pad through the light beam (MT). For the BRT, when the light stimulus appeared the subject responded by jumping back from the response pad on which he was standing, and the time necessary to make the reaction was recorded on a chronoscope.

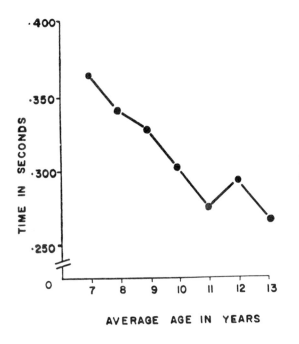

FIG. 25.   Reaction time and age for 146 boys tested annually from 7 to 13 years.

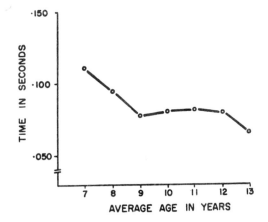

FIG. 26.   Hand movement time and age for 146 boys tested annually from age 7 to 13 years.

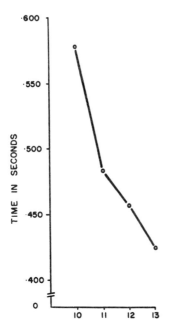

FIG. 27. Body reaction time and age for 146 boys tested annually from age 10 to 13 years.

TABLE 37. *Descriptive statistics and yearly increments in speed for hand reaction time (RT), hand movement time (MT), and total body reaction time (BRT).*

AGE in Years	HAND RT			HAND MT			TOTAL BODY RT		
	Mean (sec)	S.D.	Diff.	Mean (sec)	S.D.	Diff.	Mean (sec)	S.D.	Diff.
7	.364	.058		.111	.029				
			.024°			.016°			
8	.340	.048		.095	.019				
			.012			.019°			
9	.328	.044		.076	.015				
			.025°			.004			
10	.303	.053		.080	.022		.577	.096	
			.028°			.003			.094°
11	.275	.043		.083	.015		.483	.074	
			.007			.003			.027°
12	.282	.039		.080	.015		.456	.073	
			.011			.013°			.032°
13	.271	.032		.067	.014		.424	.057	

° Significant at the .05 level using Scheffe's test.

Source: Carron AV, Bailey DA. A longitudinal examination of speed reaction and speed movement in young boys 7 to 13 years. *Hum Biol* 1973;45:669.

Developmental Variability in Reaction Time

This study comes from the files of two of the longitudinal studies at the Institute of Human Development, University of California, Berkeley. Children in the Berkeley growth study (group 1) were tested for reaction time at yearly intervals from age 4.5 to 11.5 years. Group 2 children were measured annually in the Oakland growth study. They were originally selected from the fifth and sixth grades rather than by birth dates, so that their ages at testing range from 10 through 16 years. The number in these ages range from 15 to 76 boys and 13 to 89 girls.

Reaction time: The child's fingers were placed on a reaction board and a light pressure equivalent to 12 ounces closed the board contact. A red warning light was illuminated for 3 sec prior to the sounding of a buzzer and the signal for raising the fingers from the reaction board. A chronoscope recording in units of 1/120 sec was wired to the buzzer and reaction board. It was activated by the buzzer and deactivated with withdrawal of the fingers from the board, which broke the circuit. Ten trials with the dominant hand were administered to children 4.5 to 8.5 years; starting at 9.5 years, fifteen trials with the dominant hand were given. Group 2 underwent fifteen trials with the right hand and then fifteen trials with the left. Only data for the right-handed subjects were analyzed.

TABLE 38. *Reaction time: intraclass correlation, mean average variability, and relative intraindividual variability by chronological age and sex*

AGE (Skeletal)	MALES					FEMALES				
	N	r	M[a]	AV	RIV	N	r	M[a]	AV	RIV
Group 1:										
8	15	.313	23.03	8.30	.299	21	.401	24.50	8.00	.253
9	21	.050	22.73	7.76	.333	16	.372	21.96	7.48	.270
10	27	.243	20.00	8.41	.366	19	.135	21.22	6.71	.294
11	15	.139	20.23	6.93	.318	14	.169	19.59	5.73	.267
12	15	.204	19.32	6.82	.315	18	.259	19.80	6.59	.286
Group 2, right hand:										
13	35	.320	18.09	3.32	.151	39	.282	17.09	3.36	.167
14	51	.338	17.74	3.38	.155	45	.336	17.44	3.41	.159
15	47	.290	17.55	3.45	.165	52	.344	17.99	3.67	.165
16	25	.300	16.98	3.66	.180	41	.349	18.58	4.16	.181
Group 2, left hand:										
13	35	.330	18.36	3.82	.170	39	.322	17.31	3.42	.163
14	51	.349	17.55	3.58	.165	45	.319	17.56	3.76	.177
15	47	.385	17.25	3.65	.166	52	.331	18.16	3.71	.167
16	25	.378	16.96	3.31	.154	41	.354	18.54	3.94	.171

[a] In units of 1/120 sec.

TABLE 39. *Reaction time: intraclass correlation, mean average variability, and relative intraindividual variability by chronological age and sex*

AGE (Years)	MALES					FEMALES				
	N	r	Mᵃ	AV	RIV	N	r	Mᵃ	AV	RIV
Group 1:										
4½........	21	.19	47.00	18.59	.356	27	.23	52.71	18.63	.312
5½........	25	.31	37.99	14.93	.325	30	.33	43.08	16.84	.323
6½........	24	.28	29.70	9.31	.268	28	.37	32.13	9.15	.285
7½........	18	.36	26.81	9.15	.275	25	.34	26.54	8.11	.257
8½........	26	.23	24.56	10.80	.390	28	.39	23.18	8.05	.277
9½........	24	.20	21.98	8.30	.337	23	.27	23.13	8.02	.296
10½.......	26	.20	19.96	7.07	.317	25	.23	20.78	5.83	.246
11½.......	23	.13	19.29	7.04	.342	22	.20	19.11	5.94	.279
Group 2, right hand:										
10........	26	.65	24.58	7.63	.185	22	.38	23.16	6.05	.205
11........	66	.38	23.17	5.72	.195	77	.44	24.81	6.89	.208
12........	74	.40	19.25	4.63	.186	89	.48	19.56	5.59	.207
13........	75	.33	18.30	3.85	.173	83	.33	18.46	3.96	.176
14........	73	.36	17.58	3.24	.147	74	.36	17.89	3.63	.162
15........	52	.28	17.62	3.52	.170	62	.37	17.51	3.78	.171
16........	15	.31	16.87	4.21	.208	13	.23	19.30	4.30	.196
Group 2, left hand:										
10........	26	.69	24.63	8.85	.201	22	.47	24.62	5.81	.173
11........	66	.39	24.09	6.60	.214	77	.47	25.86	7.40	.208
12........	74	.39	19.39	5.19	.208	89	.48	19.79	5.53	.201
13........	75	.31	18.21	3.97	.180	83	.35	18.67	4.33	.187
14........	73	.52	17.27	4.09	.164	74	.35	18.00	3.66	.164
15........	52	.32	17.34	3.60	.171	62	.34	17.65	3.59	.166
16........	15	.36	16.55	3.75	.181	13	.30	19.10	4.23	.186

ᵃ In units of 1/120 sec.

Source: Eckert HM, Eichorn DH. Developmental variability and reaction time. *Child Dev* 1977;48:452–8.

Working Capacity

A total of 243 children (120 boys, 123 girls) ages 6 to 14 years who were otherwise healthy were in this study. The testing child was given a code number, and height, weight, blood pressure while sitting, and vital capacity were determined. For the work capacity test the pupil was asked to perform consecutively three different workload trials on an electric bicycle ergometer (the load was produced by a direct current generator) according to the method of T. Sjostrend and H. Wahlund (4,5). The pedaling rate was maintained between 60 and 70 revolutions per minute (rpm), and each work load trial lasted 6 min. The apical heart rate was determined by stethoscope for 30-sec periods every fourth and sixth minute of each workload. The working capacity was calculated by plotting on graph paper the heart rate versus the workload at the end of each trial. The estimated amount of work that would produce a heart rate of 170 beats per minute was then recorded as the working capacity of that individual. A straight line was then drawn through the three points, making the best fit. Working capacity correlated well with the surface area, height, weight, 3-sec end vital capacity, total vital capacity, and age. The 1-sec vital capacity and blood pressure gave relatively poor correlations.

Related References:
1. Eckbom B. Effect of physical training on adolescent boys. *J Appl Physiol* 1969;27:350–355.
2. Gilliam TB, Sady S, Thorlend WG, Weltman AL. Comparison of peak performance measures in children aged 6 to 8, 9 to 10, and 11 to 13 years. *Res Q* 1977;48:698–702.
3. Rich GQ III. Muscular fatigue curves of boys and girls. *Res Q* 1957;31:485–498.
4. Sjostrend T. Changes in the respiratory organs of workmen at an ore smelting works. *Acta Med Scand* (suppl), 1947;196:687.
5. Wahlund H. Determination of the physical working capacity. *Acta Med Scand* (suppl), 1948;215:9.

TABLE 40. *Mean values of working capacity parameters for 120 normal California school boys by age*

Age (yr)	Height (cm)	Weight (kg)	Surface Area (M²)	Blood Pressure (mm Hg)		Vital Capacity (cm³)			Working Capacity (KgM/min)	Subject (no.)
				Syst	Diast	1-Sec	3-Sec	Total		
6	121	24	0.90	101	59	990	1,210	1,290	331	10
7	127	29	1.02	102	58	1,190	1,510	1,540	368	10
8	131	30	1.06	104	61	1,260	1,640	1,720	438	11
9	140	35	1.20	110	58	1,670	2,040	2,130	472	10
10	145	40	1.31	106	60	1,720	2,130	2,230	551	9
11	152	46	1.41	114	65	2,030	2,530	2,640	650	10
12	155	48	1.45	114	67	1,940	2,850	2,905	703	20
13	160	51	1.51	118	68	2,140	3,070	3,070	739	20
14	170	59	1.68	117	65	2,290	3,600	3,600	964	20
Total										120

TABLE 41. *Mean values of working capacity parameters for 123 normal California school girls by age*

Age (yr)	Height (cm)	Weight (kg)	Surface Area (M²)	Blood Pressure (mm Hg)		Vital Capacity (cm³)			Working Capacity (KgM/min)	Subjects (no.)
				Syst	Diast	1-Sec	3-Sec	Total		
6	120	24	0.92	97	57	960	1,220	1,300	265	10
7	124	25	0.94	91	59	1,010	1,300	1,340	287	10
8	132	30	1.06	98	57	1,309	1,540	1,610	343	11
9	133	32	1.06	104	59	1,280	1,570	1,660	337	10
10	144	38	1.25	99	56	1,470	1,960	2,020	406	9
11	148	44	1.36	106	59	1,760	2,270	2,370	488	11
12	158	46	1.43	112	63	1,730	2,600	2,540	483	21
13	163	55	1.59	116	70	2,060	2,970	3,010	564	20
14	165	60	1.63	115	73	2,130	3,020	3,050	542	21
Total										123

Source: Adams FH, Linde LM, Miyake H. The physical working capacity of normal school children. *Pediatrics* 1961;28:57.

Physical Work Capacity

A total of 602 students, ages 8 to 18 years, from five typical elementary and junior/senior high schools in Philadelphia were studied. These were compared as to sex, height, weight, and strength of right and left biceps. For the latter a loop was placed over the wrist and connected to a strain gauge and a wheatstone bridge, calibrated in kilograms. The muscle contracture was isometric for all practical purposes. Manual dexterity (Carr test) was also measured. The time required to fill a board of 100 holes with three pins in each hole was recorded. Pulse response was measured at three levels. Pulse response was at fixed workloads, measured during work for 5 to 6 min on a bicycle ergometer at workloads of 300 to 600 kpm. The LPI test [Leistungs-Pulsindex, or work pulse index according to Muller (Muller EA. Ein leistungspulsindex als mass der leistungsfahigheit. *Arbeitsphysiologie* 1950;14:271.)] was done. This heart rate response to a continuously increasing workload was measured every minute over a 10-min period. The modified step test was applied; the step was adjusted according to the length of the lower extremity of the subject and in which the actual work performed (i.e., body weight × step height) entered into the calculation of the score. The pulse rate and systolic blood pressure were measured with the subject at rest in a sitting position prior to a 2-min work period in which the subject stepped up and down the step at a rate of 25 completed steps per minute. Systolic blood pressure and pulse rate were then measured as soon as possible after the end of the work period. In 26 cases maximum oxygen consumption was determined by measuring O_2 uptake at increasing workloads on the bicycle ergometer until there was a leveling off of the O_2 uptake.

TABLE 42. *Comparison of physical work capacity parameters in boys and girls by age groups*

Age Group	Sex	Height	Weight	Muscle Strength R. Biceps	Muscle Strength L. Biceps	Manual Dexterity	Pulse Response 300 Kpm/Min	Pulse Response 450 Kpm/Min	Pulse Response 600 Kpm/Min	LPI	Step Test
8	♂	130.6±0.9	29.1±0.8	9.2±0.3	8.8±0.3	12.4±0.4	171± 2	187± 2		7.2±0.3	1.94±0.13
		(50) 6.5	(50) 5.6	(50) 2.0	(50) 2.0	(50) 2.7	(50) 12	(32) 14		(50) 2.2	(50) 0.94
8	♀	128.8±0.8	28.0±0.8	8.5±0.2	8.3±0.3	12.1±0.3	175± 2	190± 2		7.5±0.4	2.42±0.15
		(51) 5.4	(51) 5.8	(51) 1.7	(51) 1.9	(51) 1.8	(49) 14	(21) 11		(50) 2.7	(51) 1.04
10	♂	140.8±1.1	35.8±1.2	13.6±0.5	13.0±0.5	10.4±0.3	162± 2	181± 2		6.7±0.4	1.74±0.09
		(50) 7.6	(50) 8.4	(50) 3.6	(50) 3.5	(50) 1.8	(50) 14	(44) 14		(50) 2.5	(47) 0.64
10	♀	140.3±1.0	35.3±1.1	11.1±0.4	10.5±0.3	10.1±0.2	170± 2	189± 2		7.1±0.5	1.82±0.09
		(50) 7.0	(50) 7.4	(50) 2.7	(50) 2.3	(50) 1.5	(50) 13	(35) 9		(50) 3.3	(50) 0.67
12	♂	152.3±1.2	44.8±1.4	16.2±0.7	14.8±0.5	9.0±0.1	147± 2	167± 2		5.9±0.3	1.39±0.09
		(50) 8.5	(50) 9.9	(50) 4.7	(50) 3.7	(50) 1.0	(50) 16	(49) 14		(50) 2.0	(47) 0.63
12	♀	154.2±1.1	45.3±1.1	14.4±0.4	13.8±0.5	8.8±0.2	163± 2	180± 2	180± 9	6.8±0.3	1.77±0.08
		(50) 7.4	(50) 8.0	(50) 2.6	(50) 3.2	(49) 1.1	(50) 17	(44) 15	(2) 13	(50) 2.1	(48) 0.60
14	♂	164.7±1.2	56.1±1.3	21.4±0.8	20.0±0.7	8.5±0.1	133± 2	142± 4	166± 3	4.7±0.3	1.31±0.07
		(50) 8.5	(50) 9.4	(50) 5.6	(50) 5.1	(50) 0.9	(50) 15	(16) 17	(34) 17	(50) 1.8	(49) 0.54
14	♀	158.7±0.9	49.3±1.0	16.2±0.5	15.7±0.4	8.1±0.1	154± 3	172± 2	181± 3	5.8±0.3	1.70±0.08
		(50) 6.2	(50) 7.1	(50) 3.3	(50) 3.0	(50) 0.8	(50) 18	(44) 15	(3) 5	(50) 2.0	(50) 0.58
16	♂	172.4±1.0	63.5±1.3	30.8±1.0	30.0±0.9	8.6±0.1	122± 2		148± 2	4.1±0.2	0.94±0.04
		(50) 6.8	(50) 9.4	(50) 6.8	(50) 6.3	(50) 0.9	(50) 14		(50) 14	(50) 1.1	(50) 0.25
16	♀	163.3±0.8	55.0±1.0	18.7±0.5	18.0±0.5	8.1±0.2	147± 2	166± 2	171±12	5.7±0.2	1.61±0.08
		(50) 5.7	(50) 7.4	(50) 3.2	(50) 3.6	(50) 1.1	(50) 15	(47) 14	(3) 21	(50) 1.5	(50) 0.54
18	♂	175 8±0.8	66.7±1.3	34.1±1.1	32.5±1.0	8.4±0.2	115± 2		140± 2	4.1±0.2	0.96±0.04
		(50) 5.7	(50) 9.5	(50) 7.4	(50) 7.2	(50) 1.0	(50) 13		(50) 16	(50) 1.1	(48) 0.30
18	♀	162.0±0.9	54.3±1.0	17.9±0.5	17.2±0.5	8.0±0.2	145± 2	164± 2	177	5.2±0.3	1.55±0.05
		(50) 6.6	(50) 6.7	(50) 3.7	(50) 3.6	(50) 1.3	(50) 14	(49) 14	(1)	(49) 2.0	(49) 0.41
20	♂	177.2±1.1	73.2±1.9	31.9±0.9	31.2±0.9	8.2±0.2	121± 2		145± 2	3.7±0.2	0.94±0.05
		(33) 6.4	(33) 10.8	(33) 5.4	(33) 5.3	(33) 1.1	(33) 14		(33) 14	(33) 1.3	(33) 0.28
20	♀	164.9±1.2	57.9±1.1	17.6±0.5	17.3±0.5	7.5±0.1	139± 2	158± 2	164± 2	5.6±0.2	1.51±0.06
		(30) 6.3	(30) 6.2	(30) 2.8	(30) 2.4	(30) 0.7	(30) 13	(28) 13	(2) 12	(30) 1.1	(29) 0.36
22	♂	179.7±1.2	75.6±3.1	35.0±1.1	33.8±1.2	8.1±0.3	119± 3		143± 4	3.5±0.3	1.18±0.07
		(19) 5.0	(19) 13.6	(19) 4.8	(19) 5.1	(19) 1.1	(19) 15		(19) 18	(19) 1.1	(19) 0.31
22	♀	163.3±1.0	59.0±1.5	19.0±0.6	18.7±0.6	7.5±0.1	140± 3	155± 3	187± 1	5.2±0.2	1.51±0.06
		(29) 5.4	(29) 8.0	(29) 3.2	(29) 3.5	(29) 0.7	(29) 14	(27) 13	(2) 1	(29) 1.3	(29) 0.35

The figures denote mean, standard error of the mean, number of observations, and standard duration.

TABLE 43. *Oxygen uptakes at different work loads in Philadelphia subjects*

	Age, Yr.	300 Kpm/ Min	450 Kpm/ Min	600 Kpm/ Min
Boys				
	10	0.85±0.02 (20) 0.09	1.11±0.03 (10) 0.11	
	12	0.97±0.03 (24) 0.13	1.20±0.03 (10) 0.09	1.53±0.04 (13) 0.16
	14	1.04±0.02 (10) 0.06	1.20±0.03 (16) 0.12	1.53±0.04 (20) 0.16
	16		1.14±0.03 (7) 0.07	1.41±0.04 (3) 0.07
	18			1.47±0.06 (10) 0.18
	20-22			1.58±0.05 (11) 0.18
Girls				
	10	0.79±0.02 (17) 0.09	1.02±0.03 (10) 0.11	
	12	0.96±0.04 (23) 0.19	1.27±0.01 (19) 0.06	1.68±0.22 (3) 0.38
	14	0.94±0.02 (20) 0.08		1.34±0.03 (19) 0.12
	16	0.93±0.05 (10) 0.17		1.26±0.02 (11) 0.08
	18	0.91±0.07 (10) 0.22		1.27±0.04 (10) 0.12
	20-22	0.87±0.02 (8) 0.07		1.35±0.07 (8) 0.20

The figures denote mean, Standard error of the mean, number of observations, and Standard deviation.

Source: Rodahl K, Astrand PO, Birkhead NC et al. Physical work capacity. A study of children and young adults in the United States. *Arch Environ Health* 1961;2:499–510.

Index to Illustrations

Index to Tables

HAND

LOWER EXTREMITY

NEUROMUSCULAR DEVELOPMENT

DATE DUE